Wellness Workbook

JOHN W. TRAVIS, M.D.,
and REGINA SARA RYAN

Wellness
WORKBOOK

*How to Achieve Enduring Health
and Vitality*

NEW
3rd edition

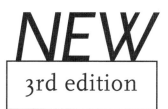

CELESTIAL ARTS
Berkeley

For Meryn, Hannelore, and Juniper.
—JWT

For Jere Pramuk, my partner and friend.
—RSR

Cover photo by Orion Press/Natural Selection
Illustrations on pages xx, xxi, xxv, xxvi–xxx, 2, 23, 28, 46, 51, 129, and 133 by Ellen Sasaki
Illustration on page 143 by Bruce Mills

Photos on pages 136, 137, and 138 by Christina Sell, Anusara Yoga instructor and owner of Prescott Yoga (Prescott, Arizona). Visit www.prescottyoga.com for her photos and descriptions of yoga asanas.

"It's All Right, Ma (I'm Only Bleeding)" by Bob Dylan. Copyright © 1965 by Warner Bros. Inc. Copyright © renewed 1993 by Special Rider Music. All rights reserved. International copyright secured. Reprinted by permission.

Harvard Pyramid reprinted with permission from Harvard School of Public Health (Cambridge, Massachusetts).

Poem 51 from *Nobody, Son of Nobody: Poems of Shaikh Abu-Saeed Abil-Kheir,* renditions by Vraje Abramia, reprinted with permission (Prescott, Arizona: Hohm Press, 2001). Copyright © 2001 by Vraje Abramian.

"Stamp Out Oughtism" reprinted with permission from Swami Beyondanada (Steve Bhaerman). Visit www.wakeup laughing.com.

Material from *The Art of Listening* reprinted with permission from Jud Morris (Boston: Industrial Education Institute, 1968). Out of print.

"Living Will" reprinted with permission from Concern for the Dying.

Library of Congress Cataloging-in-Publication Data

Travis, John W., 1943–
  Wellness workbook : how to achieve enduring health and vitality / John W. Travis and Regina Sara Ryan. — 3rd. ed.
    p. cm.
  Includes bibliographical references and index.
  1. Health. I. Ryan, Regina Sara. II. Title.
  RA776.T733 2004
  613—dc22
                                        2003021955
    ISBN-13: 978-1-58761-213-8
    ISBN-10: 1-58761-213-5

Printed in the United States

Cover design by Naomi Schiff, Seventeenth Street Studios
Interior design by Betsy Stromberg

17 16 15 14 13

Third Edition

Contents

Acknowledgements

Some of those who made it possible for me to write this book are:

My parents, Boyd and Eloise Kellogg Travis, who backed me financially when I opened a wellness center instead of pursuing a more lucrative practice of medicine;

Reverend Jack Hannum, Wilford Geiger, and the Triplett families, who showed me new horizons during my high school years, in Bluffton, Ohio;

Theodore Williams, Ph.D., my faculty mentor; "Mom" Quigley, in whose home I lived; and Diana Moseson Brown, who challenged and nurtured me during my years at the College of Wooster in Ohio;

Sally, my former wife, who supported me through medical training and helped develop my early thinking about wellness;

Angelo and Mary Ucci, and Joe and Paula Zeppieri, whose extended families welcomed me—a WASP country boy in an alien urban environment—during my medical school years in Boston;

Halbert Dunn, M.D., whose *High Level Wellness* (1961) planted the seeds for my wellness center; Lawrence W. Green, Dr.P.H., my mentor; Richard Hsieh, Ph.D., my boss at Health Services Research;

and Lewis Robbins, creator of the Health Risk Appraisal, whose innovations were my inspiration during my preventive medicine residency at Johns Hopkins University, School of Public Health;

Anne Baird, Charles Elias, the Koinonia Community, Valerie Lankford, Kim Muller-Thym, Harry Rose, Richard Yensen, and Ruth and Tony Zyna, who helped me get my act together during my transition years in Baltimore;

Mikal Baker, Lynda Berkeley, Pam Blackwell, Marina Delfino, Joy Holloway, Rosie LaRue, Kate Lynch, Annie Styron Leonard, Kenneth Maue, and Jerry Wylie—the former staff of our Wellness Resource Center—for their hugs and hassling and heartfulness;

Marty Albert, Bob Allen, Skip Andrew, Betsey Travis Angus, Don Ardell, Denny Bullens, George Cagwin, Elliott Dacher, Fran DuBois, Tom Ferguson, Terry Graves, Jutta Hagner, Chuck Hess, Dorothy Jongeward, Marc Kasky, Cissa Kelley, Marcia Travis Kilgore, George Leonard, Floyd Mann, Emmett Miller, Russ Munsell, Jeff Patterson, Kent Peterson, Dean and Cheryl Radetsky, Gaye Raymond, Ailish and Will Schutz, Jo Sherrill, Kenneth Ray Stubbs,

Elaine Sullivan, Bob Tollaksen, Dave Travis, Maria Vance, and Ibbie White—the inner circle of wonderful persons who made Wellness Resource Center and Wellness Associates so real and dear to me;

David Isaacs and Lance Hays, who pulled and pushed, humored and harassed me until I agreed to write a book;

Meryn Callander, whom I met at our final Wellness Resource Center conference in 1979, and who became my partner and wife in 1980;

Bonnie and Will Callander, the best parents-in-law a guy could have had;

George Young, at Ten Speed Press, who "got" this book when other publishers thought it should be twelve separate books; Jackie Wan, our editor for the first two editions, and Brie Mazurek, editor for this edition; and Regina, who so bravely wrestled with both me and herself to make our ideas manifest in printed form;

Hannelore Travis Barnes, my eldest daughter, who proudly carried her own copy of the 1977 three-ring-binder edition of the *Wellness Workbook* to second grade on many days and who continues to inspire me with her robust embrace of life;

Meryn's and my daughter Juniper, born as Siena Travis Callander in 1993, at home, under water, at our solar-powered forty-acre homestead in rural Mendocino County, California, whose presence has dramatically changed my life and career;

A cast of other amazing characters who have played significant parts in my life since we published the last edition and who remain sources of support and nurturance: Anne Abbott, Luana Alika, Scott Anderson, Suzanne Arms, Brad Blanton, Del Callander, Susan Campbell, Antonio Carbonnell, Jerry Cornacchio, Kristi Cowles, Rio Cruz, Rae Davies, Fred Donaldson, Jen Dudley, Vera Elliot, Bruce Erikson, Pat Frank, Lee Glickstein, Richard Heinberg, Sharron Humenick, Tina Kimmel, Joyce Knott, Kathryn Korbon, Binnie LeHew, Pam Leo, Claire Leverant, Jean Liedloff, Alan Loceff, Julie Lusk, Buffy and Chris Maple, Ellen Miller, Marilyn Milos, Sam Moon, Janet Morrow, Irv Moore, Scott Noelle, Bruce Pflaum, Patricia Raskin, Lisa Reagan, Jan Richardson, Marty Rubin, Roberta Scaer, Mary Sinclair, Jim Strohecker, Win and Bill Sweet, Bruce Terrell, Bill Thar, Lorie Vance, Maggie Watson, Amelia Williams, Susanna Williams, Cathy Wills, and Heidi Zednick;

And my mentors Bobbie Burdett and Joseph Chilton Pearce.

—JWT

Heartful thanks go to my parents, Bernard and Helene Ryan, who always held the notion that their children were smart and beautiful and capable, and who encouraged each of us to find a path for expressing that.

Thanks to all the students, friends, and associates who supported and inspired the early editions of the *Wellness Workbook*, including Lloyd Barde; Don Barley; Liz Campbell and other associates at the Association for Humanistic Psychology; Darla Grace; Anita Jordan; Terry Knob; Ben Marstellar; Greg Pickernell; Mike Richards; Bob Schellenberger; Ruth and Jim Sharon; Jackie Wan and George Young, our early mentors at Ten Speed Press/Celestial Arts; and Jim Wing.

Deep appreciation for my summer officemates for helping me stay focused on my task in this new edition, especially Kyla Haber, Jaya Hoy, Everett Jaime, Joanne Maas, Thom Shelby, and Bala and Tina Zuccarello.

Special thanks to Elyse April for her research efforts and artwork, and especially for her support and tender friendship.

Warmest regards to Brie Mazurek, gracious editor, model of patience and tact, at Celestial Arts.

Gratitude for my household members, e.e., Nachama, Lalitha, and Jim for picking up the slack and for doing their laundry at odd hours when it wouldn't disturb my work.

Admiration for Jack (John) Travis for the initial inspiration, the continued friendship, and the ongoing dedication; for Meryn Callander for editorial assistance, encouragement, and flexibility; and for both of them for their commitment to all of our children.

Thanks to the readers of the previous editions, for keeping the book alive.

Profound gratitude for my spiritual preceptor, Lee Lozowick, for his smile, his fidelity, and his compassion, and for reminding me that things are just what they are; and to Sri Yogi Ramsuratkumar, the beggar, my grandfather and protector, in whose heart I am ever blessed.

—RSR

Foreword to the Third Edition

The timing was right for the first edition of the *Wellness Workbook* in 1981, when the self-care and women's movements were calling into question the medical model of professional dominance over healthcare. John Travis and Regina Sara Ryan answered with a model of wellness that has helped a worldwide generation of people take greater control over their own health. The first edition of the *Wellness Workbook* sold over 75,000 copies.

The timing was also right for the second edition in 1988, when national health policies and the World Health Organization's sponsorship of a global health promotion movement were giving broader attention to the nonmedical aspects of health in a broader social and environmental context. Travis and Ryan answered with an alternative to the policy orientation of that movement, one that brought some focus back to people as agents of change in their own environments, their emotional and spiritual lives, and their responsibility for their own health and that of the planet. In its second edition, the book sold another 100,000 copies. And the timing is right for the third edition of the *Wellness Workbook*. Updated and streamlined, the book remains a great contribution to all health-conscious readers, no matter what their

ages. It arrives in time to greet the authors' own generation, the baby boomers, coming to that stage in life when they will face their own mortality and the need to grapple with what this book has emphasized from the beginning for all age groups: that the quality, not just quantity, of your years depends on a wellness approach to living meaningfully, not just vigorously.

As "John's Journal" hints in chapter 1, Travis began this journey when he was a preventive medicine resident at Johns Hopkins. He gravitated to a seminar on public health education that I was teaching in the School of Public Health. There, he found kindred spirits that he could find in few other corners of the Johns Hopkins Medical Institutions. He challenged us to think harder and more expansively about our definitions of health; our assumptions about causation and appropriate solutions; our tendencies to look beyond the individual and proximal social relationships to broader social and policy solutions to health problems; and above all, our persistence in calling them health "problems."

Travis and I shared a mutual suspicion of the universality and omniscience claimed for medicine, but I was also susceptible to his implicit critiques of our tendency in public health to aggregate the definition of problems to populations and to delegate solutions to higher levels of authority. Public health, like medicine, has its important contributions, but both tended to lose sight of the person, of human agency, and of opportunities to give people greater control of their health by encouraging them to take greater personal responsibility for their health.

Following the evolution of Travis and Ryan's book, as well as the international response to it, has been a source of inspiration for me, given our parallel career tracks and commitments to the concept of putting the person back into the health-and-wellness equation. They have given conceptual and spiritual leadership to the wellness movement by acknowledging the limits of medicine's focus on the immediate symptoms of illness, and by showing the way to the underlying causes over which people can exercise some control in their own lives.

While the rest of us in public health, health promotion, and health education are attempting to go upstream to get a better handle on the social and genetic determinants of health, Travis and Ryan have steadfastly looked to another stream of determinants. As they describe it, the wellness model provides a deeper probe of the lower depths of the iceberg of illness or state of health, from behavior and lifestyle, to the cultural, psychological, and motivational determinants, to the subconscious spiritual, being, and meaning levels of influence on the wellness-to-illness spectrum. This book deserves to be read at least as many times as its previous editions, but more than reading it, I commend it to all as a workbook—a bedside, chairside, and tableside companion to living well, consciously, and conscientiously.

—Lawrence W. Green, Dr.P.H.
January, 2004

Dr. Green is a health educator and the director of the Office of Science & Extramural Research, Public Health Practice Program Office, at the Centers for Disease Control and Prevention. He has been a professor or lecturer at Johns Hopkins University, Emory University, University of Texas Health Science Center at Houston, University of British Columbia, and Harvard University. He has also been a director for the Henry J. Kaiser Family Foundation, and for the Office on Smoking and Health and the Office of Health Information and Health Promotion for the U.S. Department of Health & Human Services.

Abridged Foreword to the Second Edition

The *Wellness Workbook* provides a bold new model that suggests alternative ways of living, primarily through self-responsibility and self-appreciation, whereby difficulties are resolved when more basic human needs are addressed. Instead of the typical problem-illness orientation, it offers what I would call a "possibility orientation." What if, as Regina and John suggest, you put yourself to the task of self-awareness and sensitivity; what if you laughed more; what if you really understood that the way you communicate with other people, the way you breathe, the way you express feelings, make love, pray, and especially think, all were contributing factors to your state of illness or wellness? These are among the questions raised, and the very real possibilities offered, by the *Wellness Workbook.*

The Wellness Energy System serves as the unifying principle of the book. This orientation is their special contribution to a truly holistic view of the human being. Not that they were the first, or only ones, to express the phenomenon of illness or health in terms of energy flow or energy usage. But, John and Regina have put this understanding together in such a clean and workable way as to make it irresistible. They have introduced to the public at large a profound wisdom in a form that even a child can appreciate. Most of all, I am particularly impressed by the "big picture" the book takes, in establishing a person-planet connection. No longer can we, as global citizens, consider our cancers, or even our colds, as solely our own private concerns. Our health is tied, inextricably, with the health of our environment. No longer can we neglect to examine the impact that everything—from the chair we sit in at work to the conversations we engage in over dinner—is having on our life and health. John and Regina remind and gently urge us to wake up to all of it. That's the real power of wellness as far as I'm concerned.

The *Wellness Workbook* is the most accessible, comprehensive, and certainly the most "heartful" book of its kind on the market today.

—Kenneth R. Pelletier, Ph.D.
July, 1988

Chair of the American Health Association, and clinical professor of medicine at the University of Maryland and the University of Arizona.

Abridged Foreword to the First Edition

My own search for wellness has been a long path of learning. Originally I thought someone "out there" would tell me what was wrong and what I needed to do. Some "educated" person held the power, knew the answers, had the authority to intervene on behalf of my health. The parent-to-child stance somehow seemed acceptable.

However, it was only when I took responsibility for my health, when I acknowledged my own power, when I learned to trust my own answers, when I recognized that I was the real authority about my own body, that my search for wellness brightened.

This adult-to-adult perception freed me to view healthcare professionals as resource people, to explore alternative approaches, to read, listen, learn, and grow in my own confidence. Health comes when we are total, whole people; when we have achieved a level of integration between the mind, body, emotions, and spirit; when we allow ourselves to balance. The *Wellness Workbook* is a marvelous asset. It not only gives practical information on nutrition, exercise, attitudes, and so on, but it also happily acknowledges the human spirit.

The *Wellness Workbook* holds the potential to build the confidence and to support the intelligent choices of any person on the path toward wellness. It is an act of love and caring.

—Dorothy Jongeward, Ph.D.
     February, 1981

President of Dorothy Jongeward Associates, Inc., a management consulting firm and coauthor, Born to Win: Transactional Analysis with Gestalt Experiments; *and* Winning Ways in Health Care: Transactional Analysis for Effective Communication.

Wellness is a choice—a decision you make to move toward optimal health.

Wellness is a way of life—a lifestyle you design to achieve your highest potential for wellbeing.

Wellness is a process—a developing awareness that there is no end point, but that health and happiness are possible in each moment, here and now.

Wellness is a balanced channeling of energy—energy received from the environment, transformed within you, and returned to affect the world around you.

Wellness is the integration of body, mind, and spirit—the appreciation that everything you do, and think, and feel, and believe has an impact on your state of health and the health of the world.

Wellness is the loving acceptance of yourself.

This book is about learning to love your whole self. It is about assuming charge of your life, living in process, and channeling life energy. It is about choices. It is about the *one way* to wellness— *your way*. This book is about you.

Introduction

What Is Wellness?

Wellness is the right and privilege of everyone. There is no prerequisite for it other than your free choice. The "well" being is not necessarily the strong, the brave, the successful, the young, the whole, or even the illness-free being. A person can be living a process of wellness and yet be physically handicapped; aged; scared in the face of challenge; in pain; imperfect. No matter what your current state of health, you can begin to appreciate yourself as a growing, changing person and allow yourself to move toward a happier life and positive health.

Wellness is never a static state. You don't just get well or stay well. There are many degrees or levels of wellness, just as there are degrees of illness. Nor is wellness simply the absence of disease. While people often lack physical symptoms, they may still be bored, depressed, tense, anxious, or generally unhappy with their lives. These emotional states often set the stage for physical disease through the lowering of the body's resistance. The same feelings can also lead to abuses like smoking, excessive alcohol or drug use, and overeating. But these symptoms and behaviors represent only the tip of the iceberg.

They are the surface indication of underlying human needs for such things as recognition from others, a stimulating environment, caring and affection from friends, a sense of purpose, and self-acceptance.

Diseases and symptoms are not really the problem. They are actually the body-mind-spirit's attempt to solve a problem—they are a message from the subconscious to the conscious.

Much of contemporary medical practice is involved with chipping away at surface needs. Its orientation is toward treating and eliminating the evidence of disease, and this is important. But it is not enough. It is essential to look below the surface signs to address the real needs. Wellness extends the definition of health to encompass a process of integration characterized by awareness, education, and growth.

He not busy being born is busy dying.

—Bob Dylan

The Illness/Wellness Continuum illustrates the relationship between the allopathic medical paradigm (or any other symptom-treatment system) and the wellness paradigm, which is based on self-responsibility.

Moving toward high-level wellness will involve the three steps of awareness, education, and growth. This book is designed to get you moving. In each chapter, there are exercises to help you in self-evaluation, in gaining awareness of what is working—or not working—in your life right now. Next, material is offered to assist you in your self-education. Some of it comes from others who have studied and lived it for a time. Much of it is a reminder of what you already know, but may have avoided or forgotten. In addition, each chapter includes growth options—suggestions of alternatives, invitations to stretch your limits, permission to risk, encouragement to change.

The *Wellness Workbook* is an invitation to you to consider illness and health in a bigger context: that of your connection with other people as well as with the entire planet. As we understand it, health is a result of a dynamic energy exchange between the individual and everything in creation. People cannot live well while remaining isolated from other people and things around them. We are interdependent elements in a living system. When any part is ill or healthy, it necessarily affects the energy, and changes the health, of the whole.

We think this understanding is so basic to an appreciation of wellness that we've built the entire structure and content of this book on it. So let's begin by exploring our foundation.

Illness/Wellness Continuum

Most of us think of wellness in terms of illness; we assume that the absence of illness indicates wellness. There are actually many degrees of wellness, just as there are many degrees of illness. The Illness/Wellness Continuum (below) illustrates the relationship of the treatment paradigm to the wellness paradigm.

Even though people often lack physical symptoms, they may still be bored, depressed, tense, anxious, or simply unhappy with their lives. Such

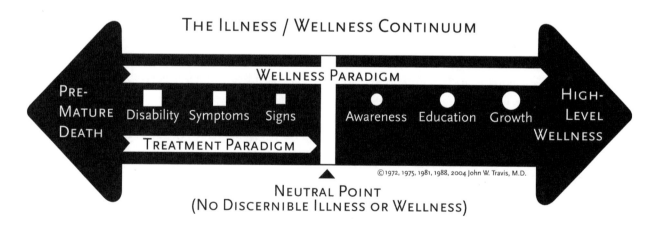

THE ILLNESS / WELLNESS CONTINUUM

WELLNESS PARADIGM

PRE-MATURE DEATH — Disability — Symptoms — Signs — Awareness — Education — Growth — HIGH-LEVEL WELLNESS

TREATMENT PARADIGM

©1972, 1975, 1981, 1988, 2004 John W. Travis, M.D.

NEUTRAL POINT
(NO DISCERNIBLE ILLNESS OR WELLNESS)

Moving from the center to the left shows a progressively worsening state of health. Moving to the right of center indicates increasing levels of health and wellbeing. The treatment paradigm (drugs, herbs, surgery, psychotherapy, acupuncture, and so on) can bring you up to the neutral point, where the symptoms of disease have been alleviated. The wellness paradigm, which can be utilized at any point on the continuum, helps you move toward higher levels of wellness. The wellness paradigm directs you beyond neutral and encourages you to move as far to the right as possible. It is not meant to replace the treatment paradigm on the left side of the continuum, but to work in harmony with it. If you are ill, then treatment is important, but don't stop at the neutral point. Use the wellness paradigm to move toward high-level wellness.

I'm sometimes alarmed by a kind of neofascism that I see in the wellness and alternative/complementary medicine movements. Covert or overt pressure is applied to get people to adhere to a particular lifestyle or dogma. There are "nutrition nuts" who want everyone to take high doses of a particular supplement or go on a certain diet. There are runners who want to make marathoners out of everyone. There are meditators who want everyone to meditate exactly as they do. Health becomes equated with a certain set of behaviors or practices, and pressure is applied to make people conform to the group norm.

While I want to get my message across, I do not want to be looked on as the expert dictating the one true way; I do not want to become part of the neofascism. The wellness paradigm calls for options, individuality, and choices freely made.

—JWT

emotional states often set the stage for physical and mental disease. Even cancer can be brought on by excessive stress that weakens the immune system. Negative emotional states can also lead to abuse of the body through smoking, overdrinking alcohol, and overeating—attempts to substitute for other more basic human needs such as acknowledgment and respect, a stimulating and supportive environment, and a sense of purpose and meaning.

Wellness is not a static state. High-level wellness involves giving good care to your physical self, using your mind constructively, expressing your emotions effectively, being creatively involved with those around you, and being concerned about your physical, psychological, and spiritual environments. In fact, it's not so much *where* you are on the continuum, but which direction you're facing. High-level wellness does not preclude periods of illness and weakness, nor does it attempt to deny that death is a natural part of life. (As you'll find in chapter 11, dying can be done from a place of wellness). Awareness of this paradox eventually led us to expand the model, but first a little background.

The Illness/Wellness Continuum was first envisioned by John in 1972, late one evening after everyone else at his office in the U.S. Public Health Service Hospital in Baltimore, Maryland, had gone home. It was a melding of the health risk continuum created by Lewis Robbins (founder of the Health Risk Appraisal) and Abraham Maslow's concept of self-actualization.

Once it was published in 1975, the continuum became an immediate success, an easy way to illustrate what this newly emerging wellness concept was all about. Health practitioners and educators began using it; soon it was appearing in books, journals, and slide presentations everywhere around the world. We naturally included it in the first edition of this book, and we continue to do so because of its visual impact. To this day it is reprinted in health and medical textbooks worldwide.

However, a simple model cannot always convey a complex concept. For a number of years we had recognized that the continuum could be misleading in one very significant area. We knew it is possible to be physically ill yet oriented toward wellness, or to be physically healthy yet functioning from an illness mentality. Our one-dimensional model simply couldn't show this distinction. For example, imagine disabled, sick, or dying people who are taking responsibility for their lives and are consciously engaged in the experience. If only the physical dimension were considered, they would fall on the left side of the continuum, but if emotional, intellectual, and spiritual dimensions are taken into account they would definitely be on the right side of the continuum.

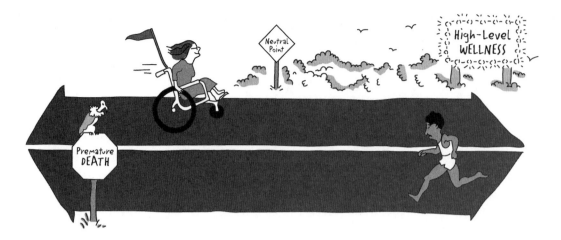

In the spring of 1986, in Vail, Colorado, John was inspired with another view of the original paradigm. Sharing his thoughts about what he had seen, Regina immediately concurred and we proceeded to flesh out the image.

What we saw was that the key difference between illness and wellness—regardless of the point on the continuum at which a person may be physically—is *the direction in which they are facing:* toward high-level wellness or toward premature death.

Think of the continuum as a pathway. People can be going in either direction on the path. A person who is physically in good health, but always complaining or worrying may be on the right of the neutral point, but definitely facing toward the left—toward premature death. Conversely, another person, whose body is handicapped physically or mentally, can still have a genuinely positive outlook, be cultivating love instead of fear and, consequently, be facing to the right, in the direction of high-level wellness.

Key Concept #2

Illness and health are only the tip of an iceberg. To understand their causes, you must look below the surface.

ABOUT ENERGY

Life is a continual dance of energy. Literally everything that we see, hear, touch, and know—including this book that you hold in your hands, and your thinking about what you are reading—is energy in one of its many forms and expressions.

Nearly all of our physical energy comes to us from the sun. Follow a bundle of sunbeams from their source across ninety-three million miles of space until they reach the earth's atmosphere. Observe their progress when they get here and you'll have a better idea of what energy transformation is all about.

As they near the surface of the earth, sunbeams warm the atmosphere, and weather is born. Winds are created, waters move, and the planet is sculpted. This is only the beginning.

Some of our sunbeams are captured by hungry green plants and put to work to grow new shoots or fruits: carbohydrates—food—ready to satisfy the lucky animal or human who happens along. The process continues.

Food sustains life, as animals and humans grow in size and strength. A big, strong adult takes a walk, or dreams a dream, cries over a silly movie, builds a monument, or makes a baby . . . and all essentially powered by sunbeams. Amazing! This is the simple magic that creates life as we know it. It's all energy dancing!

THE ICEBERG MODEL OF HEALTH AND DISEASE

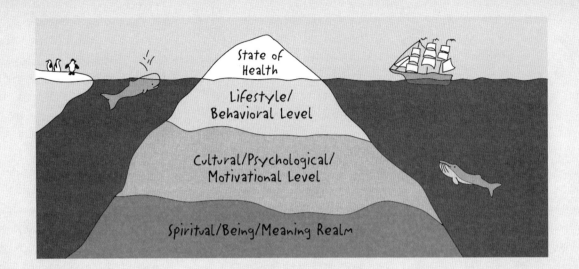

Icebergs reveal only about one-tenth of their mass above the water. The remaining nine-tenths remains submerged. This is why they are such a nightmare in navigation, and why they make such an appropriate metaphor in considering your state of wellness.

Your current state of health, be it one of disease or vitality, is just like the tip of the iceberg. This is the apparent part—what shows. If you don't like it, you can attempt to change it, do things to it, chisel away at an unwanted condition. But, whenever you knock some off, more of the same comes up to take its place.

To understand all that creates and supports your current state of health, you have to look underwater. The first level you encounter is the lifestyle/behavioral level—what you eat, how you use and exercise your body, how you relax and let go of stress, and how you safeguard yourself from the hazards around you.

Many of us follow lifestyles that we know are destructive, both to our own wellbeing and to that of our planet. Yet, we may feel powerless to change them. To understand why, we must look still deeper, to the cultural/psychological/motivational level. Here we find what moves us to lead the lifestyle we've chosen. We learn how powerfully our cultural norms influence us, sometimes in insidious ways—like convincing us that excessive thinness is attractive. We can learn, for example, what "payoffs" we get from being overweight, smoking, driving recklessly—or from eating well, being considerate of others, and getting regular exercise. We can become conscious of any psychological payoffs based on dysfunctional childhood experiences—like stuffing away our feelings as a way to gain approval from Mom and Dad.

Exploring below the cultural/psychological/motivational level, we encounter the spiritual/being/meaning realm. (Other possible descriptors include transpersonal, philosophical, or metaphysical.) Actually, we prefer to call it a realm rather than a level, because it has no clear boundaries. It includes the mystical and mysterious, plus everything in the unconscious mind, as well as concerns such as your reason for being, the real meaning of your life, or your place in the universe. The way in which you address these questions, and the answers you choose, underlie and permeate all of the layers above. Ultimately, this realm determines whether the tip of the iceberg, representing your state of health, is one of disease or wellness.

Robert F. Allen, Ph.D. (1928–1987), the founder of the Human Resources Institute in Morristown, New Jersey, pioneered an approach to wellness (long before the word was in common use) through the identification of *cultural norms*. He, and his son Judd, who now carries their work on, focus primarily on helping people to first become more fully aware of how norms may be working against their wellness and then to change the systems that support the existing norms; for example, by modifying the impact of existing modeling, rewards, and other norms.

Mainstream thinking in Western medicine has traditionally considered the state of personal health (the area above the water in the Iceberg Model) as independent of the deeper levels and acted as if this were true. We disagree entirely.

When we first wrote the *Wellness Workbook* in the late 1970s, the norms for smoking were just beginning to change. When we revised this book in the late 1980s, we were impressed with how many cities—and even states—were enacting legislation that banned smoking in public places. Today, as we revise for the third edition in the early 2000s, this shift has faded into the background of our awareness—it's hard to remember what it was like to be subjected to other people's secondhand smoke, even on international flights. The norm has changed in far less time than we ever expected. Although

many people had known for a long time that smoking affected people's health, it wasn't until the norm that condoned public smoking was changed that these behaviors dramatically decreased. Similarly, once Mothers Against Drunk Drivers created the concept of the "designated driver," that idea quickly became imbedded in our culture and has become a new norm.

But you need only watch an hour of television or peruse a single issue of a popular magazine to see that many unhealthy norms are still widely supported. Think of eco-destructive consumerism, such as people buying gas-guzzling SUVs or "disposable _____" (you fill in the blank), or the pharmaceutical industry's relentless promotion of a drug for every "problem."

Pay attention to your values and how congruent they are with the behavior of those around you. Ask yourself: How many of the advertised products that I am assailed with are really necessities? How many are downright unhealthy? What lifestyles do these commercials or ads presume and promote? Do they fit my pictures of how life really is, or should be? These advertisements are good indicators of our cultural norms.

The overwhelming power of advertising notwithstanding, greater and greater numbers of us are taking a stand and making a change. Since the mid-1970s, running and other forms of exercise and fitness have

risen in popularity to the point of becoming something of a national obsession. Other behavior-change indicators—such as greater public awareness of food addictions and eating disorders, and a massive campaign against drinking and driving—are evident everywhere. We are, at longlast, recognizing the implications that our lifestyle activities (the lifestyle/behavioral level of the Iceberg Model) have on our overall state of health. As a culture, we are finally admitting that there just may be something "below the surface."

Turning to the cultural/psychological/motivational level (one layer deeper in the Iceberg Model), we also find a number of positive signs that this level is being connected with our state of health. Witness the discussion topics on daytime TV, or the packed shelves in the psychology or self-help sections of your local bookstore. We need less convincing that our feelings and thoughts, or the abuses to which we were subjected as children—including neglect and lack of adequate touch—can contribute to our illness at least as much as germs do. We're not so dumb!

Those who study the culture, as Bob Allen did and Judd still does, generally agree that cultural norms usually lag years behind what the majority of people secretly think. This "lowest common denominator" effect serves to maintain the public mind at a level that is acceptable to everyone, even if most of us actually think it is outmoded and inadequate. Fear is usually the motivator. Quite commonly, people do not realize that their progressive beliefs are also shared by a wider segment of society. By coming together—say, in a corporate culture that they all share—they can modify the impact of their company's current modeling by changing the training, communication systems, rites, rituals, resource commitment, and relationship development that are presently the norm.

In our seminars and workshops on wellness, where it is acceptable to discuss such values openly, we would often see people stepping out of their acceptance of norms they didn't value. When people discover just how widespread their "unconventional beliefs" truly are, they are relieved and positively empowered. In the political arena, the same effect is often demonstrable. Major segments of the population in countries throughout the world are opposed to nuclear arms buildup, yet the policies of maintaining an obsolete arsenal designed for global destruction persist. Leaders of government are often afraid even to speak out, let alone act, against the supposed lowest common denominator of the cultural norm. In the social and civil-rights domain, we are more accepting of different races, different sexual orientations, and different religious beliefs—yet our legislation still often fails to reflect or support these differences.

The last major level of the Iceberg Model to achieve cultural acceptability, especially in Western societies where science and technology have been revered as the gods of progress, is the spiritual/being/meaning realm. But even this is changing. When we wrote the first edition of the *Wellness Workbook* in 1980, we were afraid to use the word *spiritual*. Instead, we used *philosophical* and *transpersonal* to label this portion of our model. The term *spiritual* was, we thought, too often confused with either the hocus-pocus of occultism or the rigidity of much formal religion, and we meant neither. To us, spirit is something much deeper, all-pervasive, and certainly not confined to one set of doctrines, experiences, or forms. Spirit, for us, means a connection with everything in creation; an animating force; the principle of unification; the shared consciousness of the one body of life. Religion, we believe, is simply one form of expressing this awareness. As such, its importance must not be undervalued.

We are far from alone in "coming out of the closet" with our acknowledgment of the spiritual nature of being. We feel a growing hunger in ourselves—and we sense the same in the people we encounter in our work—for understanding and expression of this level of reality. No longer satisfied with the testimony of professional witnesses, such as priests, ministers, and rabbis, we want to experience the spirit firsthand and integrate it into all aspects of our lives. Perhaps there is a peaceful revolution in the making. Perhaps, even sooner than we think, we will see the upgrading of the lowest common denominator in this area as well. At the same time, we recommend using caution and discernment to determine what is genuinely at the core of spirit and what is a cheap window dressing, offered by those who would attempt to package and sell us "spirit." To switch to a brand of tea that is labeled with Chinese calligraphy and called "Zen"-something is not the same as taking up a practice of Zen meditation. We can fill our rooms and cover our desks with spiritual paraphernalia, yet still not address our grasping and restlessness for more of everything.

Within or without formal religion, we believe that attunement to spirit (the foundational level in the Iceberg Model) is the ultimate source of wellbeing. Furthermore, we suggest that wellness as a way of life orients one toward greater awareness of communion with this source. These are assertions not easily explainable with words or grasped by the rational mind. In the realm of the spirit, one must read and lead more often with the heart. (See chapters 11 and 12.)

Questioning Your Cultural Norms

Which of the following are the norm in one or more groups that you belong to? Write your responses in your journal.

1. *People use their cars to go short distances even when there is no need to do so.*

2. *People are surprised when someone uses the stairs instead of the elevator or escalator.*

3. *People don't mention it if someone else's smoking bothers them.*

4. *People take on more responsibility than they can handle.*

5. *People view being slightly overweight as "natural," particularly for older people.*

6. *People drink a great many coffee and cola drinks and other caffeine-based beverages.*

7. *People persuade guests to stay for one more round of drinks or "one more for the road."*

8. *Restaurant staff expect patrons to have a drink before or during dinner.*

9. *Friends make jokes that support gender, racial, or sexual prejudice.*

10. *People act offended by public breast-feeding.*

11. *Mothers bottle-feed in the face of overwhelming evidence that it is harmful to their child.*

12. *Mothers return to work outside the home and leave their very young child(ren) in the care of random strangers.*

13. *People do not see themselves as being as capable as they really are.*

Modified, with permission, from Robert F. Allen with Shirley Linde, "Cultural Norm Indicator," *Lifegain* (Human Resources Institute, 1981).

We are all energy transformers, connected with the whole universe. All our life processes, including illness, depend on how we manage energy.

The Wellness Energy System

In 1977, Ilya Prigogene won a Nobel Prize for his theory of dissipative structures. Dissipative structures are open systems in which energy is taken in, modified (transformed), and then returned (dissipated) to the environment. A rock or a cold cup of coffee are closed systems because they do not channel and transform energy in this way. A seed, which constructs a plant from soil, air, and light, is an open system. So is a town, one of Prigogene's favorite examples. In the town, raw materials are converted into other objects by factories. These manufactured goods are then sent out into the world. Information and experience are processed in the town's schools with the end result being educated minds that are then released to make their impact on the world.

A human being is an open system, too. We take in energy from all the sources around us, organize it, transform it, and return (dissipate) it to the environment around us. The underlying theory in this book is that *efficient flow of energy is essential to wellness; disease is the result of any interference with this flow.* This is true of energy usage in all life processes, from breathing to dying.

Think of yourself as a channel of energy—energy flowing in, coursing around, and flowing out. And because you are different from every other "channel" walking around, it goes without saying that your condition (physical, emotional, mental, spiritual) is going to determine how much you take in, what it feels like inside, and how it moves out into the environment. When the flow is balanced and smooth, you feel good. When there is interference at any point—the input, the output, or in between—you can feel empty, confused, pressured, or blocked. Illness is often the result.

The process may be compared to the movement of water through a pipe (fig. 1). The source of the water, the reservoir, constitutes the *input.* The size and condition of the pipe will determine the *flow through.* The water that emerges at the other end—from your faucet, for instance—is the *output.* Ideally, it is clear, fresh, and free-flowing, as shown.

Experience tells us, however, that many things can go wrong. There can be problems at the source—the reservoir may be dry because of a long drought (fig. 2), or the water may be poisoned by industrial wastes (fig. 3).

There may be problems in the pipe itself. There could be a leak; the pipe could be blocked by accumulated debris (fig. 4), or it could be rusty. Whatever the problem, the amount and the quality of water at the faucet—the output—will be seriously affected. Overuse due to extreme need, such as putting out a huge fire, may quickly deplete the input source. Lack of use, on the other hand, may cause the water in the pipes to freeze in cold weather, or stagnate and discolor as it sits in the channel. These examples highlight interdependent systems in which changes in one part impact

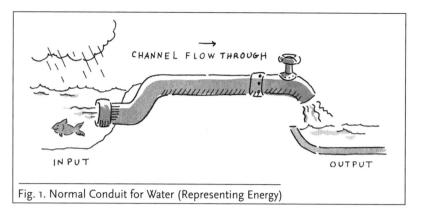

Fig. 1. Normal Conduit for Water (Representing Energy)

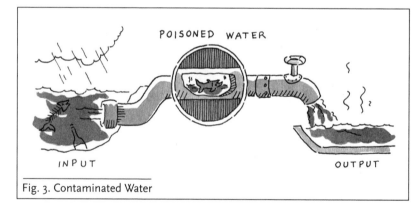

Fig. 2. Dry Reservoir

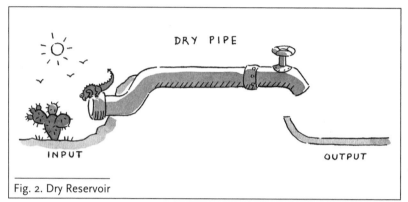

Fig. 3. Contaminated Water

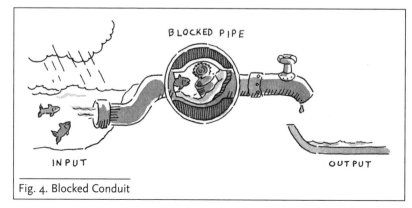

Fig. 4. Blocked Conduit

the other parts in some way and affect the operation of the whole system in general.

Keep these realizations in mind as we look at an energy-oriented systems approach for the wellness of human beings. You have at least three major sources for input around you all the time (fig. 5). These are: (1) oxygen, (2) food, and (3) sensory stimulation such as physical touch, heat, light, sound, and other forms of electromagnetic radiation. In addition, there are the less tangible inputs: emotional/spiritual information such as attention, caring, love, enthusiasm, and possibly extrasensory data.

You are the *channel* or the transformer of these energy sources. In the water pipe analogy, the flow through is dependent on the shape, diameter, and composition of the pipe. For the human organism, the list of modifiers of energy is much greater. Your sex, blood type, the pigmentation of your skin, and other racial characteristics are your genetic inheritance; there isn't much you can do about them. Over other conditions, however, you have much more voluntary control. These include your education and beliefs, previous experience, the activity of your nervous system, your flexibility, strength, body

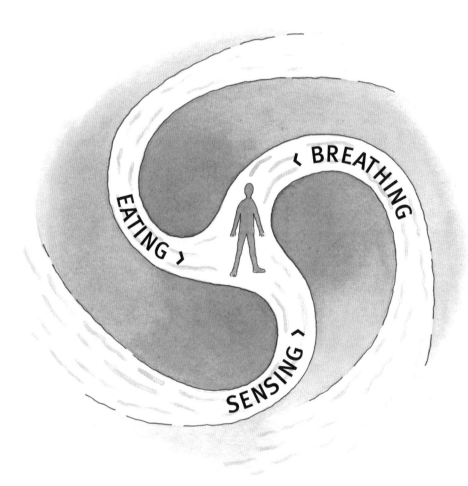

Fig. 5. Wellness Energy System: Input

weight, emotional development, muscle tension, general state of health, and functioning of organs. The less measurable factors of sensitivity, open-mindedness, and self-love are also up to you.

We use part of the energy we take in to maintain the channel—to build and repair the body itself. This is the *internal output.* At the most elementary level, we use energy to maintain a narrow internal temperature range (around 98.6°F/37°C), as circulating blood brings heat to cold areas. We secrete digestive juices for breakdown and absorption of food. We synthesize chemicals that are sent to many different organs. We produce electrochemical impulses that travel throughout the nervous system. Taking a step up in this energy transformation process, we replace worn tissue and blood cells—repairing cuts and scratches and mending bones. We move muscles that control digestion, respiration, elimination, and reproduction. And don't forget those less tangible expressions of energy—the generation of emotions, the internal dialogue of your thinking processes, your intuition, dreams, and the creation of what may be spiritual insights and altered states of consciousness.

The outside world will also be affected by the ways you transform energy (fig. 6). This is the *external output.* You radiate heat and eliminate waste products in the form of urine, perspiration, carbon dioxide, and the shedding of dead skin. The rest of us will be affected by your touching, your physical

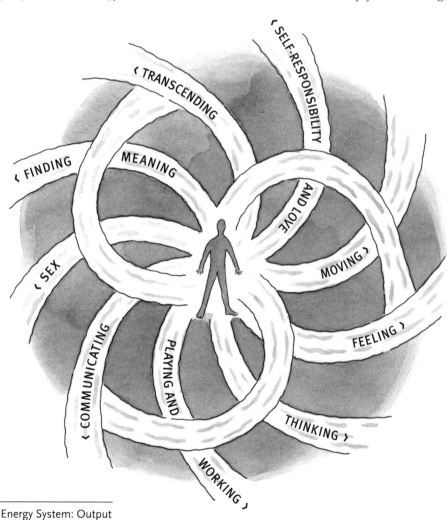

Fig. 6. Wellness Energy System: Output

work and play, your laughter and tears. We will learn about you, and ourselves, through communication, the sharing of intellectual pursuits, and the expression of creativity. You can't help but influence the planet by your interaction with the environment. Less-understood energy communications, such as telepathy and other psychic phenomena, are taking place as well. And there is no doubt that your loving energy will change us all.

Putting together the input and output, we have the complete Wellness Energy System of a human being (fig. 7). Since there are many of us, and we are all interacting and exchanging energy with each other and everything else in our environment, the picture gets more complex (fig. 8). Try looking at the world around you as composed not of separate fixed *things,* but as structures reflecting the energy that creates them—a vast dance with a myriad of participants. We have shown an idealized model of wellness based on a balanced exchange of energy. But the world is not a perfect place. Like the clogged, contaminated, or empty pipes shown earlier, we experience energy

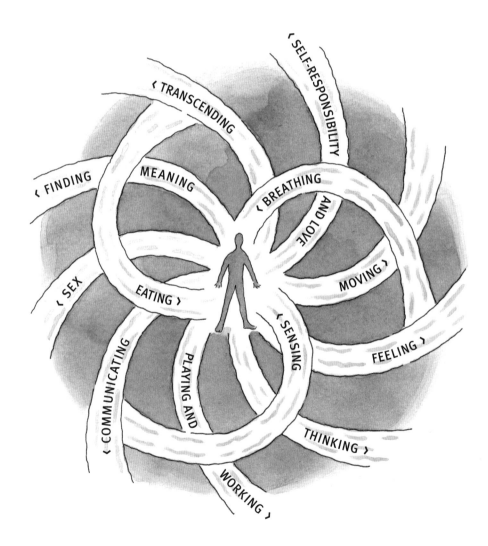

Fig. 7. Wellness Energy System: Complete
Please note that each arrow corresponds to an entire chapter of this book.

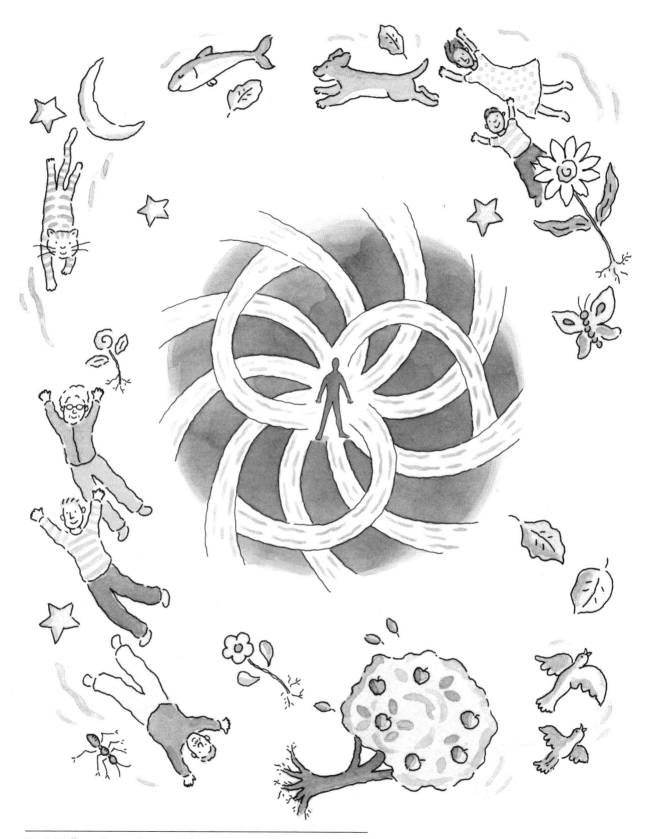

Fig. 8. Wellness Energy System: Individual and Environment Interacting

distortions that lead to imbalances in the ways we process energy. Figure 9 shows six possible distortions of energy that human beings might develop:

1. Insufficient intake of energy; for example, denying acknowledgment or compliments from other people

2. Too much of one form of energy, such as too much food

3. An intermingling, contamination, or substitution of one form of energy with another, such as attempting to use sex to satisfy a spiritual hunger

4. Blockage causing an internal buildup of unprocessed energy; for example, fear of open communication with others leading to a censoring of behavior for fear of what others might be thinking (codependency)

5. Too strong an interface with the environment; for example, an abrasive, explosive way of relating to people, which discourages further interaction

6. Too weak an interface with the environment; for example, an unfocused diffusion of energy, which shows up as a wishy-washy approach to people and commitments

These six examples do not cover all the possibilities, but they do graphically show some of the possible distortion of energy that can lead to illness.

A simpler way of representing how well your energy is balanced is the Wellness Wheel (fig. 10), which you shortly will complete as a part of the Wellness Index (next section). Each of the twelve sections of the wheel corresponds to one of the arrows in the Wellness Energy System (and to a chapter of this book). Each section represents one slice of this whole pie called wellness.

After completing the Wellness Index, your Wellness Wheel will allow you to see which areas of your life need attention. This simpler representation of your personal energy system does not show graphically, as does figure 9, what specific problems you may encounter in your own energy

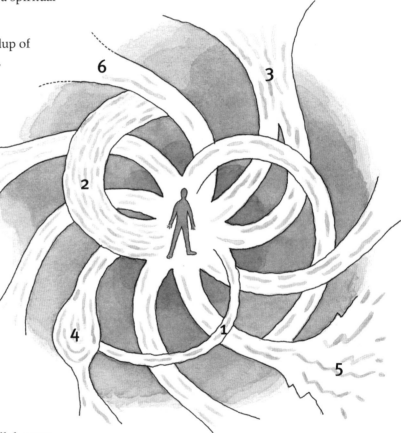

Fig. 9. Wellness Energy System: Distortions
1. Insufficient flow of energy
2. Too much of one type of energy
3. Contamination—intermingling of energy
4. Blocked energy
5. Poor interface of energy with environment (explosive)
6. Poor interface of energy with environment (ineffective)

economy. It does, however, give a good overall picture of how balanced or imbalanced your energy system is. For deeper understanding of any problem, you will need to look more closely at the specific questions in the Wellness Index whose low or high scores have produced the imbalance in your wheel. (A feature of the abbreviated, online version of the Wellness Index, the Wellness Inventory Online, is that it automatically tracks the questions that you scored lowest on, along with the level of satisfaction you indicated about your response, generating a list of your lowest scores as well as your interest in changing them. See www.WellnessWorkbook.com for more information and discounts for owners of this book.)

In the five hypothetical examples that follow, we have attempted to show some of the practical applications of using the Wellness Energy System to assess and help guide us in directions we may want to take in our lives. To test your understanding of the concept, imagine how the actual distortions of each person's arrows might look.

In summary, we have shown how the Wellness Energy System is our alternative to the usual piecemeal way of looking at health. We offer an integrated overview of all human life functions, seeing them as various forms of energy. The harmonious balancing of these life functions results in good health and wellbeing. Taken together as a whole, our picture can be no smaller than the whole planet.

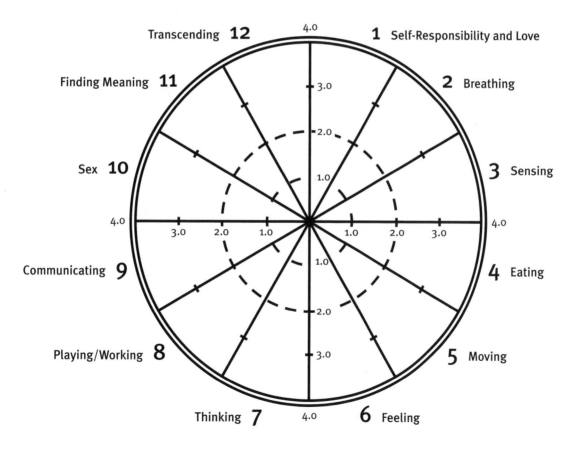

Fig. 10. The Wellness Wheel

Here are some hypothetical examples of people who have taken the Wellness Index (next section) and how they might use the Wellness Energy System as a guide to creating more vibrant health and energy in their own lives. (Before reading the examples, you may wish to take a quick look at the Wellness Index to get a feel for the statements to which the people responded.) Since the Wellness Wheel is designed for self-interpretation, each example expresses the person's first impressions, followed by more in-depth considerations about what needs attention or change. This Index and the Wellness Wheel that accompanies it offer another way in which we may take responsibility for our lives.

Example 1: Paul

Paul's impressions: "My job is a sedentary one, and I'm not much inclined to exercise. I expected low scores all around, but I'd really like to improve my overall health. I'm just not sure where to start. I'm about thirty pounds overweight now, and generally don't feel confident in myself.

"Since I was a kid I have always been the fat guy, and I hate it. No matter how much I eat, I never feel really satisfied. But I also feel guilty when I eat because I hate being so fat. I don't have many friends, and don't think I'll ever find a woman who would want to be with me."

Paul's commitments: "I think my first priority needs to be something other than a diet, since I've failed so many times before in this department. While I'm not excited about exercising, I've never really worked with a trainer or given myself the opportunity to join a gym. Lots of my friends at work are doing that now, so this would be a good way to interact with more people.

"The one part I feel sad about is the playing and working score. I don't give myself a lot of options for play. I think I miss chances to enjoy myself because I'm self-conscious, and because I've defined playing in such a limited way. I really like to play chess and bridge, but I haven't made efforts to do that for years. I think it is time to start."

Example 2: Kate

Kate's impressions: "Reading over the transcending and finding meaning sections of the Index, I recall how hungry I am to reconnect with my spiritual nature. Worry and fear tend to get the better of me, and I forget what I once knew about my relationship with God."

Kate's commitments: "I've been saying for years now that I wanted to get back into painting again. This art form has always been a food for my soul. I am praying when I am painting. When I'm fed in this way my worry and fear are so much less, and all other aspects of my life are better handled. I've been trying to meditate,

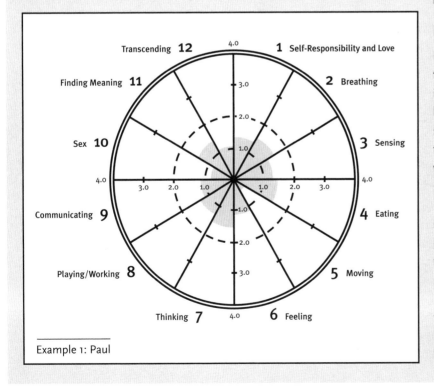

Example 1: Paul

but I'd much rather be painting. I'm going to start clearing a spot for myself in the garage, and setting up a studio again."

Example 3: Marty

Marty's impressions: "It is shocking to see how unbalanced my Wellness Wheel is. Like I'm missing half of life. I am fifty years old and when I'm out running I zoom past guys who look ten years younger than me. I run at least six miles a day, take long-distance bicycle trips on the week-ends, and am building strength and endurance. My work is so stressful that if I didn't do this much exercise I'd now be dead. I lost one job in the past year, and now have to work three times as hard, for less pay, to create a space for myself in this new company. I still make a good salary, but like everyone else, I always want more."

Marty's commitments: "My wife has been going for counseling for a year, and she wants me to join her. Our marriage is suffering. Actually, we are each suffering. I say I don't have time for counseling, but really I'm terrified. It will take a lot of energy to start to feel again. Without feeling and loving again, I'm in big trouble. I have to open my heart!"

Example 4: Ramon

Ramon's impressions: "I just turned sixty this year and have never felt bet-ter. But, my diet and eating habits are still not to my satisfaction. I want to lose about fifteen pounds and keep it off, but all that sweating and aerobic stuff is not my thing either."

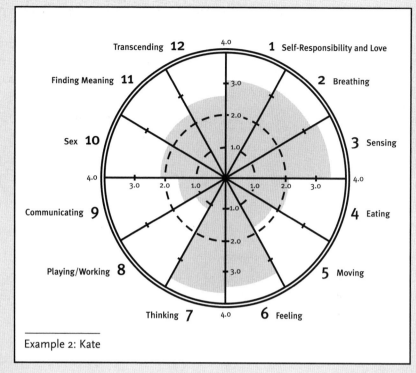

Example 2: Kate

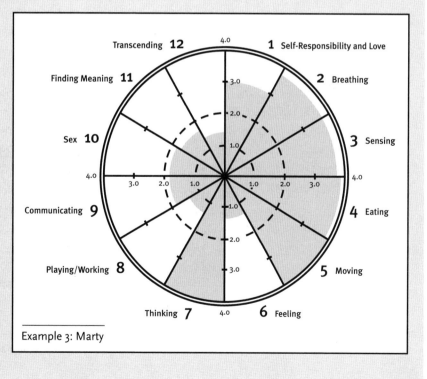

Example 3: Marty

Ramon's commitments: "I have serious bouts of indigestion whenever I eat fast, or eat heavy food, especially late at night. Constipation is also a big issue for me. I know I always feel better when I eat more fruits and vegetables. I generally like fruit, but am bored by apples and bananas, which is all my wife buys. I'm going to ask her to join me in trying other types."

Example 5: Gail

Gail's impressions: "Going to school is my life right now. If I didn't have to totally work so hard I'd be ecstatic, but I'm going to finish, no matter what! I'm not surprised that my playing and working score is lowest. I'm a perfectionist."

Gail's commitments: "I'm not going to change what I'm doing now. I'm committed to my education and know that I'll have other opportunities to do 'fun things' later, when I graduate. What I realized in doing this process was that I'm even harder on myself than I usually imagine. The area I want to give some attention to is in what it means to really love myself. I feel like a beginner in this department."

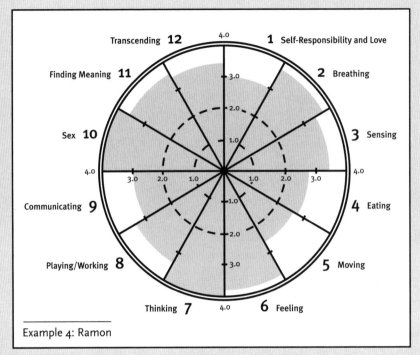

Example 4: Ramon

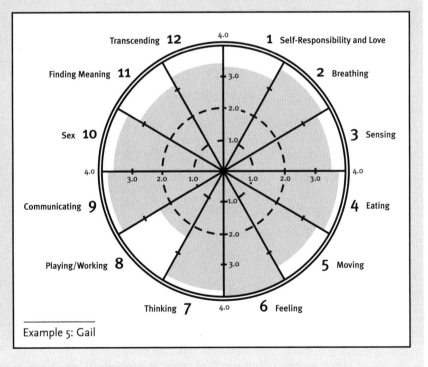

Example 5: Gail

How Best to Use This Book

Now you are ready to study each of the twelve areas in greater depth. First we suggest you complete the Wellness Index that follows. It will help you assess how well you are balancing the twelve expressions of energy and raise questions for you to explore in your reading.

The twelve chapters of the book correspond to the twelve forms of energy. The sequence of chapters approximates the order in which these forms of energy develop in human beings. In each chapter we will discuss some possible problems and diseases caused by mismanaging that form of energy. We also suggest ways to optimize the expression of each form of energy. There is overlap, of course, and it is also okay to follow your strongest interests and read the related chapters and the numbered subsections, or *modules,* within each chapter. The Wellness Index cross-references the module numbers, allowing you to explore certain questions in great depth

This book is not "nice." It does not provide ready answers. It takes you into unexpected places. It leaves you there. For logical thinkers, and that includes most of us, it will be a challenge. You may be surprised that the pages are not "neat." We have interspersed the factual text with exercises and personal examples. This may be confusing to some people, but we think it's necessary. Our intent is to address the logical, verbal parts of you, as well as to invite your participation in nonlogical processes like intuition, creativity, and feelings. This book is addressed to the whole of you—whole brain, whole heart, whole body, whole soul. So we want you to be prepared. We want you to put the *Wellness Workbook* to the best possible use for yourself—and have a great time doing so. Here are a few suggestions.

- *Master the three keys. This may sound like a riddle, but if you've read this far, the three keys are already in your hands. Simply keep them and use them as you continue exploring the chapters that follow. The keys are the three graphic illustrations of wellness that have been elaborated upon in this chapter: (1) the Illness/Wellness Continuum, (2) the Iceberg Model, and, most important of all, (3) the Wellness Energy System. If you don't clearly understand any of these, please refer back to them now.*

- *Expect more questions than answers. The philosopher Alfred North Whitehead once said: "This generation has all the answers. It's the questions that we seek." We agree. If you finish reading a chapter and find yourself with more whys and hows than when you started, we will have done our job. The Wellness Workbook is not about herbal prescriptions, or vegetarian diets, or aerobic exercise regimens, even though some of these things are considered in depth. Wellness is so much more. Wellness is about you, trusting your energy, and creating your unique and vibrant life in your own way. And that may take some serious question asking.*

- *Stay active in the process. This is a workbook to be played with, not a novel to get lost in. Stay wide awake as you read, by actively participating with us. Do the exercises. Keep lists of questions. Develop a personal wellness journal to chart your progress. Argue when you want to; write us a letter. We invite your interaction, your energy, your insights. It is important to remember that wellness is a process and that, once begun, this exploration is a lifelong adventure.*

- *Don't do it right. If there is one way to discourage learning of any kind, it is to consciously attempt to avoid mistakes. We would like you to welcome them. If you're not making any in your life now, it's probably because you aren't taking any risks. It's time to venture forth.*

Use the *Wellness Workbook* as a jumping-off point for some new experimentation, self-reflection, and reeducation, and let false starts and dead ends be your friends and teachers. Expect nothing, but anticipate miracles.

> **Be patient toward all that is unsolved in your heart and try to love the questions themselves like locked rooms and like books that are written in a very foreign tongue. . . . And the point is, to live everything. Live the questions now. Perhaps you will then gradually, without noticing it, live along some distant day into the answer.**
>
> —Rainer Maria Rilke

SUGGESTED READING

Capra, F., *The Tao of Physics* (Shambhala, 2000).

Russell, P., *From Science to God: A Physicist's Journey into the Mystery of Consciousness* (New World Library, 2003).

Wolfe, F. A., *Mind into Feeling: A New Alchemy of Science and Spirit* (Moment Point, 2000).

Young, A., *The Reflexive Universe,* revised edition (Anados Foundation, 1999).

Zukav, G., *The Dancing Wu Li Masters: An Overview of the New Physics* (Bantam, 1994).

For an updated listing of resources and active links to the websites mentioned in this chapter, please see www.WellnessWorkbook.com.

Wellness Index

We suggest that before proceeding any further, you take the time to complete the Wellness Index. It may raise many questions for you, and thereby make the following chapters more meaningful. We also suggest that you use one color of pen to record your answers as they are now, and then six months later, complete the Index again using another color. Notice any changes that have occurred.

Individual copies of the Wellness Index may be obtained from the publisher: Celestial Arts, P.O. Box 7123, Berkeley, CA 94707, www.tenspeed.com.

The Wellness Inventory, an abridged version of the Index consisting of ten questions for each of the twelve sections, is available from Wellness Associates, P. O. Box 8422, Asheville, NC 28814. The Inventory is also available in an online interactive format at www.WellnessWorkbook.com.

Instructions

Set aside an hour or two for yourself in a quiet place where you will not be disturbed while taking the Wellness Index.

For each item, rate how true the statement is for you *at this time*. Record your responses to each statement in the columns using this key:

4 = Yes/always/usually
3 = Often
2 = Sometimes/maybe
1 = Occasionally
0 = No/never/hardly ever

You will find that some of the statements cover two issues. We want you to consider the interrelatedness of the two parts, such as *awareness* combined with *action*. For example, a statement might read, "I am aware of the importance of good nutrition and eat accordingly." If only one part of the statement is true, you should mentally average the sum of your answers for the two parts of the question and record that score. This prevents getting high scores for being aware of something while doing nothing about it.

Each section contains three types of statements:

1. Statements that are explained in the modules of the chapter of the *Wellness Workbook* that has the same section number (the module number is indicated at the end of each statement).

2. Bonus questions that may not be directly addressed in any module but that are included to expand on the wellness principles covered

in that chapter (also check www.Wellness Workbook.com for more information).

3. Optional sentence completions designed to stretch your self-awareness in that area of wellness.

If you decide that a statement does not apply to you, or you don't want to answer it, you can skip it without affecting your score.

Each statement describes what we believe to be a wellness attribute. Because much wellness information is subjective and unprovable by current scientific methods, you (and possibly other authorities as well) may not agree with our conclusions. If an idea sounds strange to you, read up on it in the module referenced (or the corresponding chapter) in the *Wellness Workbook.* Keep an open mind until you have studied the information available in the *Workbook,* then determine what is true for you.

This Wellness Index is designed to *educate* and *stimulate,* more than to *test.* We've worded all statements so that you can easily tell what we think are wellness attributes—which can also make it easy to "cheat" on your score. There are no trick questions

to verify your honesty or consistency. How you rate yourself is up to you—the higher your overall score, the greater you believe your level of wellness to be. For your own sake, answer each statement as honestly as possible. It's not your score but what you learn about yourself that counts in the end.

After you have responded to all the appropriate statements in each section, compute your average score for that section, using the formula provided, and round to the nearest tenth. Then transfer it to the corresponding box in the Wellness Wheel at the end of the questionnaire.

Your completed Wellness Wheel will give you a clear presentation of the balance you have in the many dimensions of your life. If your wheel is not well-balanced or is small in size, we urge you to study the sections that concern you in the corresponding chapters of the *Wellness Workbook.* Begin with those areas that most interest you, and proceed on your wellness journey at a comfortable pace. We caution against massive and sweeping life changes. Gentle, steady progress tends to be more sustainable.

Example

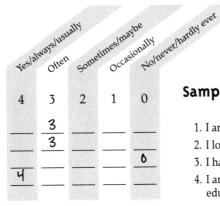

Sample Questions

1. I am a nonsmoker.
2. I love long hot baths and take them as often as I would like.
3. I have no expectations yet look to the future optimistically.
4. I am an adventurous thinker who is willing to consider new ideas in consciousness, education, and society.

___4___ + ___6___ + ___0___ + ___0___ + ___0___ = __10__ Total points for this section

Divided by __4__ (number of statements answered) = | __2__ . __5__ | **Average score for this section**

Transfer your score to the Wellness Wheel at the end of the Index.

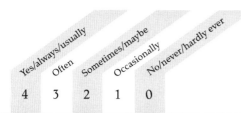

Yes/always/usually	Often	Sometimes/maybe	Occasionally	No/never/hardly ever
4	3	2	1	0

Section 1: Wellness, Self-Responsibility, and Love

1. I recognize that the responsibility for my health lies with me rather with others. (MODULE 1.1)
2. I am an active and self-responsible participant in, not a passive recipient of, any medical treatment that I receive. (MODULE 1.2)
3. I protect myself from hazards by wearing seat belts, using smoke detectors in my home, not riding in a vehicle with an inebriated driver, etc. (MODULE 1.3)
4. I check in with my body several times each day to attune to any signals it is giving me. (MODULE 1.5)
5. I am able to distinguish between accepting responsibility for a problem and blaming myself for it. (MODULE 1.6)
6. I use pain and dis-ease as an opportunity to reevaluate my lifestyle and my environment. (MODULE 1.7)
7. It is okay for me to sometimes feel out of balance, vulnerable, or in need. (MODULE 1.9)
8. I recognize that it is possible to discover wellbeing in the midst of serious or chronic illness. (MODULE 1.10)
9. I accept and forgive myself, instead of berating myself, for not being as I want to be. (MODULE 1.11)
10. I experience love for myself and for other people. (MODULE 1.12)
11. I participate in my community by voting, volunteering, contributing to worthy causes, etc. (MODULE 1.13)
12. I acknowledge that my wellbeing is interdependent with that of the planet and minimize my consumption of the planet's resources. (MODULE 1.13)

Bonus questions

13. I know my neighbors.
14. I feel financially secure.
15. When I see a broken bottle or other hazard on a pathway or in the street, I remove it.
16. If I saw a crime being committed or an emergency situation, I would report it.
17. When I see a car with faulty lights, leaking fuel, or some other dangerous condition, I attempt to tell the driver.
18. I turn off lights and appliances that are not in use.
19. I recycle paper, glass, aluminum, clothes, books, and organic waste.
20. I conserve materials and energy at home and at work.
21. My vehicle gets at least 30 miles per gallon (13 km/liter). *(If you don't own a vehicle, score 4 points.)*
22. My house has adequate insulation and, if in a cold climate, storm windows. *(Skip this question if you live in a climate that requires minimal heating or cooling.)*
23. I use a humidifier with my home heating *(Skip if you don't have central heating.)*
24. I protect my living area from fire and safety hazards.
25. I keep a dry chemical fire extinguisher in my kitchen and at least 1 other extinguisher elsewhere in my living quarters.
26. I minimize my purchases of items in excess, wasteful packaging.
27. I generate less than 1 large garbage can of nonrecyclable waste per month.
28. My domestic energy use (electricity, gas, fuel oil, kerosene, wood, coal, etc.) costs less than $50 per month per person on average.

4	3	2	1	0
Yes/always/usually	Often	Sometimes/maybe	Occasionally	No/never/hardly ever

29. I use dental floss and a soft toothbrush daily.
30. I am a nonsmoker. *(Nonsmokers score 4 points on both this and the next question.)*
31. I smoke less than 1 pack of cigarettes or fewer than 5 cigars or 10 pipes a week.
32. I am sober when driving or operating dangerous machinery.
33. When doing potentially dangerous tasks like driving or operating heavy machinery, I abstain from drugs (prescription or nonprescription) that affect my mental alertness.
34. I use the proper safety equipment (helmets, goggles, life jackets, mouth guards, etc.) when appropriate.
35. I maintain any smog equipment or safety devices installed on my car.
36. I drive within speed limits.
37. I inspect my automobile's tires, lights, brake fluid level, etc., and keep it well serviced.
38. I carry emergency flares or reflectors and a dry chemical fire extinguisher in my car.
39. I stop on yellow when a traffic light is changing.
40. For every 10 miles per hour (15 km/hour) of speed, I maintain at least 1 car length of distance from any vehicle ahead of mine.
41. I have fewer than 3 colds per year.
42. I avoid exposure to sprays, chemical fumes, or exhaust gases.
43. I purchase cleaning products and cosmetics only from manufacturers that do not test them for toxicity on animals.
44. I notice any significant changes that occur in my physical or emotional condition and seek professional advice if necessary.
45. Prior to conceiving a child, I would carefully consider my readiness to assume the role and responsibilities of becoming a parent.
46. I utilize and evaluate new or different methods of self-care.

Women only

47. I check my breasts for unusual lumps each month.
48. I have a pap test at intervals appropriate for my age.

Men only

49. I examine my testicles for any abnormalities each month.
50. If over 45, I have my prostate checked annually.

Parents only (skip any that are not appropriate for the age of your children)

51. When riding in a car, I make certain that any child weighing fewer than 50 pounds (23 kg) is secured in an approved child's safety seat or safety harness.
52. When riding in a car, I make certain that any child weighing greater than 50 pounds (23 kg) is wearing an adult seat belt.
53. When leaving my child(ren) in other people's care, I make certain they have emergency telephone numbers and that I trust their principles regarding respect for and safety of children.
54. I keep cleaning products, toxic products, medications, firearms, and other dangerous items and equipment out of the reach of children.
55. My children wear firm shoes with snugly tied laces especially when riding on escalators.
56. My children feel comfortable talking with me about sex, drugs, and other intimate or controversial issues.

Yes/always/usually	Often	Sometimes/maybe	Occasionally	No/never/hardly ever
4	3	2	1	0
___	___	___	___	___
___	___	___	___	___
___	___	___	___	___
___	___	___	___	___
___	___	___	___	___
___	___	___	___	___
___	___	___	___	___
___	___	___	___	___

57. I recognize my child as an individual and unique human being deserving of my unconditional love and respect at all stages of her/his growth.

58. I recognize and meet my child's needs for breast-feeding (exclusively for at least the first 6 months and for a minimum of 2 years thereafter, as recommended by the World Health Organization).

59. I recognize that my child's emotional needs for unconditional love, touch, and nurturing attention are as valid as any physical needs and respond accordingly.

60. I avoid the use of bribes, rewards, threats, and punishments to enforce desired behavior and instead recognize challenging situations as teachable moments or opportunities to solve a problem together.

61. I protect my child from emotional and physical neglect and abuse, including spanking, shaming, and other toxic conditions such as unmonitored or unrestricted access to television and other electronic media.

62. I recognize, respect, and support my child's unique temperament, learning styles, and abilities.

63. I seek out the information and resources (including counseling when necessary) that enable me to make informed decisions and advocate for my child's physical, mental and emotional wellbeing.

64. I respect and support the importance of my child's sustaining a healthy relationship with both my partner and myself.

___ + ___ + ___ + ___ + ___ = ___ Total points for this section

Divided by ____ (number of statements answered) = | ____ . ____ | **Average score for this section**

Transfer your score to the Wellness Wheel at the end of the Index.

Section 2: Wellness and Breathing

___	___	___	___	___
___	___	___	___	___
___	___	___	___	___
___	___	___	___	___
___	___	___	___	___
___	___	___	___	___
___	___	___	___	___
___	___	___	___	___
___	___	___	___	___

1. I wear clothing that is comfortable and loose enough to allow unrestricted breathing. (MODULE 2.1)

2. I pause during the day to notice if my posture is facilitating my full natural breathing. (MODULE 2.1)

3. I recognize that emotional states (such as fear, anger, or exhilaration) may restrict my breathing and pay special attention to breathe deeply and fully when experiencing these emotions. (MODULE 2.2)

4. I recognize cold or clammy hands, muscle tension, and high blood pressure as signs of stress and use my breath to help release my tension. (MODULE 2.3)

5. I use my breath to promote relaxation and creativity. (MODULE 2.4)

6. I use deep, rhythmic breathing as a means of helping my body heal itself of physical, mental, and emotional pain. (MODULE 2.5)

7. I use my breath as a means of centering and living fully in the present moment. (MODULE 2.6)

8. I avoid polluted environments and minimize my contribution to air pollution. (MODULE 2.7)

9. I am at peace with myself. (MODULE 2.8)

Yes/always/usually	Often	Sometimes/maybe	Occasionally	No/never/hardly ever
4	3	2	1	0

Bonus Questions

10. I get adequate sleep and awake refreshed.
11. I am limber when I awake in the morning.
12. I can easily touch my hands to my toes when standing with knees straight.
13. If under 45 years of age, I do not have deep wrinkles in my forehead.

Please complete the following sentences with the first thoughts or feelings that come to mind.

14. My breathing is _____ .
15. For relaxation I _____ .
16. My ability to relax is _____ .

____ + ____ + ____ + ____ + ____ = ____ Total points for this section

Divided by ____ (number of statements answered) = | ____ . ____ | **Average score for this section**

Transfer your score to the Wellness Wheel at the end of the Index.

Section 3: Wellness and Sensing

1. At room temperature, my hands and feet are warm. (MODULE 3.1)
2. In cold weather I keep the temperature in my home at 65°F/18°C or lower. (MODULE 3.2)
3. In warm weather I keep air-conditioning (if I have it) at 75°F/24°C or higher. (MODULE 3.2)
4. I wear natural-fiber clothing. (MODULE 3.3)
5. I use water as a means of refreshment and regeneration. (MODULE 3.4)
6. I use eye relaxation exercises to minimize eyestrain. (MODULE 3.5)
7. I avoid overexposure to midday summer sunlight, instead of relying on chemical sunscreens. (MODULE 3.6)
8. I limit my use of artificial light and use natural lighting as much as possible. (MODULE 3.7)
9. I am aware of the impact of different colors and styles of lighting on my wellbeing. (MODULE 3.8)
10. I use my sense of smell as a source of warning, healing, and pleasure. (MODULE 3.9)
11. I use music and other pleasant sounds to increase my wellbeing. (MODULE 3.10)
12. I am conscious of the negative impact of some music and sounds on my wellbeing and avoid them when possible. (MODULE 3.10)
13. I avoid frequent or extended exposure to loud noises. (MODULE 3.11)
14. I am aware of my need for touch, as well as the cultural taboos that often make it difficult to get this need met. (MODULE 3.12)
15. I receive massages regularly to increase my level of wellness. (MODULE 3.13)
16. When appropriate, I communicate with others through touch, instead of restricting myself to verbal expression. (MODULE 3.14)
17. I recognize the healing powers of touch. (MODULE 3.15)

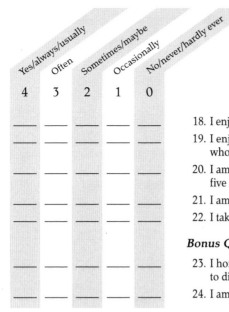

| 4 | 3 | 2 | 1 | 0 |
| Yes/always/usually | Often | Sometimes/maybe | Occasionally | No/never/hardly ever |

18. I enjoy receiving compliments, appreciation, and recognition from others. (MODULE 3.16)

19. I enjoy giving appreciation and recognition to others, and acknowledge the people who offer their appreciation to me. (MODULE 3.16)

20. I am aware of influences in my environment beyond what I can sense with the usual five senses. (MODULE 3.17)

21. I am comfortable with silence. (MODULE 3.18)

22. I take time to be alone. (MODULE 3.18)

Bonus Questions

23. I honor the changing seasons of the natural world by attuning to my body's response to differences in temperature, hours of daylight, etc.

24. I am aware of what quarter (phase) the moon is in today.

Please complete the following sentences with the first thoughts or feelings that come to mind.

25. Pleasing sights in my environment are _____.

26. Pleasing sounds in my environment are _____.

27. Pleasing smells in my environment are _____.

28. Touching is _____.

29. I nurture myself by _____.

30. I am critical of myself when _____.

31. I am pleased with myself when _____.

32. I respect the way I _____.

____ + ____ + ____ + ____ + ____ = ____ Total points for this section

Divided by ____ (number of statements answered) = | ____ . ____ | **Average score for this section**

Transfer your score to the Wellness Wheel at the end of the Index.

Section 4: Wellness and Eating

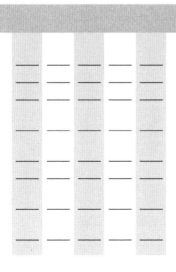

1. I know what constitutes a nutritious and well-balanced diet. (MODULE 4.1)

2. I eat at least 5 servings of raw fruits or vegetables each day. (MODULE 4.1)

3. In addition to eating well, I use a multivitamin and mineral supplement or a "superfood" supplement daily. (MODULE 4.2)

4. In my daily diet I include foods that supply cancer-fighting antioxidants, such as organic fresh vegetables rich in vitamins A, C, and E. (MODULE 4.3)

5. I drink at least 6 glasses of pure water each day. (MODULE 4.4)

6. I feel good about my eating habits and avoid using food as a reward, escape, or punishment. (MODULE 4.5)

7. I can tell the difference between "stomach hunger" and "mouth hunger" and eat only when experiencing stomach hunger. (MODULE 4.7)

8. I avoid dieting and, if weight is an issue, I address the underlying cause(s). (MODULE 4.8)

Yes/always/usually	Often	Sometimes/maybe	Occasionally	No/never/hardly ever
4	3	2	1	0
___	___	___	___	___
___	___	___	___	___
___	___	___	___	___
___	___	___	___	___
___	___	___	___	___
___	___	___	___	___
___	___	___	___	___
___	___	___	___	___
___	___	___	___	___
___	___	___	___	___
___	___	___	___	___
___	___	___	___	___
___	___	___	___	___
___	___	___	___	___
___	___	___	___	___
___	___	___	___	___
___	___	___	___	___
___	___	___	___	___
___	___	___	___	___

9. I eat slowly and chew my food thoroughly, while eating my meals in a relaxed, nurturing environment. (MODULE 4.9)

10. I am aware that my nutritional needs are unique and I attempt to learn what I can about how best to meet my body's individual requirements. (MODULE 4.10)

11. I minimize my intake of highly refined or processed foods. (MODULE 4.11)

12. I avoid chemical additives in my diet. (MODULE 4.12)

13. I buy organic produce whenever possible. (MODULE 4.13)

14. I drink fewer than 2 cups of coffee or black tea and less than 1 can or bottle of soft drink per day. (MODULE 4.14)

15. I am aware that eating fats is not the primary cause of excess weight. (MODULE 4.15)

16. I satisfy my need for protein by eating foods such as beans, nuts, eggs, cheese, fish, or chicken, and while avoiding red meat. (MODULE 4.16)

17. I read the labels for the ingredients of all processed foods I buy and am alert to misleading wording such as "enriched" or "wheat" flour. (MODULE 4.18)

18. I listen, or tune in, to my body's signals in order to recognize what foods make me feel good both physically and psychologically. (MODULE 4.19)

19. I have daily bowel movements. (MODULE 4.20)

20. While eating for wellness, I am aware of extremes and careful of absolutes, and I am patient with myself and others. (MODULE 4.22)

21. I grow some of my own food or obtain it from familiar local sources. (MODULE 4.23)

22. I am aware that vast numbers throughout the world are starving, and I make some contribution toward ending hunger. (MODULE 4.24)

Bonus Questions

23. I am aware of the difference between refined carbohydrates and complex carbohydrates and eat a majority of the latter.

24. I drink fewer than 8 alcoholic drinks a week.

25. I have no need for medications or drugs, including prescription drugs.

26. I add little or no salt to my food.

27. I have a good appetite and am within 15 percent of my ideal weight.

28. I have a well-stocked, well-equipped kitchen and I enjoy cooking.

If weight is a special concern for you, please complete the following sentences with the first thoughts or feelings that come to mind

29. Diets are _____.

30. When I binge, I feel _____.

31. Aspects of my diet that I would like to change are _____.

32. Food habits that contribute to my weight are _____.

33. My weight-related emotional issues are _____.

34. When I want to lose or gain weight I _____.

____+____+____+____+____ = ____ Total points for this section

Divided by ____ (number of statements answered) = |____.____| **Average score for this section**

Transfer your score to the Wellness Wheel at the end of the Index.

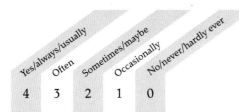

Yes/always/usually	Often	Sometimes/maybe	Occasionally	No/never/hardly ever
4	3	2	1	0

Section 5: Wellness and Moving

1. I am aware of and respond to messages from my body about its needs for movement. (MODULE 5.1)
2. I climb stairs instead of riding elevators. (MODULE 5.2)
3. I enjoy exploring new and effective ways of caring for myself through moving my body. (MODULE 5.3)
4. My daily activities include at least 15 minutes of vigorous physical effort. (MODULE 5.4)
5. I practice some form of mind-body-spirit discipline that integrates breathing, movement, and body awareness. (MODULE 5.5)
6. I engage in aerobic activity (such as running, biking, swimming, brisk walking, or other vigorous physical exercise) for at least 20 minutes at least 3 times a week. (MODULE 5.6)
7. I know how to calculate my recommended training heart rate. (MODULE 5.6)
8. I know how to take my pulse while exercising. (MODULE 5.6)
9. When exercising aerobically I keep at or below my recommended training heart rate. (MODULE 5.6)
10. I experience a natural high or altered state of mind when I exercise. (MODULE 5.7)
11. I enjoy stretching, moving, and exerting my body. (MODULE 5.8)
12. I do some form of stretching or limbering exercise (such as yoga) for 20 to 30 minutes at least 3 times a week. (MODULE 5.9)
13. I do some form of strengthening exercise (such as weight training) at least 3 times a week. (MODULE 5.10)
14. I walk or ride a bike to local destinations instead of driving. (MODULE 5.11)

Bonus Questions

15. I am aware that exercise alters brain chemistry with endorphins and I exercise to feel better when depressed, anxious, or overstressed.

Please complete the following sentences with the first thoughts or feelings that come to mind.

16. I usually engage in the following physical activities during the week: _____.
17. I am satisfied or dissatisfied with my physical activities because _____.
18. Exercise is _____.
19. I would like to change the following things regarding my body's fitness: _____.
20. After a day of little physical movement I _____.
21. After a day of much physical movement I _____.
22. My childhood experience of exercise and sports was _____.

____+____+____+____+____ = ____ Total points for this section

Divided by ____ (number of statements answered) = |____ . ____| **Average score for this section**

Transfer your score to the Wellness Wheel at the end of the Index.

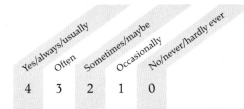

Yes/always/usually	Often	Sometimes/maybe	Occasionally	No/never/hardly ever
4	3	2	1	0

Section 6: Wellness and Feeling

1. I allow myself to experience a full range of emotions and find constructive ways to express them. (MODULE 6.1)
2. I take time to stop and ask myself "What am I feeling?" at intervals during the day. (MODULE 6.1)
3. I respect other people's differing sensitivity to and styles of expressing their feelings. (MODULE 6.2)
4. I recognize, acknowledge, and accept my fears. (MODULE 6.3)
5. I am able to feel and express my anger in ways that solve problems instead of swallowing anger or storing it up. (MODULE 6.4)
6. I am able to say no to people without feeling guilty. (MODULE 6.5)
7. My heart is open to experiencing and expressing joy. (MODULE 6.6)
8. I feel okay about crying and allow myself to do so when appropriate. (MODULE 6.7)
9. I am able to graciously accept other people's positive acknowledgments of me. (MODULE 6.8)
10. I have at least 5 close friends. (MODULE 6.9)
11. I easily express concern, love, and warmth to those I care about. (MODULE 6.10)

Bonus Questions

12. I listen to and consider other people's criticisms of me instead of reacting defensively.
13. I like myself and look forward to the rest of my life.
14. I ask for help when needed.
15. I am aware that seeking the help of professional counselors is not a sign of weakness and would do so if needed.
16. I understand the importance of grieving after a loss and allow myself to do so.
17. I see conflict as a necessary and important part of being alive and do not confuse it with violence (physical or mental) against myself or others.
18. I am willing to take important risks and do so.
19. I am aware that my feelings provide me with information about myself and use them to further my growth and evolution.
20. I am aware of the power contained in "negative" feelings and, instead of denying these feelings, draw on that power to deepen my self-understanding.
21. I accept my own worth, while appreciating my differences from others and without judging myself as innately better or worse than them.

Please complete the following sentences with the first thoughts or feelings that come to mind.

22. When I am angry _____.
23. Being angry _____.
24. When I feel sad _____.
25. Crying _____.
26. Laughing out loud _____.
27. My life is full of _____.
28. Taking risks can lead to _____.

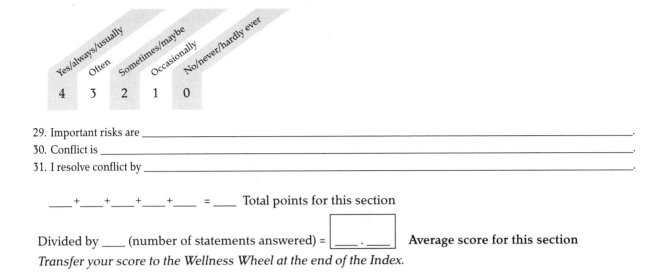

4   3   2   1   0

Yes/always/usually   Often   Sometimes/maybe   Occasionally   No/never/hardly ever

29. Important risks are _____.
30. Conflict is _____.
31. I resolve conflict by _____.

____ + ____ + ____ + ____ + ____ = ____ Total points for this section

Divided by ____ (number of statements answered) = ☐ ____ . ____ ☐   **Average score for this section**

Transfer your score to the Wellness Wheel at the end of the Index.

Section 7: Wellness and Thinking

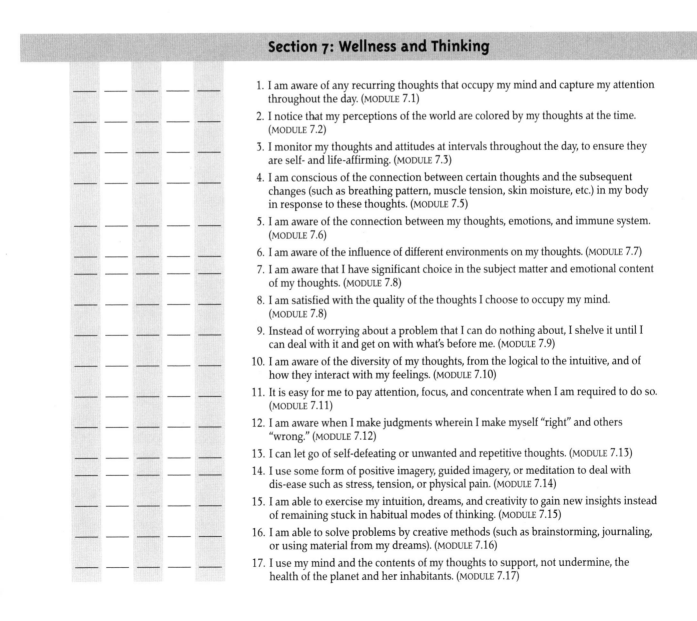

1. I am aware of any recurring thoughts that occupy my mind and capture my attention throughout the day. (MODULE 7.1)
2. I notice that my perceptions of the world are colored by my thoughts at the time. (MODULE 7.2)
3. I monitor my thoughts and attitudes at intervals throughout the day, to ensure they are self- and life-affirming. (MODULE 7.3)
4. I am conscious of the connection between certain thoughts and the subsequent changes (such as breathing pattern, muscle tension, skin moisture, etc.) in my body in response to these thoughts. (MODULE 7.5)
5. I am aware of the connection between my thoughts, emotions, and immune system. (MODULE 7.6)
6. I am aware of the influence of different environments on my thoughts. (MODULE 7.7)
7. I am aware that I have significant choice in the subject matter and emotional content of my thoughts. (MODULE 7.8)
8. I am satisfied with the quality of the thoughts I choose to occupy my mind. (MODULE 7.8)
9. Instead of worrying about a problem that I can do nothing about, I shelve it until I can deal with it and get on with what's before me. (MODULE 7.9)
10. I am aware of the diversity of my thoughts, from the logical to the intuitive, and of how they interact with my feelings. (MODULE 7.10)
11. It is easy for me to pay attention, focus, and concentrate when I am required to do so. (MODULE 7.11)
12. I am aware when I make judgments wherein I make myself "right" and others "wrong." (MODULE 7.12)
13. I can let go of self-defeating or unwanted and repetitive thoughts. (MODULE 7.13)
14. I use some form of positive imagery, guided imagery, or meditation to deal with dis-ease such as stress, tension, or physical pain. (MODULE 7.14)
15. I am able to exercise my intuition, dreams, and creativity to gain new insights instead of remaining stuck in habitual modes of thinking. (MODULE 7.15)
16. I am able to solve problems by creative methods (such as brainstorming, journaling, or using material from my dreams). (MODULE 7.16)
17. I use my mind and the contents of my thoughts to support, not undermine, the health of the planet and her inhabitants. (MODULE 7.17)

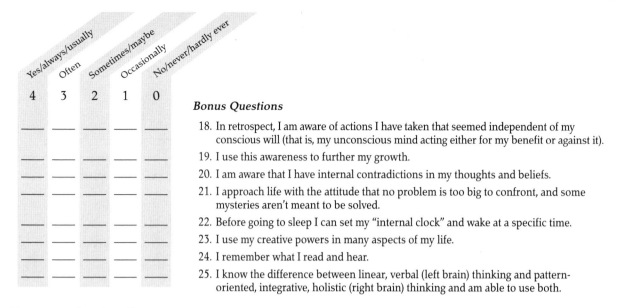

Yes/always/usually	Often	Sometimes/maybe	Occasionally	No/never/hardly ever
4	3	2	1	0

Bonus Questions

18. In retrospect, I am aware of actions I have taken that seemed independent of my conscious will (that is, my unconscious mind acting either for my benefit or against it).
19. I use this awareness to further my growth.
20. I am aware that I have internal contradictions in my thoughts and beliefs.
21. I approach life with the attitude that no problem is too big to confront, and some mysteries aren't meant to be solved.
22. Before going to sleep I can set my "internal clock" and wake at a specific time.
23. I use my creative powers in many aspects of my life.
24. I remember what I read and hear.
25. I know the difference between linear, verbal (left brain) thinking and pattern-oriented, integrative, holistic (right brain) thinking and am able to use both.

Please complete the following sentences with the first thoughts or feelings that come to mind.

26. My thoughts are _____ .
27. My mind is _____ .
28. Thinking is _____ .
29. Intuition is _____ .
30. My dreams are _____ .

____ + ____ + ____ + ____ + ____ = ____ Total points for this section

Divided by ____ (number of statements answered) = | ____ . ____ | **Average score for this section**

Transfer your score to the Wellness Wheel at the end of the Index.

Section 8: Wellness, Playing, and Working

1. I take time to nurture and strengthen myself physically, mentally, emotionally, and spiritually each day. (MODULE 8.1)
2. I approach difficult or challenging tasks from a playful point of view. (MODULE 8.2)
3. I enjoy and take time for spontaneous activities. (MODULE 8.3)
4. I balance the challenges and stresses of my life with playful and nurturing attitudes and activities. (MODULE 8.3)
5. I make an effort to play and work cooperatively, not competitively. (MODULE 8.4)
6. I am able to lighten up and avoid undue seriousness. (MODULE 8.5)
7. I laugh freely and often. (MODULE 8.6)
8. I avoid taking on unnecessary and unrealistic burdens and responsibilities. (MODULE 8.7)
9. I am aware of alternatives to my present job or work. (MODULE 8.8)
10. I use relaxation and/or visualization practices to transform any stressful or negative attitudes I have toward my work. (MODULE 8.8)
11. I value myself for who I *am*, not just for what I *do*. (MODULE 8.9)
12. The work I do enhances the wellbeing of others and the planet without taking away from anyone. (MODULE 8.10)

4	3	2	1	0
Yes/always/usually	Often	Sometimes/maybe	Occasionally	No/never/hardly ever

Bonus Questions

___ ___ ___ ___ ___ 13. I enjoy expressing myself through art, dance, music, drama, sports, etc., and make time to do so.

___ ___ ___ ___ ___ 14. I regularly exercise my creativity "muscles."

___ ___ ___ ___ ___ 15. I enjoy playing with other people and make time to do so.

___ ___ ___ ___ ___ 16. I enjoy playing on my own and make time to do so.

___ ___ ___ ___ ___ 17. I can readily think of 5 people with whom I can play.

___ ___ ___ ___ ___ 18. When appropriate, I can play before all my work is done and feel good about it.

___ ___ ___ ___ ___ 19. I can make much of my work into play

___ ___ ___ ___ ___ 20. I readily shift from a goal-oriented frame of mind to a purposeless activity when it is appropriate to do so.

___ ___ ___ ___ ___ 21. At times I allow myself to do nothing.

___ ___ ___ ___ ___ 22. At times I can sleep late without feeling guilty.

___ ___ ___ ___ ___ 23. The work I do is rewarding to me.

___ ___ ___ ___ ___ 24. I am proud of my accomplishments.

___ ___ ___ ___ ___ 25. I am playful, and the people around me support my playfulness.

___ ___ ___ ___ ___ 26. I have at least 1 activity (hobby, sport, etc.) that I enjoy regularly but do not feel compelled to do.

___ ___ ___ ___ ___ 27. I am a good worker.

___ ___ ___ ___ ___ 28. I am a good player.

___ ___ ___ ___ ___ 29. I create opportunities for my creative, intuitive self to be expressed and heard.

___ ___ ___ ___ ___ 30. I do not turn my play activities into work.

Please complete the following sentences with the first thoughts or feelings that come to mind.

31. Work is _____.

32. My work is _____.

33. Play is _____.

34. My play is _____.

On the lines below, list four of the activities that you most enjoy doing above anything else in your life.

35. _____.

36. _____.

37. _____.

38. _____.

___ ___ ___ ___ ___ 39. I allow myself to experience the activity listed in 35 above.

___ ___ ___ ___ ___ 40. I allow myself to experience the activity listed in 36 above.

___ ___ ___ ___ ___ 41. I allow myself to experience the activity listed in 37 above.

___ ___ ___ ___ ___ 42. I allow myself to experience the activity listed in 38 above.

___ + ___ + ___ + ___ + ___ = ___ Total points for this section

Divided by ___ (number of statements answered) = [___ . ___] **Average score for this section**

Transfer your score to the Wellness Wheel at the end of the Index.

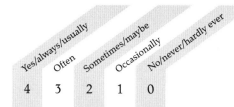

Yes/always/usually	Often	Sometimes/maybe	Occasionally	No/never/hardly ever
4	3	2	1	0

Section 9: Wellness and Communicating

1. I pay attention to how I am describing the world to myself and how I am evaluating it. (MODULE 9.1)

2. The messages I reinforce through my self-talk are focused on increasing my wellbeing. (MODULE 9.2)

3. My communications with others are clear and well understood. (MODULE 9.3)

4. I enjoy communicating and am genuinely interested in what others have to say. (MODULE 9.4)

5. I am truthful and compassionate in my communications. (MODULE 9.5)

6. I am aware that absolutes, generalizations, labels, and judgments undermine clear, mutually beneficial communications. (MODULE 9.6)

7. I assert myself in an effort to be heard and understood, and I seek to hear and understand others instead of being passively resentful of those with whom I don't agree. (MODULE 9.7)

8. I acknowledge and apologize for any mistakes I make instead of trying to cover them up. (MODULE 9.8)

9. I am a good listener. (MODULE 9.9)

10. I strive to be truthful and direct in my communications, and avoid playing manipulative psychological games. (MODULE 9.10)

11. I find out if my help is wanted or beneficial before offering it (emergencies excepted). (MODULE 9.11)

12. In my communications I strive to connect with others by relating to them as equals, instead of just trying to get what I want from them. (MODULE 9.12)

13. I respect that people of the opposite sex, different sexual orientations, or from other cultures may value communication styles that are different from mine, and I keep this in mind while communicating with them. (MODULE 9.13)

14. I am sensitive to my own and other people's tone of voice, facial expression, and body language when communicating. (MODULE 9.13)

15. I recognize that humans are not the only species on the planet that have complex patterns of communication among themselves. (MODULE 9.14)

16. I pay attention to the communications from the natural world and from my environment that offer direction in what is needed for our planet's wellbeing. (MODULE 9.15)

Bonus Questions

17. I initiate conversations.

18. I am able to communicate with strangers easily.

19. In conversation, I can introduce a difficult topic and stay with it until we reach an appropriate conclusion.

20. I enjoy silence.

21. I can communicate my limitations to others when appropriate.

22. I consider how other people are likely to react before I initiate a difficult communication.

23. I am aware when I'm merely responding to my internal "tapes" instead of acting or thinking with some degree of conscious awareness.

24. I am aware of situations when I blame others instead of accepting that I may be in error.

25. I am aware of my negative judgments of others and accept them as simply judgments, not necessarily truth.

Yes/always/usually	Often	Sometimes/maybe	Occasionally	No/never/hardly ever
4	3	2	1	0

26. I am aware of my defense mechanisms and can set them aside when appropriate.
27. I am able to listen to and objectively consider opposing viewpoints.
28. I respond to others in a conversation instead of trying to change the subject to seem more knowledgeable.
29. I am able to listen to people without interrupting them or finishing their sentences for them.
30. I am not responsible for keeping other people happy.
31. I take charge and manage a situation when it is appropriate for me to do so.
32. I let others take charge and manage a situation when it is appropriate for them to do so.
33. I cooperate with others when it is necessary for several people to take charge of a situation.
34. I am able to let go of control and allow a situation to work itself out through means I may not fully understand.
35. I can let go of my mental labels and judgmental attitudes (e.g., "this is good," "that is wrong") about events in my life and see those events in the light of what they offer me.
36. I clearly express my thoughts and feelings instead of assuming others can read my mind.

Please complete the following sentences with the first thoughts or feelings that come to mind.

37. My communications are _____.
38. People listen to my _____.
39. For me listening is _____.

____+____+____+____+____ = ____ Total points for this section

Divided by ____ (number of statements answered) = ____ . ____   **Average score for this section**

Transfer your score to the Wellness Wheel at the end of the Index.

Section 10: Wellness and Sex

1. My sexual education enables me to make responsible and caring decisions about my sexual practices. (MODULE 10.1)
2. I provide any children in my life with healthy role modeling and education about caring and responsible expressions of their sexuality and sexual practices. (MODULE 10.1)
3. I am comfortable, respectful, and appropriate in speaking about sexual issues. (MODULE 10.1)
4. I am aware of the serious nature and frequency of sexual abuse and report any such incidences to an appropriate party. (MODULE 10.1)
5. I am aware that unrealistic expectations of sex are a source of dissatisfaction and unhappiness. (MODULE 10.2)
6. I am committed to exploring my sexuality in pleasurable and positive ways. (MODULE 10.3)
7. I recognize that my sexual energy is not confined to my genitals. (MODULE 10.3)

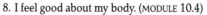

8. I feel good about my body. (MODULE 10.4)

9. I enjoy my body and the sensations of which it is capable. (MODULE 10.4)

10. It is okay to masturbate. (MODULE 10.4)

11. I am aware of a powerful mind-body connection in sex. (MODULE 10.5)

12. I am aware of, and able to attend to, my partner's needs and pleasures in sex. (MODULE 10.6)

13. With regard to my sexuality, I examine who and what are influencing my beliefs and attitudes. (MODULE 10.7)

14. I am comfortable with my own sexual orientation and gender. (MODULE 10.8)

15. I honor the rights of others to express their sexual orientation and gender in ways that are not harmful to others. (MODULE 10.8)

16. I am informed on methods of birth control and use them if appropriate. (MODULE 10.9)

17. I am familiar with methods of preventing AIDS and other STDs and use them when appropriate. (MODULE 10.10)

18. With regard to sexual practices, I strongly and clearly say yes to what I want, and no to what I don't want. (MODULE 10.11)

19. I acknowledge my sovereignty over my body, and I am able to say no to unwelcome sexual advances. (MODULE 10.11)

20. I live my life with the knowledge that as a whole person, I have within me everything that I need for my happiness. (MODULE 10.12)

21. I recognize that sex and love are natural expressions of my being, not commodities of limited supply that must be earned, won, or guarded. (MODULE 10.13)

22. I experience my sexuality as being in harmony with my spirituality. (MODULE 10.14)

23. I recognize that the wellbeing of my body is interdependent with the wellbeing of the earth. (MODULE 10.15)

Bonus Questions

24. I feel good about the degree of closeness I have with the men in my life.

25. I feel good about the degree of closeness I have with the women in my life.

26. I am content with my level of sexual activity.

27. I fully experience the many stages of lovemaking instead of focusing only on orgasm.

28. I express myself directly instead of using sexual energy as a covert means of communication.

29. I feel comfortable touching persons of my own sex.

30. I seek to resolve any upset feelings with my partner and don't try to punish or control my partner by withholding sex.

31. When I'm upset with my partner, I resolve the problem before making love.

32. I feel comfortable looking at myself nude in a mirror.

33. I desire to grow closer to other people of my choosing.

34. I am aware of the difference between needing someone and loving someone.

35. I am able to love others without dominating or being dominated by them.

36. I am able to love others to my satisfaction.

37. I am comfortable consciously abstaining from sexual activity as a way of learning more about myself.

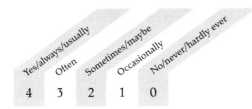

Yes/always/usually	Often	Sometimes/maybe	Occasionally	No/never/hardly ever
4	3	2	1	0

Please complete the following sentences with the first thoughts or feelings that come to mind.

38. When I want to initiate lovemaking _____.
39. My favorite erogenous zones are _____.
40. Making love is _____.
41. After lovemaking I feel _____.
42. My sexual behavior is _____.
43. To me a heterosexual lifestyle is _____.
44. To me a homosexual lifestyle is _____.
45. To me a bisexual lifestyle is _____.
46. Oral sex is _____.
47. Orgasm _____.
48. Love involves _____.
49. Loving someone means _____.
50. Without sex _____.
51. Temporary celibacy is _____.

____ + ____ + ____ + ____ + ____ = ____ Total points for this section

Divided by ____ (number of statements answered) = | ____ . ____ | **Average score for this section**

Transfer your score to the Wellness Wheel at the end of the Index.

Section 11: Wellness and Finding Meaning

1. I am aware that meanings are made up and assigned by people, not inherent in events or things. (MODULE 11.1)
2. I contemplate what is meaningful to me and regularly reexamine my values and priorities. (MODULE 11.2)
3. I listen to my own inner guidance in assigning the meaning I bring to my life. (MODULE 11.3)
4. I set realistic goals that support me in manifesting my dreams and aspirations. (MODULE 11.4)
5. I am achieving my goals. (MODULE 11.4)
6. I allocate time to focus on and further my dreams and aspirations. (MODULE 11.5)
7. I focus my awareness in the present moment, instead of living in the past or future. (MODULE 11.6)
8. My life is a mystery to be lived, not a problem to be solved. (MODULE 11.7)
9. I accept death as a normal, natural part of life. (MODULE 11.8)
10. I live in the awareness that I am dying and being reborn in every moment. (MODULE 11.9)
11. I am able to talk about my own death or the death of someone close to me with family and friends. (MODULE 11.10)

Yes/always/usually	Often	Sometimes/maybe	Occasionally	No/never/hardly ever
4	3	2	1	0
___	___	___	___	___
___	___	___	___	___
___	___	___	___	___
___	___	___	___	___
___	___	___	___	___
___	___	___	___	___
___	___	___	___	___
___	___	___	___	___
___	___	___	___	___
___	___	___	___	___

12. I have taken steps to enable me to die with the greatest amount of dignity, personal power, and conscious awareness possible at the time. (MODULE 11.11)

13. I look forward to the future as an opportunity for further growth. (MODULE 11.12)

Bonus Questions

14. I believe my life has direction and meaning, although I may not always be able to see either.

15. I have a life purpose.

16. I am prepared for my death.

17. I see my death as a step in my evolution.

18. My daily life is a source of pleasure to me.

19. I am satisfied with any counseling or growth-related processes in which I am involved.

20. My life is exciting and challenging.

21. I let my inner voice guide me instead of letting myself be moved by the expectations of others.

22. I place importance on achieving both outward (material) and inward (spiritual) goals.

Please complete the following sentences with the first thoughts or feelings that come to mind.

23. I have accomplished _____.

24. I am achieving _____.

25. I have not accomplished _____.

26. I hope _____.

27. The most futile thing _____.

28. My highest aspiration _____.

29. I am _____.

30. Death _____.

31. Problems are _____.

32. More than anything I want _____.

33. My life _____.

34. The world _____.

35. The idea of suicide _____.

36. When the odds are against me _____.

37. I look forward to _____.

38. My goals in life are _____.

____+____+____+____+____ = ____ Total points for this section

Divided by ____ (number of statements answered) = | ____ . ____ | **Average score for this section**

Transfer your score to the Wellness Wheel at the end of the Index.

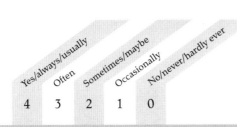

Yes/always/usually	Often	Sometimes/maybe	Occasionally	No/never/hardly ever
4	3	2	1	0

Section 12: Wellness and Transcending

This portion of the Wellness Index goes beyond the scope of most generally accepted scientific principles to express some values and beliefs of the authors. It is intended to stimulate interest in these areas. If you have beliefs strongly to the contrary, please skip the questions or make up your own.

1. I enjoy practicing a spiritual discipline or allowing time to sense the presence of a greater force moving in my life. (MODULE 12.1)
2. I experience synchronistic events in my life (frequent "coincidences" that seem to have no cause-and-effect relationship). (MODULE 12.2)
3. When ill, I am able to consciously activate and participate in my healing processes. (MODULE 12.3)
4. I am aware that my experience of the world often mirrors my beliefs about reality. (MODULE 12.4)
5. Reality appears to be subjective and may be changing as we evolve. (MODULE 12.5)
6. I live my life as a mysterious process, sometimes beyond description or comprehension, in which I have a significant role. (MODULE 12.6)
7. I am able to recognize and reframe times of "falling apart" in my life as precursors to times of "falling together," or personal transformation. (MODULE 12.7)
8. I experience myself as a part of a larger whole and am aware of my connections with people and things that seem to transcend my physical boundaries. (MODULE 12.8)
9. I use the messages interpreted from my dreams to better live my waking life. (MODULE 12.9)
10. I meditate or practice some kind of relaxation or centering process for at least 20 minutes every day. (MODULE 12.10)
11. I consciously seek to develop and trust my intuition. (MODULE 12.11)
12. I am able to accept confusion and paradox as elements in my spiritual journey. (MODULE 12.12)

Bonus Questions

13. I am curious about the nature of reality.
14. I am aware of experiencing "miracles" in my daily life.
15. I am comfortable with my intuition, or knowing things without knowing precisely how I know them.
16. I believe there are dimensions of reality beyond verbal description or human comprehension.
17. At times I experience confusion and paradox in my search for understanding of these other dimensions.
18. I am able to consciously alter my physiologic processes (such as muscle tension, circulation to a part of my body, etc.) to enhance my health.
19. When ill I am able to consciously speed up my healing processes.
20. I sing, pray, chant, or meditate with other people and experience a sense of unity in doing so.
21. The concept of god has personal definition and meaning to me.
22. I experience a sense of wonder and awe when I contemplate the universe.
23. It is okay with me if certain things are unknowable to the mind.

Yes/always/usually	Often	Sometimes/maybe	Occasionally	No/never/hardly ever
4	3	2	1	0
___	___	___	___	___
___	___	___	___	___
___	___	___	___	___
___	___	___	___	___
___	___	___	___	___
___	___	___	___	___
___	___	___	___	___
___	___	___	___	___

24. I am aware of a part of me that is greater than my mind, body, and emotions.
25. I trust and use the part of myself that has a greater wisdom than my mind.
26. I live my life with a sense of abundant expectancy rather than with specific expectations.
27. I experience a merging of my consciousness with a larger sense of consciousness, or a universal mind.
28. I allow others the freedom to believe what they believe without pressuring them to accept my beliefs.
29. I pay attention to and remember my dreams.
30. I interpret the symbols in my dreams.
31. I believe that how I think and subsequently act contributes to the wellbeing of the planet.

Please complete the following sentences with the first thoughts or feelings that come to mind.

32. The universe is _____.
33. Reality is _____.
34. When I cannot know something, I feel _____.
35. My greatest wish for my own wellness is _____.

____ + ____ + ____ + ____ + ____ = ____ Total points for this section

Divided by ____ (number of statements answered) = | ____ . ____ | **Average score for this section**

Transfer your score to the Wellness Wheel at the end of the Index.

The Wellness Wheel

Transfer your average score from each section to the corresponding box around the wheel on the following page. Then graphically display your score by drawing a curved line between the "spokes" that define each segment. Use the scale provided, beginning at the center with 0.0 and reaching 4.0 at the circumference. Finally, using different colors if possible, fill in the corresponding amount of each wedge-shaped segment.

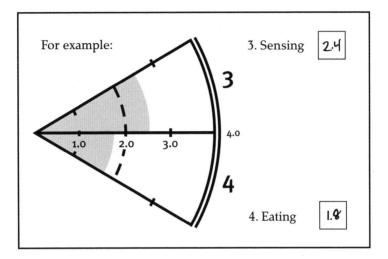

Your completed Wheel may look something like this:

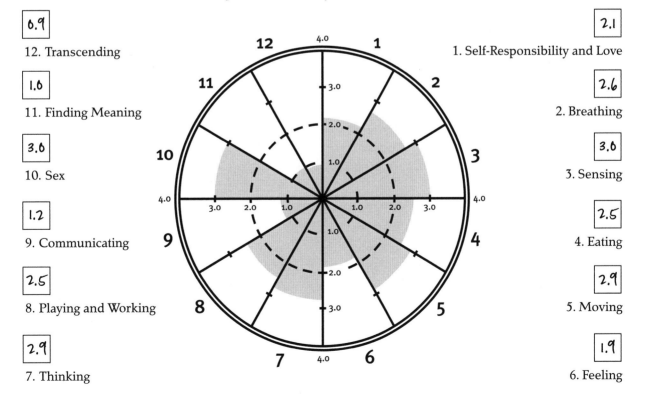

0.9		2.1
12. Transcending		1. Self-Responsibility and Love
1.6		2.6
11. Finding Meaning		2. Breathing
3.6		3.6
10. Sex		3. Sensing
1.2		2.5
9. Communicating		4. Eating
2.5		2.9
8. Playing and Working		5. Moving
2.9		1.9
7. Thinking		6. Feeling

Your Wellness Wheel

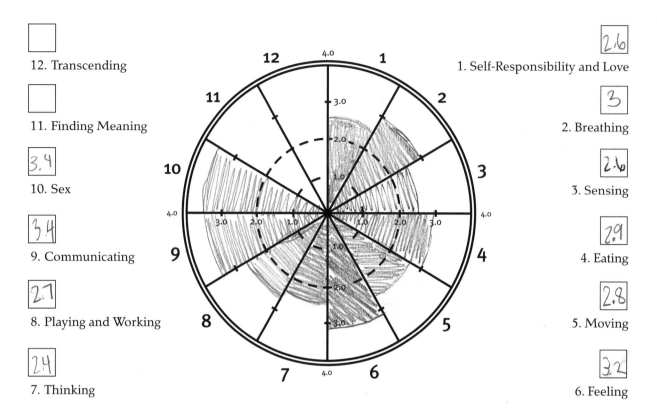

12. Transcending

11. Finding Meaning

10. Sex — 3.4

9. Communicating — 3.4

8. Playing and Working — 2.7

7. Thinking — 2.4

1. Self-Responsibility and Love — 2.6

2. Breathing — 3

3. Sensing — 2.6

4. Eating — 2.9

5. Moving — 2.8

6. Feeling — 3.2

Now that you have completed the Wellness Index, study the wheel's shape and balance. How smoothly would it roll? What does it tell you? Does anything surprise you about it? How does it *feel* to you? What don't you like about it? What do you like about it? What would you like to be different? Is there a particular section in which you would hope to make changes?

Keep in mind our caution against undertaking sweeping life changes all at once. You may first want to address the sections where you scored lowest, or you may want to begin exploring the section that excites or interests you the most or one that you can more easily handle. We recommend that you go back over the questions using colored pens or markers to indicate which ones you want to work on now versus those of lower priority. You can use the *Wellness Workbook* module references to aid you in your study of the first group of statements in each section of the Index.

Remember, every journey begins with a single step. If you can enlist others to travel with you, the journey can be a lot more fun.

Remember, too, angels can fly because they treat themselves lightly.

CHAPTER 1

Wellness, Self-Responsibility, and Love

Self-responsibility, with love and compassion, is the first form of energy in the Wellness Energy System. This creates an environment, or context, within which all other energy expressions can be better considered. Self-responsibility and love flow from the appreciation that we are not separate and individual entities, nor are we made up of separate parts. Rather, we are united in a single energy system along with everything else in creation.

It is not the strongest of the species that survive, nor the most intelligent, but the one most responsive to change.

—Charles Darwin

Wellness is like a bridge supported by two piers. Each pier is crucial to the bridge's integrity, just as the two principles of self-responsibility and love are fundamental to the process of wellness. In each case, the piers support a connection between two distant points, allowing for movement back and forth. This freedom to move between different places or attitudes, rather than rigid attachment to any particular one, is the hallmark of wellness.

Self-responsibility and love establish a life-context in which freedom and flexibility are naturally occurring states of being. They are primary expressions of life energy. Self-responsibility and love together form the foundations of wellness and encourage the free flow of all other types of energy. If either principle (or pier) is weakened, living harmoniously (or traversing the bridge) becomes more difficult. When both are strong, energy dances back and forth, and the crossing is easy.

Self-Responsibility Means

- *Developing awareness of your own processes and patterns—physical, mental, emotional, and spiritual*

- *Discovering your real needs, and finding ways to meet them directly*

- *Realizing that you are unique and the expert about yourself*

- *Making choices and living courageously in the midst of uncertainty*

- *Creating the life you want, rather than just reacting to whatever comes along*

- *Asking simply and directly for what you need and want from others*

- *Expressing yourself—both your ideas and feelings—in ways that effectively communicate to other people who you are and what you know*

- *Respecting your body through nutrition, exercise, and personal safety*

- *Creating and nourishing close relationships with others*

- *Engaging in projects that are meaningful to you; being supportive of others; and respecting your environment*

Love Means

- *Honoring your uniqueness, and enjoying the uniqueness of others*

- *Listening to your own heart—treasuring your inner wisdom*

- *Responding to life's challenges as opportunities for growth, rather than as problems*

- *Caring for all aspects of yourself—body, mind, emotions, spirit—and sharing your caring with others*

- *Exercising compassion for your weaknesses, and forgiving yourself and others*

- *Experiencing yourself as your own best friend, and remaining faithful to yourself, especially in the rough times*

- *Realizing your connectedness with all things and acting in a way congruent with that awareness*

- *Being truthful with yourself and others*

- *Celebrating the irrepressible process of life*

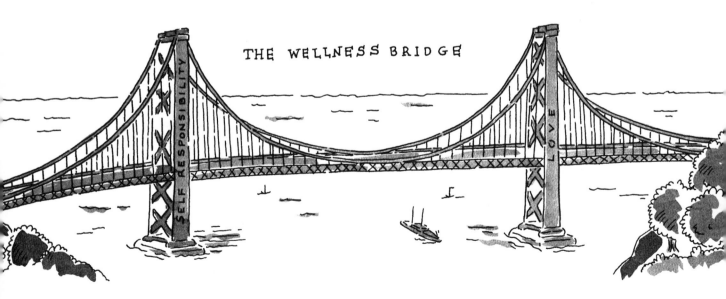

THE WELLNESS BRIDGE

With love and self-responsibility as our foundations and supports, living and wellness are synonymous.

Wellness, like life, is always a question of balance. It is a dynamic process because there are seeming contradictions to be resolved, apparent oppositions to be integrated, infinite shades of gray from which to choose. In considering the subject of health, for instance, you just don't find absolute answers to questions like: What should I eat? How should I exercise? What form of treatment is best? Rather, you must learn to balance what *you* know and what the "experts" tell you. Even though you are connected with me and everyone else you share this planet with, you are also very much alone, and you must singularly make your own life-and-death decisions. (Sounds serious. And it is!) But, if you make your life about self-responsibility and love, then the burden can be transformed into the opportunity, and the questions can become the impetus for experimentation, for learning, for trusting, for loving this magnificent and paradoxical creation—yourself.

While some types of illness are genetically determined, and others are the result of environmental or accidental factors that appear to be largely out of our control, a large percentage of the illness we experience is created when we resist the movement and flexibility that characterize life and change. Wellness offers us a bridge to cross over into new territory, to explore different possibilities, to understand the other side of any situation. When we resign ourselves to being helpless victims of disease, when we give up on ourselves, when we hold on to one system and refuse to question it even when it fails to meet our needs, we encourage sickness and death.

Wellness allows us to integrate contradictions like illness and health. It appreciates these as complementary parts of one life process. It is open to new ideas, courageous, and noncompulsive. Wellness means that we can move freely between seeming opposites, learning from each, growing from both.

The contemporary treatment model of medicine, which most of us have come to accept as the norm, is actually only one way of dealing with illness. Because we have lived with it for so long, we may never have learned that there are alternatives. Sometimes, even though it may have failed us, we have accepted its shortcomings. Because the treatment model is such familiar territory—the "home field," so to speak—we are strongly encouraged to stay there.

The Problems with Illness Care

The practice of medicine in the world today is often labeled "health care." Actually, it should be described as "illness care." It is built upon the diagnosis of disease, the repair of injury, and the treatment of symptoms—all of which are necessary and valuable services. Sometimes, it delivers just what we ask for. Oftentimes, however, we get more than we bargained for.

We've asked our medical professionals to take care of us, to be responsible for our lives. The demands come in a variety of questions and prayers:

"What's wrong, Doc?"

"Will you fix me up?"

"Just tell me I'm going to be all right!"

"I want relief now!"

"Please Doc, just let me live!"

At the same time, we've become dissatisfied with the doctor's inability to play God, threatening lawsuit or censure should treatment prove inadequate. This system also operates at an ever-increasing financial cost to the consumer and is running wildly out of control. Each of us now spends on the average $3,000 per year for such services.

Our resistance to footing such an expensive bill might not be so great if we were getting *only* what we've paid for. The fact is we're getting more than we can handle. The term for these unasked-for benefits is *iatrogenesis*. It means a condition created by the doctor's treatment. Prescription drugs, for example, have become one of the leading causes of death. In the United States, drug-related deaths rank number five on the list of killers.[1] In 1999, the Institute of Medicine's Committee on the Quality of Health Care issued its landmark report "To Err Is Human," which concluded that medical errors killed between 44,000 and 98,000 American hospital patients each year. The majority were medication errors, and given the underreporting of such errors, the number is suspected to be even larger. Moreover, the misuse and overuse of antibiotics have contributed to the development of treatment-resistant bacteria, which kill 90,000 Americans every year.[2]

The illness-care system, moreover, is often overrated. If you were to examine the list of the ten most frequent causes of death among the U.S. population in the early 1900s, you would see that we have made great strides in controlling the infectious killers: tuberculosis, diphtheria, and influenza. But in their place today we find cancer, heart disease, and stroke. We have merely substituted one set of killers for another.

As hard as it is to believe, medical science has done little to increase the potential life span of the American adult. Figures quoted about average life expectancy show an increase often attributed to the introduction of antibiotics in the 1940s and other technological breakthroughs, but this supposed increase is due mainly to a lower infant and childhood mortality rate, mostly from improved sanitation and other public health measures. More children now live out a normal life span instead of dying young; this radically affects the average statistics. Overall, we are really not living any longer than did people sixty years ago. In fact, it may be that our potential life span is being shortened by increased stresses and by poisons in the environment.

Much of the illness-care system de-emphasizes the role played by lifestyle in determining your state of health. Most illness results from choices about lifestyle, not from lack of access to health services. The excessive strains of sedentary work can encourage obesity and cigarette smoking, for example. Such work can foster depression and anxiety—conditions common among the white-collar middle class in the United States. And the mortality rates of this group during mid-life (forty-five to sixty-four) are substantially higher than those of the population at large—particularly from such conditions as cancer, heart disease, and stroke.

The cost of illness care in terms of emotional drain on the provider (the doctor) and the consumer (you) is also great. Treatment fosters dependency of the patient on the professional. The public demands a pill for every ill, and it wants relief now! The doctor (or other health professional) is cast in the role of the "Pill Fairy," a character who must possess both omnipotence and infallibility. When the pressures of this game become too great over time, professional burnout—a whole range of attitudes and behaviors, from ill temper to suicide—is the common result. The statistics for suicide, drug abuse, and heart attack among physicians reflect the dangers in this kind of situation.

The interaction between the professional and the patient often looks like the relationship between a parent and a child. Parents have power, and answers, and prescriptions. They are nurturing ("Here, let me help"), demanding ("You should do this"), and judgmental ("That's wrong"). Children have questions, feelings and needs, and compelling desires to please. They are compliant sometimes, downright stubborn and rebellious at others, and looking for both help and approval. And while this situation may be natural and necessary when one person is two years old and the other is forty, it is far from desirable, for instance, when you are fifty and your doctor is thirty.

Our current system for personal health may not be a system after all. Its orientation is toward treatment of an ailing part, a particular disease or set of symptoms, or the physical body alone. But most forms of treatment neglect to take into account that it is not a stomach that gets sick, but rather a whole person who doesn't feel well, and that human beings also have intellects, emotions, and souls, besides physical bodies. When was the last time your doctor asked you about your ability to express personal creativity in your job, your reluctance to cry or express anger, your sense of meaning and purpose in life, your awareness of the connectedness of all things in the universe?

The current illness-care system is expensive; it is risky; it discourages adults from taking charge of their own lives; it causes doctors and other helping professionals to burn out. It is limited in its perspective of life and health, and in acceptance of its own inadequacy. What it does well can be appreciated and used. What it fails to do must be assumed by another system.

This whole situation may be likened to your dealings with your automobile. You can find the best mechanics in town to fix the vehicle each time it breaks down, but they can never prevent you from abusing it and causing the next problem. A great deal of expense and effort might be saved were you to practice preventive maintenance more consistently, and exercise more care in the way you drive. There are two separate systems at work here: one for automobile repair (acute care or crisis intervention) and one for driver's education (prevention or education). Both are necessary for assuring maximum efficiency and long-term dependability of your car. The former bears a strong resemblance to the operation of our contemporary medical model; the latter represents the neglected component of wellness education. It

is the happy occurrence when one institution can perform both of these functions, but to demand this of our medical professionals, in most cases, may simply serve to increase the frustrations all around. In any case, the responsibility for prevention lies not with the doctor, it lies within each of us. It is long overdue that we recognize this and start reclaiming our personal power.

As you read on, you may wish to refer back to this chapter on many occasions. Your clear understanding of this process will provide you with a simple way to describe each dynamic that relates to your state of health. Keep in mind also that self-responsibility and love are the supports of wellness, which allow this energy flow to occur most efficiently. We need to elaborate upon these important elements. So let's talk about self-responsibility and love.

UNITED STATES: NUMBER TWENTY-ONE

When the United States is compared to other countries in terms of longevity, it does poorly. The American male ranks twenty-first and the American female ranks twentieth. Infant mortality rates are even worse at twenty-third among the twenty-nine industrialized nations—a pretty poor showing for a country that spends more on medical treatment per capita than any other country in the world.

Gerard Anderson, Ph.D., professor of health policy and management, Johns Hopkins School of Public Health, citing data from the Organization for Economic Cooperation and Development (OECD), Doctor's Guide, www.pslgroup.com/dg/448d6.htm.

1.1 Responsibility for Health

Human beings continually persist in looking "out there" for answers, formulas, and fortunes, only to discover that they had them within themselves all along. Many fables recount the adventures of a young seeker who travels the world in search of a noble truth or a priceless treasure. After years of weary searching, pain, and hardship, the aged pilgrim finally returns home only to find the object of the search in his or her own backyard.

This truth applies just as well to our desires for health and wholeness. Attempts to find the doctor, or the therapy, or the book that contains the magical solutions to all our problems and questions will end in frustration. Looking within, and assuming responsibility for what you find there, is a necessary condition for wellness.

This may be hard for many to accomplish, because from our earliest years we have accepted that somebody else knows what is best for us. As a society we have given up our personal power in many ways. To the teachers in our schools, we give the responsibility for telling us what we need to learn, and when and how to learn it; to professional mechanics, the decisions about the upkeep of our cars; to our professional politicians, the right to use our money and direct the military power of our country. Even in the area of spirituality, many people continue to allow their professional "holy one" to tell them what God demands. Likewise, we have entrusted our medical professionals with the responsibility for our health, giving them—and only them—the power to determine what our minds and bodies need.

The general attitude of "tell me what to do and I'll do it," or "you do it for me," seems easier initially.

We appreciate that the training of the specialist gives him or her a special skill. You would probably never get around to washing your dishes if you had to fix your own watch, TV, or cell phone. Experts are necessary in all aspects of life. But the problem is not that we *use* experts. The problem is that we often *shift all responsibility* to someone or something outside ourselves. When we do this, we don't have to suffer the guilt that might follow upon failure. We remember only too well the terrifying admonition: "You'll have no one to blame but yourself!"

To take charge of your own life and health implies taking calculated risks. It means recognizing that you have choices, and it carries with it your willingness to live with the consequences of those choices. For instance, in order to meet a deadline you may place yourself under prolonged stress, neglect your diet, and forget your exercise. These are your choices. If they are short-term, you will probably bounce back easily. But occasionally, they may result in a cold or some other condition that sends you to bed. Are you responsible for the cold? Yes, at some level you are. You may have no conscious awareness of it, but you created the condition that weakened your body and made it ripe for *dis-ease*. If you choose to take responsibility, you may accept the cold as an important message from your body and use it as a chance to rest and rebalance.

**Do I contradict myself?
Very well then I contradict myself,
I am large, I contain multitudes.**

—Walt Whitman

I hated medical school. "Memorize this," "Do it this way," "Don't question why they're sick, just diagnose and learn the right drugs to give." I was depressed most of the time. Depression was the way I had learned to handle anger (I found out later on). I dragged my feet and passively resisted and hurt inside a lot.

When I completed my clinical training and could see patients in the clinic at my own pace, I began to see how their lifestyle had been leading up to this symptom or disease they were now presenting to me to fix. Sometimes it looked like the pattern had been going on at least twenty years before any symptom had shown up. I would think to myself:

Here you are sick and hurting, wanting me to fix you up. That's not the problem— that's just the tip of the iceberg. The problem is in your lifestyle, yet I can't convince you of that, let alone help you change it. I'm depressed by your family (job, social, etc.) situation too. I guess all I can do is write you this prescription for a tranquilizer (or an antihypertensive, pain killer, sedative, or mood elevator). I hate to expose you to all the side effects of these chemicals, just to try to sweep something under the carpet for a while. What you really need to do is some internal vacuum cleaning, but if I sent you to the psychiatrist to help you do it, you'd either be insulted, or s/he would say you're not crazy enough and wouldn't have time to see you. There must be another way. This way simply doesn't work.

So, early in my career I decided to discontinue doing sick care and devote my life to wellness. This decision felt like a huge weight lifted from my shoulders. I focused full-time on learning ways to help people see their responsibility for their health and then consciously take that responsibility. I used the psychological training and body therapies I'd been learning, and much more. It was in 1972, during my preventive medicine residency, that I found the 1961 classic *High-Level Wellness* by Halbert Dunn, M.D., for $2 on the clearance table at the Johns Hopkins Medical Bookstore. I thought "wellness" was a silly word that would never catch on, but he put ideas together in a way I'd never seen before.

Most importantly, I continued to use myself as a laboratory, learning how to express anger more effectively, becoming less passive, and practicing dealing with my problems more directly. The sore right foot I developed during my fourth year in medical school was nearly crippling me as I began my residency. It seemed to be my body's way of resisting walking, to avoid stepping into more of this stuff that didn't feel good. It cleared up when I began enjoying my work.

My belief that the only way I could be OK was to follow in my dad's footsteps and become a family physician came to an end. I took on a new area, wellness, and despite my initial pessimism that it would ever become a viable concept, thirty-plus years later it's an everyday word.

—JWT

I.2 Responsibility for Medical Treatment

We resist self-responsibility when we assume we are helpless in the face of a "foreign invader." The belief that germs *cause* disease is still widely accepted. Disease is viewed as that something "out there" that "happens to" us poor, unsuspecting victims. We are told that our ancestors lived in terror of evil spirits and called upon the magical incantations of shamans to drive them away. An important element in any healing that took place as a result of these incantations was the shaman's easing of his "patient's" fears, thereby creating a healthier internal state. Given that modern-day placebos are sometimes almost as effective as the drugs to which they are compared, many of *today's* medical regimens may be promoting healing through easing our fears as much as (or more than!) through their actual physiologic effects. In fact, there is now a resurgence of interest in shamanism, faith healing, and other age-old forms of intervention that have fewer side effects than allopathic medicine.

Regardless of the modality, many of us are reluctant to take responsibility for our illnesses because we have lost touch with our reservoirs of knowledge and intuition, our physical body signals (both internal and external), and our gut-level, emotional responses. We mistrust ourselves and turn instead to the others who *really* know. The end result is a diminishment of personal freedom, a weakened self-concept, and a power-robbed existence—a high price to pay.

To accept responsibility for your health in no way implies that you should never seek the help of a doctor or a healer. To assume this is to misunderstand the concept completely. Your doctor, your counselor or therapist, a spiritual advisor or friend, a nutritionist or bodywork specialist—many others can be incorporated into a health team to work with you in moving toward wholeness. Each person can likely be a fine resource, offering valuable experience and knowledge that you do not have. It is up to you, however, to spearhead the formation of such a team, to assert your rights as a consumer in the medical economy, to ask questions, to seek other opinions, and to accept that you know yourself better than anyone else does.

And finally, there is just good common sense. Call it awareness, call it care—it is about self-responsibility. It shows itself by exercising safety with respect to ourselves, our homes, our automobiles, our children and loved ones, our environment. Sometimes, it is as simple as wearing a seat belt or removing poisons to a place that children can't reach. Sometimes it is more involved—a plan of escape in case of fire in your home.

[People] must begin to change from passive recipients of medical care to active, self-responsible participants; otherwise our goal of developing an adequate national health system cannot be realized.

—Elmer E. Green, Ph.D., Menninger Foundation

I.3 Safety

While the illness-care system de-emphasizes the role played by lifestyle in determining the state of health, the truth is that our health is much more in our own hands than in those of our doctor. Most illness in this country results from the everyday choices we make about how we live our lives, rather than from lack of access to health services. No training is needed to put on a seat belt in the car or to buckle up young children in a car seat, but these simple gestures can save lives and dramatically decrease the chances of severe injury. It takes only a minute to ask your doctor or pharmacist to check your prescription and over-the-counter medications for possible adverse drug interactions, or to double-check that what has been prescribed is exactly what was placed in the bottle.

From 1992 to 2003, the FDA received about 26,000 reports of medication errors—that's about 200 errors a month. But most experts believe that thousands more go unreported. The reasons for these errors are many, but improper labeling and confusion over product names are the most common. Among the elderly, hospital admissions for incorrectly used prescription drugs is extremely high, and drug errors within hospitals also pose a problem. Many patients are taking multiple drugs when they enter the hospital, and when new drugs are administered, some can adversely affect others. The Institute of Medicine, of the National Academy of Sciences, has estimated that drug errors alone may account for about 7,000 deaths each year in the United States.

You already know many ways to prevent accidents, since most of this is basic good sense; for example, making sure the smoke detector is working in your home or using a designated driver. Yet the complications and pressures of modern life may cause you to put these safety precautions low on your list of priorities. Many of us also know that some foods are de-energizing us, increasing our stress levels, and ruining our teeth, yet we like them, we are addicted to them, or they are convenient, and so we keep eating them instead of transitioning to a more wholesome diet. The world around us can be dangerous, but there are many practices and devices that can make it safer. Commonsense safety is easily overlooked as an integral part of a personal wellness program.

Self-responsibility in this domain may start with a slow "walk" through and around your home, your workplace, and your car, looking for safety hazards. Look over the list below and ask yourself what you already know about safety and wellness in each area.

- *Home fire extinguishers*

- *Icy sidewalks and steps*

- *Use and maintenance of stairs and handrails*

- *Slippery floors and movable area rugs*

- *Wet, slippery surfaces, especially bathtubs*

- *Children's access to prescription or over-the-counter drugs*

- *Out-of-date prescriptions or over-the-counter drugs*

- *Seat belts and air bags*

- *Automobile tires, wiper blades, and antilock brakes*

- *Car seats for children*

- *The speed limit*

- *Operation of machinery under the influence of alcohol or drugs*

- *Escape plans in case of fire both at home and away*

- *Overloaded, improperly fused electrical outlets*

- *Poorly protected electrical wires*

- *Use of electrical equipment near water*

- *Space heaters*

- *Storage of cleaning products, medicines, and poisons in homes where children live or visit*

- *Use of household cleaning products and pesticides that contain toxic substances*

- *Emergency phone numbers*

- *Accessibility of first-aid supplies*

- *First-aid skills for choking, burns, shock, and the like*

- *Protection from high sound or noise levels*

- *Safe disposal of paints, paint thinners, gasoline, oil, and so on*

- *Children's toys*

Depending upon where you live, you will have many other items to add to this list. In Arizona, where Regina lives, the creation of "defensible space" around homes is critical during the long dry seasons when the risk of forest fires is extreme.

The next major advances in health of the American people will come from the assumption of individual responsibility for one's own health and a necessary change in lifestyle for the majority of Americans.

—John H. Knowles, M.D., former president, Rockefeller Foundation

---

Once upon a time, long ago, when life was still very young, the Pill Fairy arrived on her first official visit to the people of planet Earth. She came on an errand of mercy. Her job was to help end the reign of pain and suffering that kept people from enjoying the full fruits of their labors. And so she set to work.

Assuming many disguises and dispensing her gifts in various forms—sometimes as magical chants accompanied by ritual dancing, often as strong-smelling brews concocted from the herbs and roots of fields and forest, frequently as salves spread lavishly over the body—there seemed no end to the ways of her magic. She was honored and sought after everywhere.

Slowly, however, the people began to suspect that hers was a temporary power. Though sometimes lasting for many weeks, her interventions often brought only a short-term release. Sooner or later the people had to seek her out again, queuing up on longer and longer lines to receive her healing potions or magical charms. But what else were they to do?

As time passed, some of the people began to question, to voice their doubts, to accuse her of playing favorites or of trying to take them under her spell to gain power. Was she *really* such a good fairy after all? they wondered. Wasn't there a better way?

The Pill Fairy still lives today. No longer dwelling in caves, or

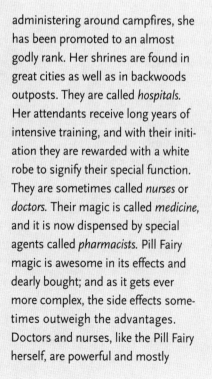

administering around campfires, she has been promoted to an almost godly rank. Her shrines are found in great cities as well as in backwoods outposts. They are called *hospitals*. Her attendants receive long years of intensive training, and with their initiation they are rewarded with a white robe to signify their special function. They are sometimes called *nurses* or *doctors*. Their magic is called *medicine*, and it is now dispensed by special agents called *pharmacists*. Pill Fairy magic is awesome in its effects and dearly bought; and as it gets ever more complex, the side effects sometimes outweigh the advantages. Doctors and nurses, like the Pill Fairy herself, are powerful and mostly

benevolent, laboring long hours to help the suffering masses who expect them to have a prescription or a procedure for every pain. Recently, less-invasive procedures, such as body therapies, and less-toxic substances, like herbs and homeopathic remedies, have become popular, but the model under which they are used remains similar to that of the Pill Fairy.

More and more, even doctors and nurses have begun to wonder if there is, perhaps, another way. But then the people still need them so desperately, and reward some of them so handsomely, that they have little time to look elsewhere.

1.4 Self-Responsibility = Self-Trust

You don't trust what you don't know. It is paradoxical that a culture like ours, which promotes an almost pornographic obsession with the appearance of the physical body, could encourage a pervasive ignorance and mistrust of it. Sex education, or the lack of it, provides an excellent example. This subject is still controversial within most school districts in the United States today, despite dramatic increases in teenage incidence of HIV and other sexually transmitted diseases. Need another example of the lack of awareness about the body? Ask a number of people where the pancreas is. You may find yourself directed to a local restaurant down the block.

What can you say about a population that may know more about the structure and the function of the automobile than it does about the workings of the human body?

It's hard to love when you feel guilt and shame. For all of our scientific sophistication, the sad fact is that many of us sense that our bodies are somehow inferior to our minds. Some parts of the body are felt to be shameful; some of its processes considered "dirty."

Young children know nothing of shame and guilt. But once learned, these feelings will surface throughout life. It takes some active involvement to overcome these influences, to reestablish a trust, a love, a sense of reverence for the body. After all, the human body has, over the past two hundred million years since mammals first appeared on earth, developed into a truly amazing vehicle.

Where's the Pancreas?

Match the letter to the number (not all are shown)

1. Pancreas _____   7. Adrenals _____

2. Pituitary _____   8. Stomach _____

3. Thymus _____   9. Pineal _____

4. Ovaries _____   10. Testes _____

5. Spleen _____   11. Parathyroid _____

6. Thyroid _____

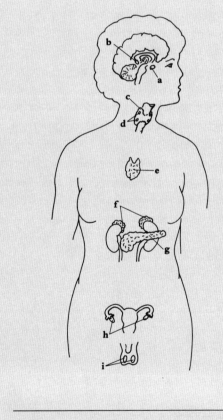

Answers: 1G, 2A, 3E, 4H, 5 (none), 6C, 7E, 8 (none), 9B, 10I, 11D

1.5 Body Awareness

Twenty-four hours a day, throughout your entire life, you make use of your body's built-in feedback system. Too hot—take off your coat. Too cold—put on a sweater. Hungry—eat. Thirsty—drink. Headache—take a painkiller. These are the easy ones. There are many more, however, that are suppressed or disregarded because you have more important things to do. You are neither ready nor willing to do anything about them. Tired muscles, sore throat, congested head? Swallow a cold capsule and keep on pushing! That knot in your stomach as you walk into the office each morning? Have another cup of coffee and start working! Light up a cigarette and begin coughing? Decide to quit as soon as this project is over! The list of examples goes on and on. This most sensitive machine, the body, is constantly trying to tell you something. It will do its best to keep a molehill from developing into a mountain, but most of us simply will not listen to its messages. We are only too quick to anesthetize pain and alleviate symptoms, forgetting that these are only warning signals, not the real problem. If we are to be well, we need to start listening to the entire body, then providing it with the best conditions possible so that it can continue healing itself. And that is something the body knows how to do. All the medical technology at our disposal does not really "cure" anything. *Only the body-mind heals itself.*

One of the most important principles of wellness is learning to call upon our innate body-trust or self-trust. Consider its opposites—ignorance, shame, fear, neglect, and the tendency to praise or blame something out there for what's happening in here—and you will find the primary components of this kind of trust.

Body-trust means learning about how your body works and at the same time loving and respecting it for the magnificent and powerful creation it is. It means attuning to its signs and signals, both internal and external. It includes listening to yourself to discover what you want to change. Most importantly, body-trust or self-trust involves a new way of thinking based on (1) the knowledge that healing occurs from within, but only when you are ready to be healed, and (2) the realization that patience and compassion are the key attitudes to facilitating that process.

A Conversation with a Body Part or Symptom

Getting prepared: Phase 1

1. *Take pen and paper and this workbook or your journal.*

2. *Move to a quiet place where you will be uninterrupted for at least twenty minutes.*

3. *Close your eyes and rest for about three to five minutes, breathing deeply.*

4. *Open your eyes.*

(continued)

Setting the stage: Phase 2

1. Using pen and paper, or talking aloud to yourself, or simply tracing in your own mind, recall the history of the problem as if it were the personal "life story" of a person you have known:

   When was the problem born?

   How and where did it grow?

   What have been the high and low points in its life?

   When does it come to visit you?

2. Rest with your eyes closed for a few minutes.

The conversation: Phase 3

1. Imagine the problem sitting in a chair across the room from you.

2. Give it a name.

3. Write as fast as you can, without editing and without rereading, a conversation between yourself and the problem:

   Regina: Headache, I hate you.

   Headache: You hate me? You hate yourself!

   Regina: . . .

   Continue for as long as you feel inclined. Expect nothing. When finished, reread what you've written.

The wrap-up: Phase 4

What this experience has taught me:

_____

_____

_____

_____

_____

_____

_____

Try this same procedure, with the same problem, on several different occasions. Compare, contrast, learn from the results.

1.6 Responsibility versus Blame

We waste much of our valuable life energy by burdening ourselves with guilt and blame ("I should have done this . . ." or "I shouldn't have said that . . ."). It is a currency of our culture, used to manipulate and control people, usually when they are young and small. It is the stuff of which many religions are made, and many of us are so enmeshed in our feelings of shame and guilt that it is hard to see a situation objectively.

Taking responsibility for choices that may have resulted in an illness or injury does not mean taking on blame. There is a big difference. With blame, you berate yourself for not being perfect, or burden yourself with guilt that creates more stress. In taking responsibility for a problem, you accept that while you may not have intentionally engineered your present life situation, and you may, in truth, be able to point to this or that "external" as a contributing factor, you alone are responsible for how you choose to *respond* to the situation. Regardless of how difficult the challenge that you are facing may be, if you can accept, with love and compassion, that there is a lesson—even a gift—to be found, you can release blame and embrace the process.

This issue may be one of the most difficult ones you will encounter in learning how to increase your wellness. Blame and guilt get mixed in with responsibility from an early age. Having heard, at a tender age, an angry voice question "Who's responsible for this mess on the floor?" you may intimately link the concept of responsibility with a message of blame. These connections may go so deep, and originate so early in your life, that the word "responsibility" may carry some negative charge regardless of how conscious you become. Becoming aware of how such messages have been wired into your thinking will set the stage for change.

1.7 Dis-ease as Feedback

Disease is not really the problem. It is more likely the body's attempt to solve the problem—a feedback of sorts that says "something isn't working properly." That "something" is probably much more than cramped, disfigured fingers, or a headache over the right eye. As the metaphors in a poem, or the images in a dream, these body signs can often be interpreted at many levels. The most apparent says, "I've got arthritis" and "Mother had it too." Reflecting more deeply, however, you might realize that all your life you've swallowed anger and clenched your fist behind your back. With this awareness, the focus of attention changes radically. Instead of determining how many painkillers you can safely continue to take, you ask what other, more direct ways there are for expressing your feelings. Then you're ready to take the road toward high-level wellness, generously reinforced with the self-compassion and love that will encourage your continuing success.

1.8 Love and Compassion

If you were going to climb a mountain, you would make a number of necessary preparations. An important one might be to consult with those who have taken the trip already. Then you would carefully pack the minimal amount of essential gear, checking and double-checking to make sure everything was in good working order. Only then would you set out on your adventure.

The journey toward higher levels of wellness poses a similar challenge, and requires similar preparation. The equipment is less tangible, so it may be easy to neglect what is most essential. In remembering knowledge, self-trust, safety, and perseverance, you might forget love and compassion. Yet these form the knapsack that carries all your other resources.

Compassion is an attribute of love. It means an empathic consciousness of weakness or distress, together with the desire to alleviate it. Any attempt at change that lacks it is doomed from the start. It is just that important!

Bodily Symptoms—Trackdown on Deeper Meanings

Illness, pain, and accidents are often signs of deeper needs that are going unmet. Perhaps this trackdown method will help you to get in touch with what some of these needs are.

Trackdown Steps	Regina's Example: Tension Headache	Your Example: _____
1. It feels like:	A knife over my right eye	
2. It happens when:	I've been pushing myself hard for several days	
3. It prevents:	Reading, feeling excited about life	
4. It encourages:	More sleep, less work, admitting my weaknesses	
5. It provides the reward:	Relief from overwhelming demands	
6. It may indicate the deeper need for:	Reorientation of work and self-care priorities	
7. A more direct way to meet this need might be:	Asking for help rather than trying to do it all myself	

1.9 Being Out of Balance, Vulnerable, or in Need

From our earliest years we have been rewarded for being strong, for achieving. We got attention in the form of touch, acknowledgment, and rewards for being what others defined as OK. As a result, we often assumed that our self-worth depended upon "doing the right thing." Needing this attention in order to live, we set about trying to accumulate more of it, only to be disappointed and frustrated when our best attempts sometimes failed. We were often weak, unprepared, and misinformed, and we accepted that this meant that we were "not OK," or "not good enough." An interesting paradox then emerged. Some of us learned that by getting hurt, through accident or illness, we got even more attention. Perhaps we were soothed with candy and ice cream, or permitted to stay home from school while Mother brought hot soup and the TV set to our bedside. And so the pattern was reinforced. If we couldn't get sufficient attention with our achievements, we could get it by our sicknesses. The seeds planted in our childhood continued to flow as we moved through adolescence and into adulthood. They are with us today and will be as we advance to old age.

The comedian on a popular late-night talk show remarks about his eighty-two-year-old mother: "She loves her new therapy. The doctor is all the time touching her, touching her!" We laugh, knowingly, because most of us recognize how readily people use suffering to get the attention or touch they haven't gotten through other means.

You can accept this insight and resign yourself to it as "the way things are." You can criticize the hypochondriacs of the world or of your own household and resolve to steel yourself to their needs. Or you can examine your own life to see why this tendency shows itself, and you can resolve to do something about it. What would it be like to arrive at a place where you could ask for the attention, the touch, the caring you need, *when* you needed it? Suppose you start viewing your own illness as a need for attention or connection in some broader context of your life? Imagine the many lessons you would learn, and the growth you could achieve, if you used the experience of disease as an opportunity to reevaluate your lifestyle and environment. What answers might surface if you posed yourself the question "Why might I need this problem at this time?" Could you possibly relax enough to enjoy the rest that an illness may afford? Are you willing to honor and respect yourself in the midst of your weakness, rather than in spite of it? Can you believe that it is OK to be weak, in need, out of balance at times; that it is basically OK to be just as you are—a glorious series of contradictions?

The process of high-level wellness does not preclude an occasional bout with illness. If we view sickness as an evil to be eliminated under all circumstances and at any cost, we make death the ultimate enemy. This attitude can lead to the support of the quantity of life above its quality.

Our culture emphasizes independence and self-sufficiency, overlooking the reality of our interdependence. Many diseases actually result from the isolation and loneliness that are fostered by this mistaken view of reality. The supermom or Mr. Perfect, who appear to have no needs of their own, are frequently the ones who get cancer or have a heart attack without warning.

The problem with trying to give more than you receive is that the balance of give-and-take is upset—there have to be enough people willing to receive in order for people to be able to give. We can practice becoming part of the great give-and-take, practice receiving graciously rather than appearing to have no needs. These are skills that, as you acknowledge your vulnerability and interdependence as a member of our species, will weave you more strongly into the web of our shared lives and hence will enhance your wellness.

How I Learned to Be Sick

As children, we all received messages about illness and health from many different sources—our parents, teachers, movies, books, TV, the Internet. Often these communications are so strong that we adopt them and carry them with us for years. If indeed we learned illness behaviors and associations, we can unlearn them too. This exercise will refresh your memory about how you learned to be sick.

List the names of persons you knew as a child, or cite experiences you remember as a child, then explain what messages you received from them.

Person/Experience	Explanation	Messages You Remember Receiving about Illness and Health
Example: Mom	She took lots of aspirins every day to cope with the pain of her arthritis.	"All the women in our family have arthritis." "Tall people always have low-back pain."

Remembering a Childhood Illness

Past experiences shape your responses to the present, although the carryover is not always immediately apparent. Recalling childhood illness experiences, and reflecting upon them, may help you better understand yourself and how you interpret illness/wellness today.

Write about an illness experience you remember having as a child. Describe it in as much detail as possible—unpleasant symptoms, your sickroom, any medicines, how long it lasted, how your parents responded, the "goodies" it provided, and so on.

_____

_____

_____

_____

_____

_____

_____

_____

_____

_____

_____

_____

_____

_____

_____

_____

_____

_____

_____

_____

_____

As you read over your description, look for carryovers to your present situations.

1.10 Wellness in the Midst of Illness

Wellness describes the quality of natural health or wellbeing that is fundamental to human beings. This quality of wellness is *not* dependent on physical wellbeing for its expression. It is an unconditional state of being that may be *obscured*—but not *destroyed*—by illness. It is therefore possible to discover wellbeing in the midst of a serious or chronic illness. Although this may seem simple and obvious, it is a major statement that sets the wellness approach apart from the more common treatment approach that measures only our state of physical health.

One aspect of self-love and self-acceptance is allowing disease to be an instructive and positive life force. The lessons that accompany it are essential to the fully functional human being. Since we are all going to die anyway, the test seems to be how we deal with our illnesses rather than how well or how long we can avoid them.

One day years ago, Regina fell on the ski slopes and broke her leg. It was right in the middle of a very pressured period of work. The situation forced her to slow down, to rest, to struggle with her general reticence to ask for help from someone else. It became an opportunity rather than a problem. She used the time to write a new book, *After Surgery, Illness, or Accident: 10 Practical Steps to Renewed Energy and Health,* about how to make optimal use of the recuperation period.

History is filled with examples of individuals who experienced personal transformations as a result of serious disease or crippling handicap. For instance, the writings of Helen Keller and the music of Ray Charles have inspired millions of people all over the world. More recently, Christopher Reeve's advocacy for the handicapped provides another notable example. Wellness may be encouraged by a physical handicap as much as by a vigorous exercise program or a pure diet. Of themselves, none of these things automatically leads to wellness. When used as tools for self-exploration, for education, for growth, everything leads to wellness.

Be Your Own Doctor

Many of us wait until our doctor delivers an ultimatum about our health before we make changes in our habits and lifestyle. Often, the doctor's recommendations are simply reiterations of what we already know we should be doing—but for which we don't want to take responsibility.

In your journal, make a list of at least ten things that you already know will increase your wellness but that you currently overlook or avoid. Be as specific as possible (for example, "Getting seven to eight hours of sleep, instead of my usual five").

Look your list over carefully. Choose one item to do today and promise yourself you'll do it.

I.II Forgiving Yourself and Others

> **Making a mistake and then judging yourself harshly is like paying compound interest on a bad investment.**
>
> —Doc Childre and Howard Martin

Most of us tend to be unduly critical of ourselves, and a great deal of valuable life energy is wasted in burdening ourselves with this negativity, guilt, and blame: "I should have done this . . ." or "I shouldn't have said that . . ." Some things simply cannot be changed. The question then becomes, "Can we accept these things—and ourselves?" If the media is presenting us with an image of beauty or health based on youth and an unrealistic standard of perfection, it is often hard to feel good about ourselves. Instead, we berate ourselves when we don't measure up. If we can shift the focus from comparing ourselves to others to self-appreciation for who we are, we will be building a foundation of love, inspiring ourselves to change what we can and when we can.

> **THE SERENITY PRAYER**
> **God grant me the serenity**
> **To accept the things I cannot change,**
> **Courage to change the things I can,**
> **And the wisdom to know the difference.**
>
> —Reinhold Niebuhr

The willingness to accept things as they are is the first step toward lasting change. Without the compulsiveness of "have to's," changing can be a joyous adventure.

Acceptance is often confused with resignation, but the two are not the same. At its best, resignation may be a necessary preliminary step toward acceptance. But resignation is more often dry, passive, and lifeless. It is frequently an attitude of defeat. Real acceptance, on the other hand, is a choice, an active and lively process that requires your participation.

You can't rush this acceptance that leads to compassion and forgiveness. You can't force yourself to forgive yourself or others. Any life change, positive or negative, entails some grief, some letting go of what was. And grieving takes time. Acceptance and forgiveness are generally the results of adequate grieving, although sometimes they are simply experienced as an unexpected infusion of pure grace! One minute you feel hatred for someone, and the next you are struck by their pain and forgive them on the spot.

To forgive means to be willing to refuse to hold onto the past; to release grievances; possibly even to reconcile, although this won't always be possible when another person is involved. Forgiveness includes the willingness to look below the surface of behaviors or feelings. Here we find the essence of the precious being, which is ourselves, or another. When you stay connected to that essential "one," forgiveness is so much easier.

Forgiveness of yourself or others often brings with it a relaxation in the body, and peace of mind. This harmony is the essence of health and the heart of wellness.

GUILT VS. REGRET

It's important not to confuse guilt with regret. Guilt results from doing something that we knew was "wrong" *at the time*. Regret comes from *later* learning that we could have done something better. When we understand the difference between guilt and regret, we can move beyond blaming ourselves for what we didn't know or weren't able to do at the time (like taking drugs whose side effects were unknown at the time).

We are all products of our time and culture, as were our parents and their parents before them. We cannot be expected to act on information that we didn't have.

Even when we have the correct information, sometimes cultural and economic conditions limit our ability to implement what we know would be the best course of action. Making this all-important distinction can often help us to reduce our guilt load to what it really is—regret. We can transform that regret into motivation to be more conscious about future decisions we may make.

SELF-ACCEPTANCE

When we were writing the first edition of this book, John and I both had difficulty with the fact that I was a cigarette smoker, and our book was about wellness. What would people think? Should we tell them? In working out this problem, we realized that it was more important to accept each other as we were than to try to fit other people's expectations. His acceptance of me, and my willingness to go outside when having a cigarette, led to his writing a little piece like this about the process. He also shared some of *his* "vices."

We have each received more comments about those three paragraphs than about almost any other part of the book. Smokers were relieved. Nonsmokers were touched. The whole process of dealing, personally and together, with our inconsistencies has inspired patience and compassion for ourselves and for others.

Come to think of it, I've learned a lot about patience and self-acceptance in the years since then, and all of it motivated by seeming crises. In 1981, while traveling in India, I contracted hepatitis and spent eight weeks sick and alone in a foreign country. Here was an opportunity to face my deepest fears of death and abandonment—which I did. Years later, I fell on the ski slopes and broke my left leg in three places. Four months of greatly restricted mobility were the result. The "monsters" met this time were dependency and self-recrimination. I went through a "dark night of the soul"— sometimes called "depression"—for a chunk of time, and the compassion for the suffering of others that it taught me is inestimable. Will the lessons never end? Not as long as I'm alive, I suppose.

I consider myself a "well being," yet I've probably been laid up more than most people I know. But then, my definition of wellness has more to do with learning and loving than it does with sickness and health.

By the way, I stopped smoking cold turkey in 1988 as I stood in a parking lot in a small town in Germany. I stopped that day because I finally saw myself as a hypocrite, hiding my smoking from some people and allowing it with others. The hypocrisy was too much to take. Not only was this a step in the direction of better health, but it was importantly, for me, a step in personal integrity.

—RSR

Here I Am #1

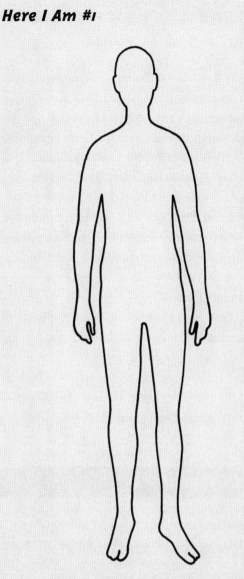

Imagine that the outline above is you as you are right now. Color or write on it or around it, commenting on each part of you, head to toe (for example, short, curly hair—OK; stomach—flabby; feet too big—shoes hurt). Remember to comment on your insides (heart, lungs, brain, and so on) as well.

Here I Am #2

Now imagine that this is your ideal self. Write all over or around the outline, commenting on yourself as you would like to be (for example, 20/20 vision—no more glasses; 120 pounds— looking good; lungs—clear, asthma gone).

Compare your two selves. You may find you are unduly critical of yourself. Some things simply cannot be changed—accept them. Focus on your positive points instead, or on those aspects that can be changed.

1.12 **Love and Wellness**

In fact, being in love is what it's all about. As you fall in love with yourself, you naturally get healthier. All the do's and don'ts of health education can only build a house of straw unless love is the foundation. When you see love in operation in a relationship, you see trust, acceptance of the uniqueness of each person, understanding of differences, and forgiveness of failings. To love yourself is to love your body, your emotions, your intelligence, your spiritual nature. It is to trust, accept, understand, and forgive yourself. The challenge is to remember that love is all around you, and to open yourself to receive it. Love is not *out there* waiting to be found; it is within you, wanting to be recognized. All things in the universe are connected; all things in the body are connected as well. There is simply no place where the body starts and the mind stops; no place where the universe starts and the individual stops.

Finally, love means being compassionate with yourself. As you begin to realize how many things affect your state of wellness, you may at first be overwhelmed, thinking that you have to *do something* about each of them. But the connectedness of all things actually makes this whole business of living wellness a lot easier. As you breathe better, you move better, and digest your food better, and relax more deeply, and develop greater self-awareness, and . . . the associations multiply. When this happens, we appreciate one of the basics of wellness—that it's all one process.

The challenge of living well is the challenge of becoming the clearest, most loving, most aware channel of energy you can possibly be. To do so means to become a natural alchemist in the highest sense of the word. It is to become a transmuter of energy. It is to transform yourself.

NATIONAL "LOVE YOUR BODY DAY"

Since 1999, the National Organization for Women (NOW) has sponsored a national Love Your Body Day, highlighting the need to speak out and raise people's awareness about the many ways in which ads and images of women are offensive, harmful, and disrespectful. This creative program suggests numerous activities that encourage self-appreciation as well as ways that schools, organizations, groups, and individuals can take action in this regard.

Although this event is essentially about women's bodies, men can certainly profit by applying the same types of awareness and action against the exploitation and disrespect of men's bodies. Since body image is an important factor in self-esteem, and self-esteem is an important factor in health, the subject of loving and honoring the body is a core issue for everyone.

Learn more about the program and how you can participate at www.nowfoundation.org/issues/health/lybdkit.

1.13 Wellness and the Planet

> **Think globally, act locally.**
>
> —Anonymous

Moving one step beyond personal/familial wellness issues, we come face-to-face with our responsibility for the neighborhood, the city or town, the county, the state, and the country in which we live. One vote does make a difference! And many votes can make a bigger difference. The more we express consciousness and accountability in our own lives, the more we will see and enjoy our interdependence with one another. A beginning may be as simple as getting to know who our neighbors are, which easily extends to working together in protecting our shared, local environment from overdevelopment and pollution.

Beyond participating in our local community, the awareness that planet Earth is a finite entity can strengthen our willingness to conserve resources and energy. About 20 percent of the world's population uses 80 percent of the planet's resources, much of it very wastefully. The other 80 percent have noticed this wastefulness, as we've made our greed obvious via our TV and movies, which are seen by more people in other countries than in our own. They want the same standard of living that we have. It's doubtful that the planet can support that much waste, so it's up to us to start reducing our energy claims so that we are only taking our fair share.

We can see the consequences of our greed as we become aware of the planetary changes that affect everyone—for example, global warming, increased UV radiation from damage to the ozone layer, damage to the oceans and their plant and animal life, and the acid rain that kills forests.

There are many actions we can take: We can choose to downsize—to live in a smaller home (and to insulate it well and keep the thermostat cooler in winter and warmer in summer). We can choose to use public transportation or carpool to work; to plan ahead when we go shopping to avoid extra trips. We can ask "Do I really need this?" before making a purchase; we can buy products that are not unnecessarily disposable or wastefully packaged. We can act on the fact that it is much more effective to reduce, rather than to reuse or recycle. Once we begin to view our daily decisions in the light of our awakening sense of responsibility, we learn that almost every individual choice we make is a choice for the rest of humanity as well. When we make our choices with this level of awareness and responsibility, we are promoting planetary wellness.

All of this has been leading up to a definition of one of the general principles governing the approach to wellness taken in this book. It is sometimes called *body-trust,* sometimes simply *self-trust.* Turn around ignorance, shame, fear, neglect, and the tendency to praise or blame something out there for what's happening in here, and you have its components.

LIVING LIGHTLY

"Living lightly on the planet" is an expression used by people who are conscious of their "energy footprint" and are attempting to minimize it. Americans, on average, require twenty-six acres (10.5 hectares) of land per person to support their lifestyle, compared to a worldwide average of seven acres. Developing nations average three to five acres.

People who live lightly on the earth consciously evaluate their behaviors with regard to how they may enhance or disrupt the natural balance of all things. They are aware that exhaust gases from cars and industrial pollutants are painting a brown haze across the horizon, and that chlorofluorocarbons may be destroying the planet's ozone layer, exposing us to harmful radiation. They realize that unrestricted urban sprawl is wantonly eliminating our green space; herbicides and pesticides are poisoning our soil and, consequently, our food. Greed and waste are the characteristics of a population that has lost touch with itself.

Take some time to reflect on your own lifestyle and the ways in which you touch the earth, the water, the air. Your wellness, our wellness, and that of our children depend upon this.

SUGGESTED READING

Capacchione, L., *The Creative Journal: The Art of Finding Yourself* (Newcastle, 1989).

Dadd-Redalia, D., *Home Safe Home: Protecting Yourself and Your Family from Everyday Toxics and Harmful Household Products in the Home* (J. P. Tarcher, 1997).

Dossey, L., *Healing Beyond the Body: Medicine and the Infinite Reach of the Mind* (Shambhala, 2003).

Jampolsky, G., *Good-Bye to Guilt: Releasing Fear through Forgiveness* (Bantam Books, 1985).

Levey, J., and M. Levey, *Living in Balance: A Dynamic Approach for Creating Harmony and Wholeness in a Chaotic World* (Conari, 1998).

Moss, R., *How Then Shall We Live?* (Bantam, 1996).

Muller, W., *Sabbath: Finding Rest, Renewal, and Delight in Our Busy Lives* (Bantam, 2000).

Weil, A., *Health and Healing* (Houghton-Mifflin, 1998).

For an updated listing of resources and active links to the websites mentioned in this chapter, please see www.WellnessWorkbook.com.

NOTES

1. DrugIntel, "Adverse Drug Reactions, Adverse Drug Events, and Medication Errors Are a Leading Cause of Preventable Death in USA," www.drugintel.com/pharma/cause_of_death.htm.

2. U.S. Food and Drug Administration, "Battle of the Bugs: Fighting Antibiotic Resistance," www.fda.gov/fdac/features/2002/402_bugs.html.

CHAPTER 2

Wellness and Breathing

Breathing is synonymous with living. It is basic to our energy-transforming metabolism. In the Wellness Energy System, breathing provides the first energy input. The oxygen that breathing provides is needed for the production of the high-energy chemical bonds that result when it combines with our blood sugar within every cell of our body. Our breathing invokes more-subtle energies not presently recognized by most of Western science—the prana, *or life force.*

Air is the first food of the newborn.

—Edward Rosenfeld

The human body is remarkably adaptive and resilient. Human beings can survive for many weeks without food, for several days without water. But without air, life ceases in only a matter of minutes. Every cell in the organism requires a continuous charge of oxygen in order to carry out its function. Breathing supplies this energy to the bloodstream, but since it has been happening automatically for every moment of your life, you've probably given very little attention to it. Yet without it, everything stops. So this is where we will begin our investigation of wellness.

When the air is clear, your lungs strong, your body relaxed, and your mind at peace, you experience total wellbeing.

Unfortunately, this ideal is seldom realized. In the language of the Wellness Energy System, the input source—the air—may be polluted in some way. Or perhaps there just isn't enough of it available. High-altitude climbers must carry their own oxygen, or risk unconsciousness and even death around 24,000 feet. Being in an overcrowded room without proper ventilation will have a similar, albeit less deadly, effect. The channel (which is you) may have breakages (poorly functioning organs, illness, accident), or be blocked by foreign objects, by the restriction of muscles created from emotions such as fear, anger, and grief, by tight clothing, or by chronically poor posture. It may also be contaminated by the poisons of nicotine and tar accumulated in lung tissues.

The resulting output—your general metabolism, and your ability to work, play, and communicate with others—will depend upon these factors *and* upon how effectively the energy has been used.

The Process of Breathing

Breathing may be likened to the functioning of the old-fashioned blacksmith's bellows. Lift up the handle, opening the bellows, and air is sucked in. Let go, the bellows collapse, and the air rushes out.

The components of the process are volume and pressure. As the volume of the bellows increases, the internal pressure decreases, creating a vacuum effect that draws in the outside air. When the bellows collapses, the volume decreases, and the increasing internal pressure forces the air back out again.

The bellows at work within your body consists of the lung tissue's elasticity as well as a number of fascinating muscles. The most active of these is the diaphragm—a dome-shaped muscle located at the base of the rib cage and above the stomach. It contracts during inhalation and pulls down on the bottom of the chest, increasing the volume inside the chest cavity. At the same time, the chest capacity can be further increased by elevating the ribs slightly and moving them outward and upward. When all is working smoothly, what results is maximum volume and minimal pressure. Air is drawn in—you are "inspiring." Relax these muscles and the elastic property of the lungs causes them to contract. The diaphragm is pulled back up, ribs move back in and down, the pressure builds, and the air is exhaled. The illustration at right further clarifies this.

Adult human beings breathe an average of 16,000 quarts of air each day.

The Importance of Breathing

Some excellent examples of the positive and therapeutic uses of rhythmic breathing and breath awareness come from such diverse activities as childbirth and sports. Many women today are choosing natural or drug-free childbirth, focusing on using a variety of breathing techniques to reduce anxiety and pain, as well as to assist the normal bodily processes involved in birthing a child. The father, or another supportive person, may serve as a coach to encourage the woman to regulate her breathing as the infant moves down the birth canal.

In sports, controlled breathing in swimming is absolutely essential in maintaining a steady, smooth movement through the water. Observe weight lifters going through their paces and you will see the results of much practice in the coordination of breath and movement. In dancing, skiing, yoga, and running, breath control plays an important part. Whether or not you participate in such recreational activities, you can profit from breath awareness in whatever you do.

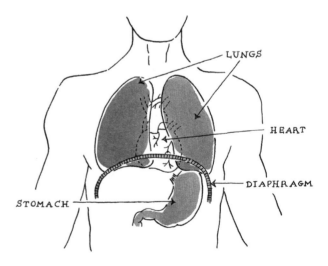

2.1 Breathing Freely

Physical posture is one of the main factors that determine whether our breathing is free or restricted. How can the diaphragm possibly do its job of expanding if the abdominal muscles that support it are weak, or if the midsection is caved in on itself in a way that makes it difficult for any abdominal or diaphragmatic movement to take place? The body will compensate by breathing exclusively from the upper chest, never fully filling the lungs. The result is only a half breath, or less.

Our furniture, our cars, and our clothing often encourage poor posture, leading to poor breathing. Years of adapting to unhealthy environments leads to habits that are difficult to change. Recall the cramped school desks that some of us sat in so many hours a day, over twelve or more years of our lives—desks that forced us to double over at the waist, or to strain our neck.

Pause for a moment and check your posture as you read this. Does it enhance your natural breathing, or restrict you to a shallow, constrained intake of air? Those of us who work at sedentary occupations may suffer a whole range of health problems, including low-back pain, headaches, hemorrhoids, stomach and intestinal maladies, congested sinuses, and other respiratory complications. Without proper oxygenation, we tire easily, start to feel foggy, and may soon lose interest in the task at hand. We think we need time out for a caffeine break (coffee, cola, chocolate), when what we really need is more oxygen!

People today are spending more and more hours behind the wheel, as they drive to work on crowded freeways or navigate a stop-start dance through traffic-choked city streets. Even if the car we drive has an ergonomically designed seat, the stress or fatigue we endure as we drive can aggravate conditions leading to poor posture and poor breathing. Cars without such design features compound the negative effects, discouraging the relaxed but aligned posture that best serves breathing. Cramped legs, strained low back, and tense arms and shoulders are common, even on short trips. Truck drivers and others who frequently drive long distances often suffer more serious problems.

If you are engaged in office work, examine the position of your desk, worktable, or computer station, as well as the kind of chairs you use—both for work and for relaxation. Become more aware of the posture you most frequently assume when you work. Evaluate how these elements are affecting your ability to breathe fully. If you work for a company with an ergonomics expert, ensure that your workplace is ergonomically sound.

Clothing design may also discourage freedom of movement and restrict breathing. Our culture prizes the flat belly and continues to invent torturous means of ensuring it. Figure-controlling pantyhose and tight-fitting jeans are big business, and not easily dismissed. If you artificially tighten the abdomen to flatten the belly, this activity generally involves holding your breath, which cuts off vital energy flow. You may also tighten the genitals and anus in the same motion, blocking the flow of sexual energy as well. Tight waistbands and tight collars are also offenders in promoting poor breathing habits.

If you note the alignment of the spine of a relaxed, standing child, you'll see what a natural, healthy posture looks like. The "hanging gut" that so many adults experience is not the same, however, as a relaxed but strong belly or midsection. Lack of muscle tone in the core muscles of the abdomen, buttocks, thighs, and genital region is the result of lack of exercise, poor diet leading to overweight, and the long-term patterns of sitting (as mentioned above) or lounging in ways that encourage a lack of tone in the midsection. A weak middle is one of the primary reasons for low-back pain as well as insufficient intake of oxygen. The remedy for this weakness is not to artificially suck in the belly—this immediately causes you to hold your breath, exactly the opposite of what is needed. Instead, try lifting your sternum while rolling your shoulders up, back, and down, bringing your shoulder blades downward. Notice how this alignment naturally creates more breathing room while naturally toning the belly. The optimal remedy is to strengthen the core muscles while at the same time learning to breathe more fully and consistently.

The diaphragm physically separates the lungs and heart from the abdomen. Additionally, above the diaphragm is the domain of the intellect, the rational mind; below it is the emotional realm, the "gut," the pleasure centers and reproductive organs. Breathing then becomes the harmonizing force, the integrating process that unites and balances us, head with heart with belly.

WORKPLACE ERGONOMIC SUGGESTIONS

Adjust your workstation as follows:

- Ideally, your computer screen should be an arm's length away from your eyes. If you wear bifocals, you may need to get special lenses so you can look at your screen comfortably without neck or eyestrain.

- Adjust your workstation (screen, keyboard tray, and chair seat) so the top of the computer screen is at eye level. This will help keep your neck relaxed.

- Situate your screen to avoid glare. Use window curtains, blinds, or shades if needed.

- The screen is a dirt magnet and a dusty display is tiring to your eyes, so wipe it off on a regular basis.

- Choose a chair that is padded and firm; the seat should be wider than your thighs, with a waterfall edge. Adjust it to fit your size and support your back and legs properly.

- Face your work directly and keep your things within easy reach.

- Place your document holder at the same height as and distance from you as the screen to minimize shifting your head and neck back and forth constantly and to reduce eyestrain.

Adjust your posture as follows:

- To avoid stress and strain on your arms and wrists, position the computer keyboard at elbow level. Your upper arm and forearm should form a right angle (90 degrees), with your upper arms comfortably close to your sides and your forearms parallel to the floor.

- Keep your wrists straight; use a wrist rest for support. Avoid resting your wrists or arms on sharp edges.

- Your back should be kept in an "S" shape, not a "C" shape.

- Your thighs should be parallel to the floor and not touching the underside of your workstation (you may need to remove the drawer).

- Keep both feet flat on the floor; use a footrest if your legs are short or your chair cannot be lowered.

- If you spend much time on the phone, use a headset.

- Take regular breaks. Walk around and stretch as often as possible.

Adjust your workspace as follows:

- If possible, reduce the amount of unnecessary noise in your area; excess noise is jarring to the nervous system. Could you close the door, move a loud printer or copier, or adjust the volume on the intercom or music? You may also want to take your breaks in a quiet place.

- Decorate your area with some beautiful plants. Not only will they add some life, they will help remove carbon dioxide from the atmosphere and improve air quality.

Inspired by Julie Lusk, *Desktop Yoga* (Penguin, Putnam, Perigee Books, 1998).

Oxygen taken into the lungs is a life force—called *prana* by the yogis of India. The red blood cells moving through the lungs pick up oxygen and proceed to carry it throughout the body, charging every muscle, bone, nerve, and organ. Quite an impressive process, especially when you consider that it has been going on day and night from your first moment in the world. Fortunately, it happens without need for your conscious direction.

Breathing is not something you *do*. Rather, it is something that you *allow*. Left alone, the body will do what it needs to do, and most efficiently at that. Then why devote so much attention to it?

The answer is that we *don't* allow our breathing to happen smoothly and naturally. We continually do things that restrict it. Changing this tendency requires, at least initially, that we pay attention to it. Rather than adding something new, observe how you currently breathe and then find ways to remove the obstacles, the conditions, that are blocking your breathing and consequently depriving you of a full life.

I've got to keep breathing. It'll be my worst business mistake if I don't.

—Steve Martin

Experiencing a Full Breath

While it is not possible or necessary to fully expand the lungs with every breath, to heighten awareness it is vital that you experience how a really complete breath feels. Used periodically, this exercise utilizes the lungs to capacity and extracts great amounts of "life force" from the air.

Try this exercise sitting, standing, and lying down. Through the nose:

1. *Exhale deeply, contracting the belly.*

2. *Inhale slowly as you expand the abdomen.*

3. *Continue inhaling as you expand the chest.*

4. *Continue inhaling as you feel your collarbones lift.*

5. *Pause briefly. Don't hold.*

6. *Exhale in reverse pattern, slowly. Release the shoulders, relax the chest, contract the belly.*

7. *Repeat.*

This exercise requires gentle practice to make inhalation and exhalation smooth and balanced. First, practice breathing so the inhalation and exhalation are of equal duration. Next, allow the exhalation to become a little longer. Breathe in this manner as long as it's comfortable.

Remembering to Breathe—Allowing Natural Breathing

As you go through a day, there are many occasions during which you block breathing by your posture or level of tension. Use this exercise to remind yourself to check your breathing and to remove factors that may be restricting your natural breathing.

Purchase some self-adhesive colored dots at a stationery store. Go through your house, your office, your car, your wallet, and your purse, and place these dots in prime locations. Each time you see one, use it as a cue to remind yourself to allow breathing.

Variation: Make signs (perhaps using sticky notes) that say things like BREATHE or WAKE UP or REMEMBER and put them around where you are sure to be surprised by them regularly. Change your computer's screen saver so it says BREATHE. When you notice these reminders, attune to your breathing or lack of it. Allow it.

P.S. When people ask about the dots or the signs, use this as an opportunity to breathe again, and to spread the good word!

Breathing for Balance

As you breathe, the air traveling through the nasal passages stimulates the sensory nerve linings and consequently affects your brain. Involving both nostrils more fully will assist your body in its great balancing act. Use this exercise to increase awareness of imbalanced breathing and bring breathing into balance, as well as to relax and energize your whole system. Short daily practice periods will enable you to make your breathing smooth and balanced.

1. Begin by exhaling completely, using both nostrils.

2. Press your thumb or forefinger against the right nostril, closing it completely, then inhale slowly and easily through the left one alone.

3. Hold the inhaled breath for a few comfortable seconds, then close the left nostril and exhale through the right nostril. Hold while comfortable.

4. Inhale through the right nostril, then release your finger from your left nostril, close off the right, and exhale through the left nostril. Hold. Inhale left . . .

5. Continue for five to sixteen cycles, then stop. Allow breathing through both nostrils.

This is a simplified version of an ancient yogic technique.

2.2 Emotional States and Breath

> **No one ever told me that grief felt so like fear.**
>
> —C. S. Lewis

Fear, grief, anger, and even exhilaration are emotional states that produce physical changes in the body. These changes increase overall body tension and restrict breathing. Any excess tension will upset the balance and interfere with normal breathing.

Marjorie experienced an asthmatic attack when she noticed the flowers on her doctor's desk. She panicked. Her mind issued a "red alert" to her body, and she responded by sweating and gasping for air. The flowers, she later learned, were artificial. But the pain she felt was real. Whether the danger is real or imaginary makes little difference. Fear will create tension, and tension will affect the ability to breathe. What we perceive, believe, trust, and fear in our minds will spill over into the body and manifest in some way. There is simply no place where the mind stops and the body starts and vice versa.

Recall a recent fearful event in your own life and reflect how your breathing was affected by it. Perhaps you have had a near accident in your car. No impact or injury, but upsetting nonetheless. Suppose you narrowly miss hitting a child who has run into the street. A few moments later you pull over—because something has knocked the wind out of you. That something is fear. You take some slow, deep breaths, and pinch yourself in relief that you are still in one piece. Your fast-beating heart begins to slow to its normal rhythm, and you proceed on your way.

Retelling the incident, or waking from a dream about it, you experience the same breathlessness that accompanied the event itself. Once again, you pause to get your breath to complete your story, or to fall back to sleep again.

The inability to breathe fully is also one of the most common reactions to grief. People experiencing great sadness at the loss of a loved one often describe a feeling of steel bands binding the chest. The heart has been wounded or broken in the figurative sense, but the physiological reaction is literal. The muscles associated with respiration tighten in an attempt to protect this vulnerable region from further injury. Shallow breathing serves the self-protective function of cutting off feeling, and this is often temporarily necessary. Holding, stroking, and massaging the grieving person may give the feeling of security again. This contact, and the acceptance it symbolizes, can encourage the crying and deep sighing necessary in working through a loss experience. Releasing grief breaks the vise-like grip around the rib cage and allows breathing to happen normally again.

> **Not everything that is faced can be changed; but nothing can be changed until it is faced.**
>
> —James Baldwin

Holding in emotions such as fear, grief, or anger restricts breathing; the conscious use of breath can be an invaluable tool in learning to express emotions appropriately.

2.3 Releasing Tension

The link between states of tension or relaxation and the rate and depth of breathing is clear. Whether sensing danger from external stressors or from disturbing thoughts within, the body reacts to protect itself. The instinctive response has been called the "fight, flight, or freeze" mechanism. First described by Hans Selye, M.D., one of the leading authorities on stress, this mechanism involves a whole range of automatic reactions. These serve to energize the body to do battle or to run away, whichever seems right at the moment. A surge of adrenaline raises blood pressure and increases heart rate, blood flow to muscles, and general metabolism. The rate of breathing becomes faster, more shallow, and arrhythmic.

There are other measurable changes that characterize the fight-or-flight response. Some very tense individuals commonly have hand and foot temperatures below 70°F/21°C when they are in a room-temperature environment. (And despite the old saying, cold hands have nothing to do with warm hearts.) Palms and fingers may become moist with small amounts of perspiration released by the adrenaline discharge. Such clammy hands are another sign of chronic tension. Similarly, muscle tension increases throughout the body; this may show up as morning stiffness or excessive facial wrinkles. These wrinkles are caused by the constant stretching and bunching up of skin due to overactivity of the underlying musculature. If you notice any of these symptoms with regularity, you can be sure your body is aroused excessively—and unnecessarily.

As an occasional and temporary condition, this "alarm" state serves the whole organism well, but when it characterizes your general approach to living, you sap huge energy reserves that are needed for other purposes. Sooner or later the results will show up in some destructive way, in the body as well as in the spirit. Selye has indicated that stress plays some role in the development of every disease. The constructive, conscious use of the breath can break this pattern of stress as a way of life.

Stress is not all bad. It is, in fact, a necessary component of most life situations. Death is the only stress-free condition. For example, a tensionless state—the limp handshake—is far from desirable. But equally discomforting is the tight, rigid grasp. What we're looking for is a balance between these extremes—the firm yet relaxed handshake; the supportive yet gentle embrace. This happy combination is seen in the performance of the dancer and the movements of the accomplished skier, and heard in the music of the masterful pianist.

The problem is, most of the time we fall far short of this ideal state of relaxed tension. We use excessive amounts of energy in striving for perfect form. The result is often loss of balance, early fatigue, and accidents. Many of us live an uptight existence, absorbed in and surrounded by anxiety-producing situations. We end up with headaches and stomach problems. We can begin releasing this vise-grip approach to life by paying conscious attention to our breathing.

"I Am Relaxed"—A Simple Form of Relaxation

1. Sit comfortably and quietly.

2. Tell yourself that you are going to use the next five, ten, or twenty minutes to rebalance, to heal, to relax yourself.

3. Surrender the weight of your body, allowing the chair or floor to support you.

4. Close your eyes, gently cutting out visual stimulation and distraction.

5. As you inhale, silently say to yourself: "I am . . ."

6. As you exhale, silently say: ". . . relaxed."

7. Continue to breath normally, not trying to change it in any way. Just watch it happening and continue to repeat: "I am" with inhalation; "relaxed" with exhalation.

8. As your mind begins to wander, gently bring it back to the awareness of your breath and your statement "I am relaxed." Be compassionate and loving with your "leaping frog" mind that wants to be anywhere but here.

9. Continue doing this for as long a time as you have established.

10. Notice any changes in your experience.

11. To conclude, discontinue the phrase and slowly stretch your hands and feet, your arms and legs, your whole body.

12. Open your eyes a sliver at a time—like the sun coming up in the morning.

13. Continue on your way.

2.4 Breathing and Stress

The way you breathe is the way you live your life. Actually, the words for spirit, meaning life force and breath, are the same in many languages. For example, in Sanskrit it is called *prana;* in Hebrew *ruach;* in Greek *pneuma;* in Latin *spiritus.* In English, to *inhale* is to *inspire*—that is, to take in the spirit. To *exhale* is to *expire*—to release the spirit. The word *conspire* literally means "to breathe together." All of life can be observed as a taking in and giving out, as movement and rest, as controlling and letting go.

Experienced body therapists report dramatic changes in people who start to practice full breathing. Breathing heightens awareness and encourages the release of long-held tensions. Tears, deep sighs, and the recollection of old and painful memories commonly accompany deep massage or manipulation of the muscles involved in respiration.

A psychologist described a game he used to play as a child. He had practiced the ability to control his respiration so completely that he used to challenge his brother to detect any movement that would indicate breathing. He was trying to make himself invisible—to insulate himself from hurtful emotional situations. As an adult, he found that this self-protective approach had become a source of great sadness, of joylessness. Now that he has become aware of what he has been doing, he frequently checks whether he is breathing fully, and he uses daily exercise to encourage richer breathing. He claims that his whole vitality is richer as a result.

How do you breathe? How would you describe your general approach to living?

"I knew I was back in the driver's seat in my life," reported a prominent college professor, "when I smiled at the elevator in my office building." He went on to tell the story about this slow, unreliable elevator, which had become such a great source of stress and frustration to him over the years. Day after day he waited for it, pacing anxiously, checking his watch, cursing it. One day, he became involved in a research experiment on the campus and learned a simple technique of relaxation. This involved a short, daily practice of rhythmic breathing and the repetition of a positive word—a *mantra.* The discipline was enjoyable, and the study intriguing, so he kept it up. The morning that he found himself smiling at the elevator, he woke up to a whole new appreciation for life. He credited the change to the relaxation practice, and has stayed with it ever since.

Stories of this nature are becoming commonplace in the literature about relaxation and consciousness development. Nearly all of the relaxation techniques include the use of breath control or breath awareness. No longer the sole privilege of spiritual adepts, these practices are being encouraged, and adopted, by educational and industrial groups because they show results. Educational consultants train classroom teachers in relaxation methods that serve to both reduce stress and encourage creativity in children. Biofeedback/neurofeedback training, which relies heavily on slower, deeper breathing, is receiving acceptance throughout the medical community. Large companies are incorporating workshops in stress management and meditation for their employees because they find it beneficial. Many of these stress-reducing techniques include using breathing for relaxation.

As a society we are constantly exposed to anxiety-producing circumstances that cause excess tension. Driving our car to work; the pressures of job production, deadlines, term papers; the noise of technology; the music on the radio—all of these can set us on edge so easily that we tend to lose touch with what life would be like without them.

If you have recently found yourself in a situation in which you were threatened—a near accident, the start of an important examination—you may recall that breathing came with some difficulty. Anger, fear, sedentary work, the pace of fast-food restaurants, and the nightly news—to name a few—may cause a dramatic change in your breathing. Slowing down, attuning to the breath, taking a few deep inhalations and exhalations will assist you in releasing the unnecessary distress that builds up so easily.

Cleaning House . . . Waking Up . . . Calming Down . . .

When you feel foggy and tired—whether from the atmosphere in a smoke-filled room, accumulated carbon dioxide stored during sleep, or tense, sit-down work—you can use these exercises to help clear out your head and wake up your body, as well as to calm down by releasing tension.

Exercise 1

Stand up. Relax your knees and muscles around your anus and genitals. Place your hands on your upper thighs. Bending from the waist strains and stresses the back—instead, use "hip-hinging" by bending at the crease between the legs and the torso.

> *Inhale deeply through your nose.*
> *Exhale forcefully through your mouth while pulling your navel back toward your spine.*
> *Push all the air out of your lungs.*
> *Repeat.*

Exercise 2

Stand up. Raise your arms above your head. Begin to jump up and down rhythmically as if you were jumping rope.

> *As you jump up, inhale quickly.*
> *As you land, expel the air from your mouth with the sound of "hu."*
> *In the beginning, continue for about thirty seconds; increase gradually at each session, up to a five-minute session.*
> *Stop. Allow your breath to come naturally.*

Exercise 3

Stand up. Inhale through your mouth as you raise your arms above your head. Pretend that you are trying to grasp the stars. Get up on your tiptoes. Reach even higher, inhaling all the way. Release. Go limp. Exhale vigorously. Bend from the waist and let your head and arms dangle like a rag doll's. Stop. Breathe normally.

2.5 Breath and Healing

Left alone, the body knows best how to heal itself. The technical word for this is *homeostasis,* meaning the natural tendency to reestablish balance. With illness, energy is blocked—the balance is upset. The state of "dis-ease" is the result. Breathing is a primary method for correcting this disharmony.

Breathing deeply and rhythmically will assist your body in healing itself. Good respiration provides the oxygen needed by every cell, every muscle, bone, and organ. When part of you is ailing, the whole organism is thrown out of balance. Vigilant red blood cells rush to the aid of the injured or diseased part. Since it is the oxygen you inspire that provides the energy to the cells, it naturally follows that these cells need to be charged to their fullest potential in order for healing to occur.

It has long been known that pain is intensified by the anxiety that accompanies a threatening situation. Fear causes the body to tense itself, a spontaneous reaction to the need to fight or run away. So what we have is a two-stage process—fear giving rise to tension; tension increasing pain. Using the breath to manage tension will help to quiet both the fear and the pain. The intuitive wisdom used by parents of young children provides us with an excellent example. The child who has been crying and gasping for breath is cautioned to "take a deep breath" and "calm down." Mother knows that the scare and the sight of blood worsen the child's pain. Panic reactions generally involve this same gasping or fast, shallow breathing pattern. Bringing their breathing to the attention of the injured party can immediately change the level of anxiety. To use this reminder for yourself in a crisis situation, it helps to be attuned to your breathing on a regular basis.

Life means rhythm!—With its first breath the newborn baby enters into the rhythm of life; with its inhalation and exhalation, it begins to experience the flow of life in its alternating positive and negative phases, pulsating within it like an alternating current. Life is thus an uninterrupted chain of rhythmic breaths, in and out, until with his last breath man "expires," i.e., "breathes out," and closes the final link in the chain.

—Selvarajan Yesudin and Elizabeth Haich

What is true for the relief of physical pain is also applicable to mental and emotional pain. Sadness, depression, and boredom can frequently be turned around by a change in breathing. So, as you reach for the aspirins, the antacid tablets, or the telephone to call your doctor, remember to breathe as well. Singing can be a great help—producing full-bodied energy. In breathing well, you let go of the restrictions to the natural healing process.

Breathing with Every Cell—For Healing

Part 1

Sit in a comfortable position (but not slouching), with arms and legs uncrossed. Surrender the weight of your body, allowing the chair or floor to support you.

Softly close your eyes.

Bring your attention to your nose and imagine what air looks like as it enters here. Follow its path down into your lungs, observe it swirling around, and see it moving back up and out. As it leaves, tell yourself that it is carrying away tension, pain, and disease.

Do this for one or two minutes.

Part 2

Bring awareness to the center of your belly. Imagine a tiny opening here through which you are breathing.

Visualize the oxygen coming in, swirling around in the abdomen, lower back, anal and genital regions, and then flowing out.

Tell yourself that it carries away tension and pain as it leaves.

Continue breathing from here for another one or two minutes.

Part 3

Now focus at a point in the center of your chest, close to your heart. Visualize a tiny door opening here.

As you inhale, draw air into your chest and upper body, and into your heart as well.

Watch it swirling around, and carrying away tension as it departs.

Do this for one or two minutes.

Part 4

The point of breathing now moves to the center of your forehead.

Breathe from here, releasing tightness in all the muscles of your face and clearing out the cobwebs in your brain. Again, continue for one or two minutes.

Part 5

Repeat this process in other areas, especially those that are diseased or in pain.

Breathe from the palms of your hands, the tips of your big toes, the undersides of your knees, the base of your spine, and so on.

Part 6

Now breathe with every cell of your body.

To conclude

Complete your directed imagery. Breathe naturally. Begin to stretch. Slowly open your eyes. Notice the sensations in your body and any changes in your breath.

2.6 Breath and the Moment

Your breath is a built-in alarm clock that rings an average of ten to sixteen times every minute, reminding you that you're alive, right now! But as with so many habitual cues in your environment, you become so accustomed to the ringing that you don't hear it any more. Ruminating about the past and anticipating the future, you neglect the *right now* that is slipping away before you can stop to enjoy it.

Failing to live in the present can be a source of great sadness and dissatisfaction with life. A well-to-do psychiatrist was once asked the secret of his success. His patients praised his methods, and his waiting room was always filled with people. "It's easy," he remarked. "I simply tell them to do one thing at a time, and to do it as if it were all they ever had to do in the world." That's part of what is meant by awareness.

The use of breath can help you to achieve an expanded sense of awareness in your everyday life. You start the practice of cueing in to the process of breathing in all different circumstances (waiting for the bus, watching the sunset). The inhalation reminds you to open yourself as fully as possible to what is happening *now*.

What is my body doing? Where are my thoughts taking me? What am I feeling? Who is this person I'm talking with? What does this food feel like in my mouth? Why is my shoulder feeling so tight?

The exhalation allows you to let go of worrying about the past and the future. The inhalation opens you again.

In its purest form, this awareness is the silent appreciation of the way things are—the experience of just being with the flower, the other person, the movement of your body as you dance. This is the stuff of which awestruck moments and peak experiences are made. Coming back from such a high, a normally gray world is seen in full color and words fail to communicate the experience.

It is easy to misinterpret awareness training as a methodology for neglecting rational planning and goal-directed behavior. "Don't think about the future, just chill!" Nothing could be further from the truth of what real awareness is about. Instead of living only *for* the moment, awareness encourages living fully *in* the moment. And this moment may be devoted to designing a new strategy for environmental protection, planning for your retirement, or studying for tomorrow's biology exam. The point is that you choose consciously to address yourself to each issue. You immerse yourself in the task at hand with energy and concentration. You attune yourself to all the input—at the rational, emotive, physical, and even psychic levels. You do it with passion—knowing that you are doing it!

Try the simple experiment of eating a piece of fruit with awareness. You take the first bite. The texture excites your mouth. You start chewing, experiencing the exquisite flavor, the sweet juice. Before you can swallow, you realize that you've checked the time, picked up a magazine, looked out the window, decided to call a friend, and wondered if you need to get your videos back by this afternoon. Not such a simple task, this eating with awareness. As you begin to practice it, you are often overwhelmed with how unconscious so much of your life has become. This is when you offer yourself compassion. Then you can relax into the experience and laugh at how much learning you still have to do, without judging yourself harshly for not yet being fully aware.

Various forms of meditation use the breath to aid in relaxing, concentrating, and attuning to the deeper, spiritual, creative self—these will be addressed further in chapter 12.

Using breath attunement on a regular basis will aid you in maximizing your body's built-in feedback system—those constant messages it offers you are its attempt to regain balance. Responding to those messages will create that state of relaxed awareness that your body most wants to have.

Three Breaths

Take three long deep breaths. As you continue to inhale and exhale, you may add a few words, such as these from Thich Nhat Hanh:

Breathing in I smile,
Breathing out I relax.
This is a wonderful moment.

Or even simply:

In, out,
Slow, deep,
Smile, release.

AIR POLLUTION AND YOUR HEALTH

The gist of the scientific studies and the clinical evidence can be summed up briefly: Air pollution is related to human sickness and sometimes to premature death; people of both sexes and all ages can be affected, but the danger is greatest for the very old, the very young, and people already sick with certain chronic ailments.

Air pollution probably causes and certainly aggravates all these conditions:

- Diseases of the respiratory (breathing) system: nose, sinuses, throat, bronchial tubes, and lungs. All these organs have direct contact with inhaled air.

- Diseases of the heart and blood vessels. Pollutants can pass through the lung membranes into the blood.

- Cancer, especially of the lungs. Airborne cancer-causing agents can enter the body through the skin as well as the lungs and be carried by the blood to any organ.

- Skin diseases, allergies, eye irritation.

U.S. Environmental Protection Agency, www.epa.gov/airnow.

2.7 Breathing Pure Air

Breathing polluted air not only causes coughing, chest tightness, and eye irritation, but actually impairs lung functioning and weakens the ability of white blood cells to fight infection. Thus affected, the respiratory system may become the weak link in the body's chain—and a receptive environment for diseases such as influenza, bronchitis, and pneumonia.

Emphysema, which is principally linked to smoking, occurs when the lung tissues lose their elasticity. The lungs are no longer able to expel air on their own, so breathing becomes more difficult and even impossible. Since we generally use less than a quarter of our lung capacity in normal breathing, a heavy smoker may become aware of lung damage only when exercising. The slow, subtle progression of this disease makes it more serious because it may not be detected until it is too late. Emphysema is a major cause of death in the United States.

Asthma is another condition that affects the ability to breathe. It is a reaction triggered by allergenic substances as well as by threatening emotional situations.

The whole planet is breathing—through its lakes, forests, mountains, and fields. The planet's needs are identical with those of human beings—a clear and ready input source and an unrestricted channel. It's not easy to be a healthy fish in a polluted lake. It's hard to remain a healthy person while breathing polluted air. And the sad fact is that the planet is gasping. Air pollution has reached crisis proportions. Where will the planet turn for help in releasing its tensions? Where can it go for some fresh air?

If all things are connected, and all beings are literally breathing the same air, then self-responsibility means social responsibility. We are all dependent upon one another. We need to examine many of the details of our lifestyle with this realization in mind. With respect to the environmental crisis created by air

THE PLANET NEEDS AIR

Tropical rainforests support the exchange of gases such as carbon monoxide, carbon dioxide, methane, and oxygen in the atmosphere. The forests are a dynamic part of our hydrologic cycle (rain and water systems), and they even act as a global air conditioner—by storing and absorbing carbon dioxide from the air, storing the carbon, and giving us fresh, clean oxygen. Excess carbon dioxide is the primary factor in global warming, which is heating the planet and threatening our future. Excess carbon is released into the atmosphere with our use of fossil fuels (such as driving cars) and from cutting and burning of wood or vegetation. Uncontrolled logging and burning in tropical forests accounts for one-third of our carbon emissions, making global warming far worse. Responsible forestry helps us to turn down the global thermostat. By stopping the destruction of mature (old-growth) forests, we prevent a huge amount of carbon from being released into the atmosphere; by promoting Earth-friendly planting and management of young forests, we promote the absorption of large amounts of atmospheric carbon.

pollution, we must weigh our decisions about the size of the car we drive and how much we drive it. We need to look at the type and quantity of the fuel we use in heating our homes. We can involve ourselves in local efforts to improve the environment in which we live, as well as voice our support for political candidates who represent a consciousness about pollution-control issues.

Keeping yourself balanced will help you focus on your own *real* needs and those of the planet on which you live. Despair, panic, and compulsiveness in approaching any problem only serve to intensify it—and often divert you from the real issues.

Remember the basic principles of wellness: trust, compassion, self-responsibility, and the positive value of "illness." Well used, these can bring about health for yourself and for the entire planet as well.

HOW'S THE AIR OUT THERE?

(PSI) Pollutant Standards Index Value	PSI Descriptor	General Health Effects	Cautionary Statements
500 400 300	Hazardous	Premature death of ill and elderly. Healthy people will experience adverse symptoms that affect their normal activity.	All persons should remain indoors, keeping windows and doors closed. All persons should minimize physical exertion and avoid traffic.
200	Very unhealthful	Premature onset of certain diseases in addition to significant aggravation of symptoms and decreased exercise tolerance in healthy persons.	Elderly and persons with existing diseases should stay indoors and avoid physical exertion. General population should avoid outdoor activity.
100	Unhealthful	Significant aggravation of symptoms and decreased exercise tolerance in persons with heart or lung disease, with widespread symptoms in the healthy population.	Elderly and persons with existing heart or lung diseases should stay indoors and reduce physical activity.
50	Moderate	Mild aggravation of symptoms in susceptible persons, with irritation symptoms in the healthy population.	Persons with existing heart or respiratory ailments should reduce physical exertion and outdoor activity.
0	Good		

U.S. Environmental Protection Agency, www.epa.gov/airnow.

2.8 Inner Peace

The ultimate result of learning to deal creatively and constructively with stresses, of using your breath to relax and center yourself, is inner peace. This doesn't mean perfection, but rather acceptance of your limitations and an ability to forgive yourself and others for shortcomings. Inner peace is also more likely if you can accept any limitations of circumstance or environment, changing the things you can and accepting the things you can't.

Ultimately, inner peace comes from being sufficiently relaxed and balanced within your self that you can feel your connectedness to your family, friends, community, the planet, and any transcendent reality you may experience.

SUGGESTED READING

Ballentine, R., S. Rama, and A. Hymes, *Science of Breath* (The Himalayan Institute Press, 1998).

Benson, H., *The Relaxation Response* (Avon Books, 2000).

Davis, M., *The Relaxation and Stress Reduction Workbook* (New Harbinger Publications, 2000).

Farhi, D., *The Breathing Book* (Owl Books, 1996).

Goldstein, J., *Insight Meditation: The Practice of Freedom* (Shambhala, 1992).

Hendricks, G., *Conscious Breathing: Breathwork for Health, Stress Release, and Personal Mastery* (Bantam, 1995).

Hittleman, R., *Yoga: 28 Day Exercise Plan* (Workman Publishing, 1975).

Kitzinger, S., *The Complete Book of Pregnancy and Childbirth* (Alfred A. Knopf, 2003).

LeShan, L., *How to Meditate: A Guide to Self-Discovery* (Little, Brown, 1999).

McKay, M., M. Davis, et al., *The Relaxation and Stress Reduction Workbook* (New Harbinger Publications, 2000).

Ram Dass, *Journey of Awakening: A Meditator's Guidebook* (Bantam, 1990).

Ramacharaka, Y., *Science of Breath* (Kessinger Publishing Company, 1997).

Rozman, D., *Meditating with Children* (Integral Yoga Distribution, 2002).

Siler, B., *The Pilates Body* (Broadway Books, 2000).

For a catalog of excellent audios for breathing and relaxing, contact Emmett Miller, M.D., Deep Healing Tapes and CDs, P.O. Box 6028, Auburn, CA 95604; (800) 528-2737; www.drmiller.com (see appendix A).

For an updated listing of resources and active links to the websites mentioned in this chapter, please see www.WellnessWorkbook.com.

CHAPTER 3

Wellness and Sensing

Sensory information (light, heat, touch, sound, odor, taste, movement, and so on) is the second form of energy input in the Wellness Energy System. Vast amounts of energy are received from our environment and channeled by our physical senses (and possibly through other senses that are less well understood). These energies are necessary for our protection and survival, and they serve as our most basic form of communication.

If the doors of perception were cleansed, man would see things as they are, infinite.

—William Blake

It is through the senses—seeing, touching, smelling, hearing, tasting, temperature, movement (kinetic and kinesthetic senses), and others—that we come to know and enjoy the world. Our ability to work, to feel pleasure, to communicate with others, and to impact the world is directly related to our efficient use of sensory energy. In the context of wellness this means appreciating the senses, taking care not to abuse them, and using them more creatively.

Everywhere there is sad evidence that many of us have "lost our senses." You probably know people who burn their skin, allow it to blister and peel, and then go back for more in an attempt to look "healthy" and "sexy" in their summer clothes. The noise of dishwashers, air conditioners, power tools, trucks, and loud music invades everywhere, making us irritable, angry, listless, or unable to sleep. Loud sounds from machinery and music can actually damage our delicate hearing mechanisms and cause headaches and hearing loss. When it comes to tasting, many of us tax our digestive systems constantly with food that is too hot and beverages that are too cold, ending up with burnt tongues and stomach pains. We move apathetically through an environment filled with chemical pollutants, hoping that we're not absorbing too much nuclear radiation from the power plant upwind. The more we abuse our senses with these types of overstimulation, the more we dull ourselves to their subtle warning signals—the body's cries for help, for balance.

The flip side of this sorry state of affairs is the withdrawal from sensory stimulation. Our fears cause us to freeze up when we are being touched. With depression and boredom, we turn inward and often neglect our need for sunlight and fresh air. With grief, we numb ourselves to the outside world as we attempt to cope with a loss. Studies of young mammals clearly indicate that early deprivation results in lowered activity, improper physical development, and many failures in sexual functioning.[1]

Your senses are marvelous instruments that require vigilance to keep them in tip-top operating condition. Becoming a skilled technician in their care and creative use is one of the foundations for wellness. This chapter is your owner's manual for the senses. It will deal with touch, movement, temperature, sight, sound, and smell (taste is covered in the next chapter). This chapter is about coming to your senses.

Warm Hands and Good Health

By relaxing and focusing on warming your hands, you can raise your hand temperature as much as 20°F/11°C in five minutes. The result of hand warming is usually a deep state of relaxation or one of the altered states of consciousness experienced in meditation. It is an effective stress reducer and can be used in the control of migraine headaches. It helps the body to carry out its self-repair.

Sit in a relaxed position. Place your hands on your lap, palms facing up, fingers easy.

Begin to slowly say to yourself: "My hands are getting warmer."

Repeat five to ten times or more, maintaining a relaxed mood. Three to five minutes of focused attention will generally start to yield results.

Combine the repetition of the words with a mental picture that suggests warm hands. For instance, see your hands being bathed in warm water; imagine that you are holding your hands up to the sun; visualize someone rubbing your hands to encourage circulation; see rivers of warm energy flowing from the trunk of your body into your hands. In your mind's eye, surround your hands with a glowing yellow light. Feel them getting gradually warmer.

3.1 Wellness, Stress, and Cold Hands

Of all the forms of energy we can sense, the most fundamental is thermal energy. Given this basic source of energy, our bodies are able to function and sense a myriad of other stimuli: electromagnetic radiation (particularly visible light); vibration of air, which we experience as sound; physical contact, which we experience as touch; and chemical stimuli, which we experience as taste and smell.

The human body maintains a very narrow temperature range—averaging 98.6°F/37°C—and generally is equipped to handle temperature fluctuations in wonderfully adaptive ways. Our senses are geared to detect a lack of thermal energy or a surplus. If it is cold, the blood vessels constrict, breathing increases, and circulation in the extremities slows down to conserve heat energy in the central portions of the body. If it is warm, we breathe less. As we metabolize the food we eat, and when we exercise, we create large amounts of internal heat. This is used to maintain our temperature, with any excess being released to the environment.

The way your body generates and uses heat reflects your overall wellbeing. More heat is generated in the trunk of the body and distributed to the limbs and head through the flow of blood. Hands and feet, ears and scalp act like radiators. When you are hot they help dissipate heat; when you are cold their blood vessels constrict and send heat back to the center of the body. This happens not only in response to the temperature around you, but in emergency and chronic stress conditions as well. Faced with a life-threatening crisis, this diversion effect is helpful in providing a maximum amount of energy to the heart, lungs, brain, and muscles. Over a longer period, if stress becomes chronic, this adaptation can be more harmful than helpful. It leads to a retention of energy and is manifested by cold hands and feet. An extreme example is seen in the disorder known as Raynaud's disease, in which hands become painfully cold. Many people have a less serious form of this condition without even being aware of it. The first manifestation is consistently cold hands, even when the temperature outside is above 70°F/21°C. Later complications include migraine headaches, blood-sugar problems such as hypoglycemia or diabetes, menstrual problems, and depression.

If you have this tendency, you can learn to consciously make your hands warmer, using methods such as visualization processes and temperature biofeedback/neurofeedback (see page 46). You can monitor your hand temperature by touching your lips—a stable reference point—to note whether your hands are warm or cold. Soaking in a hot bath or taking a sauna produces relaxation in a similar way by encouraging blood to flow to the body's periphery. When this happens, your tissues expand with more blood and you experience pleasure.

3.2 Wellness and Temperature

Despite our technological sophistication, we are still subject to the powers of wind and rain and sun. Living well includes a rekindled respect for the natural rhythms of things—and an attempt to harmonize ourselves with the changes, both internal and external, that weather brings.

Today it is almost possible to ignore the weather, as we move from heated or cooled homes to heated or cooled automobiles to heated or cooled offices, schools, department stores, and supermarkets, then back again. These luxuries have brought with them negative effects on life and health. Summer colds are frequently the result of air-conditioning that creates January in June, upsetting the body's equilibrium in the process. As we move in and out of these artificially cool environments, we repeatedly chill and dry the mucous membranes of the nose and throat. Our mucous glands must work overtime, often to the point of exhaustion, pumping extra fluids and then slowing down dramatically. The lungs are shocked by differences in temperature of sometimes twenty or thirty degrees as we leave an air-conditioned car or building to walk across the street. Humidity fluctuations may be even greater. In this tenuous state, the body is ripe for hosting some confused virus. It's the summer cold!

Winter brings its own unique stresses. Many North Americans suffer colds and other more serious respiratory problems during the winter. The dryness that central heating produces in the air plays havoc with the whole respiratory tract. The extremes experienced in moving from the overheated home into the stabbing cold outside create similar unbalancing effects.

Because the body's need to generate and conserve heat is greater in the cold season, the heart, especially, works harder at this time. Heart failure and other coronary fatalities occur more frequently in winter than at any other time of year. The same individual who rakes leaves or exercises vigorously without difficulty in the gentle autumn weather may suffer a heart attack when shoveling snow from the front walk in near-freezing temperatures.

If body-trust, self-responsibility, and moderation are your governing principles, you can celebrate the changing seasons in good health. Here are some simple suggestions:

- *In warm weather, keep air-conditioning no lower than 75°F/24°C.*

- *Keep humidity generally between 40 and 50 percent; if you live in a dry or cold climate, use a vaporizer or humidifier in areas of your house where you spend a lot of time.*

- *Acclimatize yourself with outdoor exercise as soon as the seasons start to change.*

- *In cold weather, keep the temperature in your home about 65°F/18°C.*

- *Loose clothing over tight forms a natural air insulation and keeps you warm.*

- *Check your heartbeat occasionally (see page 129). If it's too fast, rest from your work or exercise.*

If necessary, make your needs for comfort and health known to those who control the thermostats. As the seasons change, your body slowly adapts. Learning to respect your internal rhythm during seasonal transitions is an important aspect of wellness. Don't be too hard on yourself. Work during hours that support your personal efficiency rhythm. Rest or "goof off" when work energy wanes. Nourish yourself throughout the year, but particularly during the transition times between seasons.

3.3 Wellness and Clothing

Anthropologists report that people who wear little or no clothing show much greater skin sensitivity than do people who are usually clothed. Observations of infants verify this. Babies who are almost always covered are less active and less sensitive than those who are generally lightly clothed or naked. There is little chance that nudity will ever become the social norm, but we can still learn how to *use* our clothing rather than be used by it.

The skin must be allowed to breathe if it is to remain healthy. Many skin disorders are the results of irritation and improper ventilation caused by clothing. Popular synthetics, such as nylon, Dacron, and polyester, are made of smooth fibers that can be very tightly woven. These fabrics are often favored because they resist wrinkling, but they don't "breathe." Our bodies invisibly eliminate a substantial portion of waste products through the skin, and it is best to allow these to pass out via the open weaves of natural fibers such as cotton, silk, and wool. The first nylon pantyhose were discovered to promote vaginal infections because they trapped heat and moisture, making an ideal environment for infection. This necessitated the addition of breathable cotton crotch panels.

If they want to see me, here I am. If they want to see my clothes, open my closet and show them my suits.

—Albert Einstein
(upon being asked to change his clothes
to meet an ambassador)

People who wear skintight clothing might cause a sensation, but they may do so at a cost to their skin. For ages, religious ascetics used coarse fabrics and even hair shirts to subdue the flesh as a method of penance and self-discipline. If you have to wear tight, coarse materials in uniforms or suits because of your work, you can minimize their restrictive or numbing effects by wearing soft natural-fiber undergarments (cotton or silk) next to your skin and by changing into something more comfortable after work.

Fashion is a form of ugliness so intolerable that we have to alter it every six months.

—Oscar Wilde

As you look over your wardrobe today, consider these questions:

- *How many of your clothes are constructed of natural fabrics?*

- *How many contain synthetics?*

- *What differences in mood and behavior do various textures produce in your body?*

- *Do you want more of your clothes to be comfortable—soothing to the skin, loose enough to provide for freedom of movement, enhancing of sensual pleasure?*

- *Does your clothing really reflect you—your moods, your personality, your ideals of how you want to be?*

You might want to try going without clothing, whenever appropriate, in order to air your skin. This will enhance its sensitivity and promote its health. Even Inuits who live in snow huts sleep nude under thick furs.

3.4 Wellness and Water

Being in water is a healthy experience. Water stimulates every cell of the skin as it relaxes tightened muscles and promotes healing. It wakes you up, calms you down, and washes away the problems of the day along with the dirt.

More people every day are enrolling in health spas, swimming year-round, and installing whirlpool baths and spas in their own homes. It has always been difficult to get children out of the water—and now the same is sometimes true for adults.

The Japanese have championed communal bathing for centuries. An entire family shares the intimacy and pleasure of being naked together, as each fulfills the basic needs for personal cleanliness and relaxation. Our reticence to accept such a practice in the West reflects our fear of the physical body and its functioning.

There is more to bathing than promoting cleanliness. Water has always been a religious symbol because of its connection to purification, refreshment, and regeneration. We all come from the water—evolving from the creatures of the sea, floating in the uterus of the mother. Water, like air, has the capacity to touch us all over, in every crack and crevice of the body. Immersing yourself in it is one of the greatest and simplest pleasures known to human beings. The security of being surrounded in it can be a source of great healing. And the possibilities for its creative use are limitless:

- *Drinking it. Water is an important source of minerals and serves to wash out wastes. The standard advice to drink 6 to 8 glasses of pure water daily may be more important than ever in a world filled with more and more toxins and pollutants (see chapter 4), for more about this life-enhancing elixir).*

- *Showering. Take a shower using hot water for thirty seconds, followed by cold water for thirty seconds, followed by hot, and so on. This type of shower is great for stimulating your circulation.*

- *Bathing. Fill the tub with hot water and a mild bubble bath. Light a few candles. Put on your favorite music or take in a good book.*

- *Soaking in a hot tub or bath. Whirlpool jets soothe and untangle the knots in tired muscles.*

- *Sweating in a sauna, steam bath, or sweat lodge. Follow up with a short, stimulating cold shower.*

- *Having a water fight. Remember how hard you laughed?*

- *Swimming. Even if you don't know how, just get in there and splash out your frustrations. Surrender to the healing touch of the water.*

- *Exercising. Water aerobics is a good way to get a low-impact workout.*

- *Soaking your feet. Fill a basin with hot water and mild soap or baking soda. Experience your whole body relaxing as your feet do. Finish off by drying them with a coarse towel. Then give yourself a foot massage.*

- *Visiting a hot springs. If you don't live near any natural hot springs or mineral springs, check into them on your next vacation. Often they are not well advertised. The curative powers of these waters have been praised for ages.*

- *Making medicine. Some Native American healers have long used water to cure a variety* of ailments. We know that polluted water can be poisonous, so why shouldn't energized water become medicine? At the least, it wouldn't hurt to try. Fill a glass or bottle with water and place it on a windowsill where it will receive the first rays of the rising sun. Before you go to bed, sit with the water, telling it what you need for your increased health and wellbeing. In the morning, drink the whole glass.

• *Cleansing your energy field.* Compose a ceremony in which you use water to symbolically cleanse your body (or the body of a loved one), and your mind and soul from illness, darkness, "sin," and painful memories. Make it a beautiful occasion. Take a new or additional name to signify your new life. Be at peace.

Beginning in 1994, Japanese medical doctor Masaru Emoto began an in-depth research study into the life energy present in or absent from water. (The energy of life is *hado* in Japanese and *chi* in Chinese.) Taking hundreds of samples of water from both pure and polluted sources, he froze the water and then photographed the resulting ice crystals. His results were both awe-inspiring and terrifying, as the photos clearly showed that some water was literally dead, devoid of life force or energy, based in the deformed or chaotic patterns of its crystalline structures. Other water was vibrantly alive—its crystalline structure was beautiful, growing, dynamic! This is an important discovery when you realize that both the human body and the earth are primarily made up of water. To learn more about Emoto's work, visit www.hado.net.

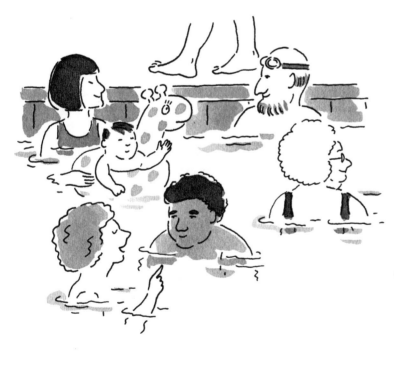

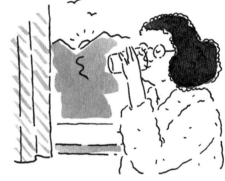

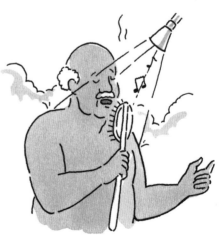

3.5 Wellness and Seeing

Adults receive the majority of sensory stimulation through their eyes. The ability to learn, to navigate, and to communicate depends upon visual input. So strong is the connection between seeing and knowing that the words have become synonymous in our language.

Few people in our overstressed culture escape problems associated with sight. Can you name ten friends who do not use glasses or contact lenses? Can you name five? Some degree of near-sightedness, far-sightedness, or other refractive error is experienced by the vast majority of people in the industrialized countries of the world. If we are to experience greater wellness, we need to address the real reasons behind this epidemic of poor eyesight. We need to maintain the health and strength of our eyes, since it is with them that we feed our souls.

Like breathing, seeing is not something you need to *do;* rather, it is something that you allow. Most people, however, do not appreciate that seeing is essentially a passive process. They strain to count the stars in the sky, to read the tiny print of newspapers, and to keep awake while studying organic chemistry long into the night. The conditions of civilized life place our minds and bodies under continual tension that blocks our ability to let seeing take place naturally. Poor vision, like so many other dis-eased conditions, is not something that invades, or happens to us. Rather, it is something that we encourage by our lifestyle. The traditional treatment has been to prescribe corrective lenses. While these serve to correct an imbalance, they also keep the condition in a relatively static state—something like using a crutch to compensate for a broken leg.

The idea that poor eyesight is primarily a result of stress was pioneered by ophthalmologist William Bates, M.D. The solution to our vision problems, according to Bates, is not to stop reading, or looking at the stars, or studying for an exam, but rather to relax the mental strain that causes the imperfect functioning of the eye in both close and distance vision. Aldous Huxley was one of many who have had some degree of success in doing this. Relaxation is the key.

Bates himself was rejected by his colleagues, who preferred to think of refractive errors as static problems unrelated to lifestyle or habit and to treat them only with lenses. The approach to treating them with stress reduction exercises is a slow and time-consuming process that few are likely to carry out, but Bates's relaxation exercises are worthwhile even if your vision does not improve. To relax your eyes is to relax your whole body.

Relaxing the Eyes

Resting

Since so much of our sensory input is visual, temporarily closing off this channel will almost immediately cause the rest of the body to slow down. Brainwave patterns change to a lower frequency as soon as the eyes are closed. Resting your eyes is an important way of reestablishing balance throughout the system and reducing unnecessary strain.

Palming

This is a technique developed by Bates for relieving eyestrain.

1. *Sit or lie down and take a few moments to breathe deeply.*

2. *Now gently close your eyes.*

3. *Place the palms of your hands over your eyes, with your fingers crossing over your forehead.*

4. *Use memory and imagination to realize a perfect field of black. See it so black that you cannot recall anything blacker.*

5. *Do not try to produce any experience. Simply allow the blackness to happen.*

6. *Continue for two to three minutes, breathing easily.*

7. *Remove your hands from your eyes and slowly open them.*

8. *Do this several times a day, or whenever you need to relax.*

3.6 Wellness and Ultraviolet Light

Every schoolchild knows that sunlight reaching our skin should be our primary source of vitamin D. This vitamin is essential for the development of tissues, bones, and teeth, as well as for regulating the level of calcium in the blood. Inadequate amounts of vitamin D lead to rickets, a disease resulting from the body's failure to assimilate calcium and phosphorus and characterized by softened and deformed bones. It is seen dramatically in neglected children who have been kept in dark rooms for many years. Their bodies are underdeveloped.

But too much sunlight creates other problems. Ultraviolet radiation from the sun, while beneficial in small quantities, can be hazardous or even fatal in large doses. The cultural message that a deep, dark tan makes you more attractive is a dangerous one. An important controversy, and one that receives remarkably little attention, concerns the effectiveness of sunscreens to prevent the most lethal of skin cancers, melanoma. While sunscreens clearly prevent ultraviolet rays from burning the skin and seem to protect against the more common but less fatal basal cell and squamous cell carcinomas, the manufacturers of sunscreens (formerly called "tanning lotions") have never suggested that they prevent melanomas. This fact is overlooked by most consumers and health authorities alike.

Melanomas were virtually unheard of before the introduction of tanning agents in the 1940s. Since then, the rate of melanoma has risen faster than any other cancer type. Meanwhile, parents slather sunscreen over their children's bodies and send them out into the sun, believing that they are "safe." Similarly, adults seek a tan, believing it's "healthy" as long as they are "protected" with sunscreens. To the contrary, there is evidence that sunscreen use may actually *cause* melanomas. Researchers counted the nevi (pigmented skin moles) in 631 kids, then interviewed their parents about their sunscreen use. After adjusting for latitude and skin type, those who used the most sunscreen had the most moles, while those who used the least sunscreen and instead wore protective clothing had the fewest.[2]

Ozone depletion may play some role in the higher melanoma rate, but the rate began to go up long before ozone depletion became an issue. Recently manufacturers have touted "broad-spectrum" sunblocks, which reflect more of the rays that penetrate more deeply into the skin, but no claims or studies have been made that suggest that melanomas can be prevented in this way. Meanwhile, most dermatologists, epidemiologists, and sunscreen makers continue to remain mute about the connection between sunscreens and melanoma. With a multi-million-dollar market at stake, the sunscreen industry in particular has an interest in keeping these facts out of the public eye, and little research is being funded.

The only true protection is found in avoiding the sun, especially during the middle of the day (10 A.M. to 4 P.M. during daylight savings time). If you must venture out, stay in the shade or wear a hat and other protective clothing.

3.7 Natural and Artificial Light

As light enters the eyes, conveying images to be registered by the brain, it also affects the pineal and pituitary glands—the master controllers of the endocrine system. Any change in endocrine balance will cause major alterations in body chemistry and physiology and will affect both health and behavior.

Experimentation with animals is showing us the relationship between the presence or absence of light and hormone secretion in the body. A Wisconsin research team found that they could increase both weight and milk yield in cattle by 10 to 15 percent simply by increasing the number of hours of light the animals received. The normal nine to twelve hours of light exposure was raised to sixteen hours per day. No additional consumption of food was necessary to accomplish these gains. The entire effect seems to be the result of the manipulation of the light.[3]

Industrialized egg farming has relied on the same techniques for years. Confined to their cages inside large, light-controlled buildings, the chickens readjusted to a rhythm motivated by the increased light. The result was increased production of eggs (although quality may be adversely affected).

During the 1940s, while perfecting the process of time-lapse photography, John Ott, Ph.D., discovered that plant growth was significantly altered in greenhouse conditions. Sunlight passing through glass was being filtered, eliminating the near-ultraviolet (near-UV) portion of the light spectrum. The plants suffered from this deprivation. He found a similar problem in the animal kingdom. A friend's colony of minks was not breeding properly. Raised in a basement where they received only artificial light, the animals' normal breeding patterns were seriously affected by a lack of near-UV light.

For millions of years, life on planet Earth has evolved while bathed in a sea of radiation from our sun. Like plants in greenhouses, or minks in basements, humans, too, are bound to experience some detrimental effects from living most of their lives within walls. When we fail to get a healthy, safe dose of natural light on our bodies every day, we cut ourselves off from a very important source of input energy.

Ott reported that the brightness, buzzing, and flickering of fluorescent lights contribute to irritability, inattention, and impulsive behavior. Spurred by Ott's pioneering work, the National Cancer Institute found that ordinary fluorescent lights were causing mutations in the chromosomes of hamsters and could possibly stimulate cancer growth. Fluorescent lights also have been linked with hyperactive behavior of some children who are exposed to these lights for long periods of time over many years.

In 1984, Norman Rosenthal, M.D., of the National Institute of Mental Health discovered and named seasonal affective disorder (SAD), also called "winter depression," and pioneered its treatment with bright light in the early morning, which fools the body into thinking the day is longer. The existence of this phenomenon is further proof of how sensitive we are to the light in our environment.

Unfortunately, this area of wellness has also been largely ignored, but we suggest that you may increase your wellness by installing full-spectrum incandescent lights at your workplace and getting outside for some part of every day. At the same time, you should protect your skin and eyes from too much shortwave ultraviolet radiation by staying out of midday sunlight during the summer months and by wearing protective clothing.

3.8 Wellness, Color, and Electromagnetic Energies

Visible Light

Sight is more than a useful way to keep from stepping into holes. If our needs for safety and survival are provided for with care and attention, we can nourish a sense of joyfulness and wonder by using light and sight to feed our souls and heal our bodies. The aesthetic senses are high on the scale of human needs.

Light and color have long been used in physical and mental therapies. From ancient times, the Egyptians and later the Greeks used colored minerals, salves, and dyes of various colors and painted their healing sanctuaries in differing shades, all for the purposes of healing. It was obvious to these early practitioners that color and light were intrinsic to the creation of balance within the body. In the Middle Ages, the Arab physician Avicenna used red to move the blood, yellow to reduce pain, and so on, and the famous alchemist Paracelsus also used color and light extensively for healing.

Color therapy today is based on increasing scientific findings about the effects of various colors on the brain. In the 1940s and 1950s, for instance, it was confirmed that the color red stimulates the sympathetic part of the autonomic nervous system, while blue stimulates the parasympathetic part. In 1990, reports were made at the annual conference of the American Association for the Advancement of Science on the successful use of blue light in treating psychological problems, including addictions, eating disorders, impotence, and depression. Other highly practical applications of color therapy have been made in some prison systems. Notably, pink is the color chosen for many holding cells, as it is observed that this color immediately reduces violent and aggressive behavior and even temporarily reduces muscle strength.

One need only look at a variety of contemporary advertisements to see how particular colors have been chosen to elicit a mood that is conducive to the product being sold. Most of us appreciate the mood-setting qualities of dimmer switches, track lighting, and high-intensity spotlamps. In the industrialized world, indoor lighting has become a huge artistic industry that many businesses are utilizing effectively. Restaurants have always done so. Often rated on "atmosphere" or "ambiance," restaurants have long paid attention to the quality of their lighting.

Light Pollution

Your ability to see the stars is one of your inalienable rights and that right is being taken away. The amount of outdoor lighting is increasing every year. You can see the sky clearly in the mountains or out in the country because the amount of outdoor lighting in the vicinity is at a minimum. There are no more stars over the country lane than there are over the city street, but as light pollution spreads, city dwellers can see fewer and fewer stars.

You used to be able to go up in this valley and see Mount Baldy fifty miles away. Now you can't even see the stars at night because of the smog.

—An elderly native of a Los Angeles suburb

Electromagnetic and Nuclear Radiation

Besides visible light, we live in a sea of other electromagnetic frequencies (EMFs). At one end of the spectrum, we experience the extremely low frequencies generated by interactions of the earth's atmosphere with the thousand or so lightning storms going on at any given moment worldwide (this is known as Schumann resonance). In the middle of the spectrum, we are affected by the light from the sun and by the solar "wind" of other frequencies of radiation. And at the other end of the spectrum, we are bombarded with high-energy cosmic rays coming to us from deep space. Besides these natural sources of radiation, we have tremendously increased our levels of EMF exposure with our increasing demands for new forms of technology. A wide range of electromagnetic frequencies are now being artificially generated through the transmission of power and used for long-distance communication (radio, TV, cell phones, and the like).

Our lives begin to end the day we become silent about things that matter.

—Martin Luther King Jr.

While most of us can't consciously sense these forms of radiation, individual cells in our bodies may be harmed by them—another form of sensing. Controversy over the effect on humans of nearby power lines and transformers has been raging since the 1970s, with no resolution in sight. Radiation from computer processors and video displays is another common source of constant exposure for people who work with them. Cell or mobile phones emit far more radiation than the cordless phones commonly found in homes. For years, cell phones have been suspected of causing cellular damage, especially when held close to your head for long periods. But the little research that *has* been done on this issue has failed to make a significant difference in getting people to change their habits. We recommend keeping the phone as far from the body as possible (not in your pocket or on a belt) and using headphones with a graphite ring to suppress the cord from acting like an antenna and carrying EMFs to your head.

While people have always been exposed to some nuclear radiation from the natural environment, an increase in exposure due to technology is a growing concern. The residues from nuclear testing, the buildup of nuclear wastes, and nuclear accidents, along with land-contaminating practices associated with weapons development and recent wars, are all stressing your body's already overtaxed resistance. Our health and the health of future generations may depend upon greater awareness and some serious political action in this domain. The smaller the dose of human-made radiations we are exposed to, the healthier we are likely to be.

EMFS

Visit these websites for important information about EMFs:

www.mercola.com/article/emf/emf_dangers.htm

www.clarus.com/shared/emf2.shtml

www.equilibra.uk.com/emfsbio.shtml

www.infoventures.com/emf/hrpt/AboutHRPT.html

3.9 Wellness and Scents

The sense of smell is generally one of our most neglected forms of energy input. Our ancestors, like the animals, depended on their noses to warn them of approaching danger. Yet most of us in the Western world have not developed our sense of smell to any great degree. It lies dormant. Other than detecting a skunk on a country road, a cloud of fumes from a passing bus, or the odors of rotting garbage, we pay little attention to the constant subtle input of olfactory information.

The sense of smell is designed to serve as both a source of warning and a source of pleasure. Food is probably the most common and most pleasurable stimulus to the sense of smell. Most of what we assume to be our sense of taste is actually our sense of smell. The six basic taste sensations of sweet, sour, bitter, salty, astringent, and pungent are combined with the wide range of smells to provide us with the sensations we experience while eating.

The olfactory portion of the brain is closely tied to the limbic system—that ancient and primitive part of the brain where emotions are felt. Often, strong feelings associated with childhood experiences can be triggered by a whiff of a long-forgotten scent. Recall the smell of your grandmother's house? Of the incense or candles in church? Of a new car? We often respond to smells of food cooking with emotional intensity and strong memories. Food on the grill? A slow-simmering soup? Sometimes a smell will generate an emotional response even though we are unaware of the specific memories associated with it.

Almost every living thing emits a scent. Along with water vapor, the skin is constantly secreting unnecessary by-products. These odors produce each individual's unique body scent. Although these scents change with emotional state, diet, and season, they remain chemical signatures. An animal mother detects her baby from a group of many similar babies based on scent.

In some cultures, it is only when two persons are within smelling distance of each other's bodies that they feel themselves to be making meaningful contact. This is an essential part of their social interchange. Sexuality is also closely tied to the sense of smell.

In our ultrahygienic culture, organic body odors are usually abhorred. We go to great lengths to cover them up with artificial scents and deodorants for underarms, genitals, or mouth—in the same way that we deodorize the bathroom, kitchen, or trash can. In our obsession with eliminating natural odors, we have surrounded ourselves with a host of new, unnatural ones made from synthetic chemicals. Many people are becoming allergic to these ubiquitous chemical scents and finding it very hard to avoid them. Symptoms can range from mild nausea to near collapse. An entire medical specialty (environmental medicine) has arisen to diagnose and treat the victims of this culturally induced malady.

As we move toward high-level wellness, we often experience our sense of smell becoming more acute. On the unpleasant side, smoke that didn't bother us before becomes offensive. If the fumes from a single car passing us on a deserted road smell horrible, imagine what effect the thousands on the freeway must be having on our bodies. We taste the sodium benzoate in bread. We are overpowered by the smells left in clothing from the scented detergent and the lingering smell left on our clothing and skin from hugging a perfumed person. When we detect these warning signals, we can choose to suffer and be discouraged that things are getting worse, or we can choose to minimize both the amount of artificial chemicals in products we choose and our exposure to these chemicals in our environment.

On the pleasant side, we can become aware of the unique scent of each of our loved ones and of our own bodies, the wonderful scents of flowers and trees calling out to us from afar, and the subtle aromas of food. A fuller appreciation of the natural fragrances of life is one of the benefits of wellness.

AROMATHERAPY

Because the perception of odors—whether conscious or unconscious—can have a major impact on memory and emotions, and therefore on thinking and feeling, it stands to reason that the olfactory sense could be used more wisely in supporting wellbeing. Plant substances have been used for centuries to calm the nerves, aid digestion, or lift the spirits. *Aromatherapy* is the name for the contemporary practice of using essential plant oils—from flowers, herbs, grasses, shrubs, and trees—for their therapeutic effects. Similar to herbal therapy principles, essential oils are phytochemicals with particular biological properties. Lavender, for example, is calming and sedative; basil, rosemary, and peppermint are uplifting and stimulating; and jasmine and ylang-ylang can promote euphoria.

With aromatherapy, essential oils are used in a variety of ways. Some can be safely applied directly to the skin, like precious perfume. Warmed by the body's heat, soon their soothing or energizing aromas are inhaled. Certain oils can even cause vasodilatation, which in turn warms the underlying muscles. This is why analgesic balms for sore muscles are often so aromatic. Massage therapists commonly add a few drops of essential oil to their basic massage formula in order to enhance its effects. When added to a vaporizer or to steaming water and carefully inhaled, some oils—like eucalyptus—can help relieve respiratory congestion. Even a few drops of oil applied to a soft facial tissue and then sniffed offer an effective way to use essential oils while traveling.

Essential oils are frequently diffused into the air by adding two to five drops to a small amount of water, then heating it. These methods employ a nebulizer, diffuser, or scent pot; many varieties of these tools can be found at your local health-food or department stores. Essential oils can also be sprayed into the air (five to eight drops to one ounce of water), or added to a bath (five to ten drops).

Because aromatherapy has become big business, the word is being used to sell many products—such as highly perfumed soaps, lotions, room deodorizers, and candles, and potpourri mixtures—that contain mostly petrochemical-based ingredients, to which increasing numbers of people have become allergic. As with reading the labels on your foods, we recommend that you read the labels on your cosmetics and the other products that the body will absorb. Remember, if you inhale it or put it on your skin, your body is absorbing it and will be affected by it, for better or worse.

Approach aromatherapy with common sense and personal discrimination. Always start with a very small amount and determine your own tolerance. We recommend that you use only the purest-quality essential oils. This can be challenging to determine, because the practices of refining essential oils and then diluting them are so widespread. If you are unsure, ask a knowledgeable person at your local health-food store about the most reputable brands (which are rarely the less expensive ones), or educate yourself about this wonderful art and science.

3.10 Healing Music and Other Healthy Sounds

In the Greek myth of Orpheus, we find a powerful testimony to the power of music. Throughout his journey in the underworld, Orpheus played his lyre and sang. His music pacified the dark forces, bringing tears to the eyes of the gods and softening their hearts. Music does stir emotion. It is no wonder that it has been called the language of the soul. Music can soothe, or energize, or enervate, or fan the passions. You've no doubt experienced the emotional effects of music at some point in your life—perhaps at a wedding, a graduation, or a funeral. In every culture, spiritual or religious ritual is accompanied by music, whether it involves the rousing drumbeat of a tribal dance, the mournful strains of a medieval requiem, the awakening call of the cantor, or the joyous chorus of hand-clapping gospel singers.

Music alters the body and the mind. Just as loud, harsh sounds can cause injury to the eardrums and set the nervous system on edge, so, too, music and other sounds, such as the ocean or your own heartbeat, can enhance deep relaxation, supply you with new energy, stimulate creativity, and even transport you into other states of consciousness. When used consciously, music is a form of healing. So, when you are particularly stressed, or feeling sick or in pain (with a backache, arthritis, or a bothersome cold, for instance), try using a little music therapy on yourself. Plants grow better with certain types of music—why shouldn't the same be true for you?

The key to using music for healing is to allow yourself to let go into it. Many people will listen to music critically, identifying the interactions of the various instruments or comparing the selection with other pieces. This is listening with the mind, whereas therapeutic listening is done with the whole body. You literally drop your attention from your head to somewhere lower in your body—you imagine that your heart is listening; you allow your abdomen to be filled with the music; you let the music come in through your hands and feet; you breathe it. You keep letting go into the music, as if the sounds were waves or clouds carrying you away or supporting you.

Depending upon the type of music you choose, this method of listening can be either deeply relaxing or highly energizing. Listening with this degree of openness will alter the frequency of your brain waves, your rate of respiration, and your blood pressure. It can stimulate imagery, evoke memories, release emotions, and dissipate tension.

Other Creative Uses of Sound for Wellness

- *Sing. Open your mouth, your eyes, and your throat. Sing at the top of your lungs, or quietly hum under your breath. Use singing to lift your spirits and to breathe more fully. Chant or hum to get your energy vibrating. Use the repetition of the same sound or phrase to relax you, or to raise your consciousness, or to literally reprogram your body to a health-inspiring message.*

- *Play an instrument. Maybe it's time to dig out that old guitar, recorder, or drum, or to start taking lessons. For many people, music playing is both a form of energy release and relaxation and a means of creative expression. Drums are particularly good for this and can be used without any instruction.*

- *Listen to the movement of air through your nostrils and to other natural sounds in the environment. Use wind sounds in combination with visualization to help you clear certain conditions, such as headaches or a sense of confusion. Use water sounds to encourage relaxation. The sound of birds chirping is excellent for inspiring hope and joy. Be creative. Make up your own uses for natural sounds.*

Build Your Repertoire

Perhaps you have plenty of musical favorites to choose from already—different selections to help you to relax or to release built-up frustration. But if you don't, it may be time to start accumulating a music library of pieces that you can use for winding up or winding down. Many large music stores have a section of so-called new age instrumental music where you can find many interesting selections. Classical music offers unending possibilities as well. See appendix A for help in getting started.

The Mozart Effect

Are you ready to expand your sensory awareness and appreciation of music, or to experience the healing effects? Music- and sound-healing expert Don Campbell, author of The Mozart Effect, *suggests that you spend ten minutes of dedicated listening time a day for five days. (For more about the Mozart effect, see appendix A.)*

On the first day, pick out a piece of favorite instrumental music from your collection. While it plays, sit back or lie down with your eyes closed. Breathe. Notice whatever you notice.

The second day, do some ordinary activity as you listen to the same piece, like washing dishes, opening your email, or writing out checks.

The third day, listen and also act out conducting the music, as if you are a famous maestro.

The fourth day, listen to the same piece of music as you eat a meal.

On the fifth day, do the same relaxation method as on day one. Notice the difference in appreciation or effect from day one to day five.

3.11 Wellness and Loud Sounds

We need, expect, and appreciate sound. The sound of music, of rain, of wind in the trees—these are the food of the soul. Imagine what your world would be like without them.

On the other hand, excessive sound input can cause serious complications, and this is a growing problem in our industrialized world. The insidious background noise in our environment, which many of us have come to take for granted, has been increasing by about 1 decibel per year, on average.

We have known for a long time that hearing loss is one of the occupational hazards of being around noisy equipment. In reporting on the causes and treatment of deafness, one doctor wrote in an 1831 issue of *The Lancet:* "The blacksmiths' deafness is a consequence of their employment; it creeps on them gradually, in general at about forty or fifty years of age."

These losses are due to prolonged exposure to sound levels of between 90 and 100 decibels. Because these levels damage nerves, the losses cannot be reversed. Hearing aids are largely ineffective in remedying the condition. Realizing the magnitude of this problem, the U.S. Department of Labor publishes occupational safety and health standards that include guidelines for the levels of noise allowable in industrial and business establishments. The Environmental Protection Agency makes recommendations for acceptable levels of noise in the environment at around 45 to 55 decibels.

Hearing loss is not the only problem associated with noise. Noise increases stress and irritability and may be a factor in even more serious emotional disturbances. People who live near airports have shown a higher rate of stress disorders than those in similar economic areas farther away from airports.

Awareness and self-responsibility in regard to noise pollution may be as simple as using a set of acoustic earmuffs or earplugs to protect yourself when working around loud machinery. Attending certain concerts or parties where loud music is played will require some conscious action on your part. Many musicians who use amplified sound suffer from severe irreversible hearing loss before middle age. The sound levels at some clubs have been reported to average about 100 decibels. Some are even blasting away at up to 140! Headphones can create even more damaging levels of sound. The more

NOISE AROUND OUR HOMES

Noise Source	Sound Level for Operator (in dB)
Refrigerator	40
Floor fan	38 to 70
Clothes dryer	55
Washing machine	47 to 78
Dishwasher	54 to 85
Hair dryer	59 to 80
Vacuum cleaner	62 to 85
Sewing machine	64 to 74
Electric shaver	75
Garbage disposal	67 to 93
Electric lawn edger	81
Home shop tools	85
Gasoline power mower	87 to 92
Gasoline riding mower	90 to 95
Chain saw	100
Stereo	up to 120

Ecological Living, "Noise Pollution," www.ecological-living.info/ecoliving/noise.php.

you stay in these environments, the sooner your ears and your whole nervous system will become accustomed to the amplified sounds. The noise may no longer seem to bother you, but physiological damage to your hearing is occurring while you are simultaneously drugging yourself with a form of sensory overload. It will then take greater amounts of input to stimulate you, at the same time that you lose an appreciation for the subtleties of sounds.

Hearing loss is not always physically caused. Some losses may result from the desire to avoid hearing something or the wish for distance in a relationship. Sometimes the event that triggers it occurs long before the actual hearing loss is detected.

Care and consciousness; moderation and body-trust; self-responsibility and love—these need to be the guiding principles in exercising respect for the magnificent sense of hearing.

SOME HELPFUL HINTS FOR A QUIETER HOME

- Use carpeting to absorb noise, especially in areas where there is a lot of foot traffic.
- Hang heavy drapes over windows closest to outside noise sources.
- Put rubber or plastic treads on uncarpeted stairs (they're safer, too).
- Use upholstered rather than hard-surfaced furniture to deaden noise.
- Install sound-absorbing ceiling tile in the kitchen.
- Use wooden kitchen cabinets; they vibrate less than metal ones.

- Put a foam pad under blenders and mixers.
- Use insulation and vibration mounts when installing dishwashers.
- Compare, if possible, the noise outputs of different makes of an appliance before making your selection.
- Install the washer and dryer in the same room with heating and cooling equipment, preferably in an enclosed space away from bedrooms.
- If you use a power mower, operate it at reasonable hours and use a slower engine setting—it will operate less loudly.

- When listening to a stereo or TV, keep the volume down.
- Place window air conditioners where their hum can help mask objectionable noises, but avoid locating them facing your neighbors' bedrooms.
- Use caution in buying children's toys that can make intensive or explosive sounds—some can cause permanent hearing injury.

Ecological Living, "Noise Pollution," www.ecological-living.info/ecoliving/noise.php.

SOUND LEVELS AND HUMAN RESPONSE

This decibel (dB) table compares some common sounds and shows how they rank in potential harm to hearing. Note that somewhere between 70 and 90 dB is the point at which noise begins to harm hearing (it varies with the length of exposure). To the ear, each 10 dB increase seems twice as loud.

Sounds	Noise Level (dB)	Effect
Air-raid siren	140	Painfully loud
Jet takeoff (200 feet)	120	Maximum vocal effort
Thunderclap	120	
Auto horn (3 feet)	120	
Rock concert	120	
Pile driver	110	
Garbage truck	100	
Heavy truck (50 feet)	90*	Very annoying
City traffic	90	Hearing damage after 8 hours
Alarm clock (2 feet)	80	Annoying
Hair dryer	80	
Noisy restaurant	70	Telephone use difficult
Freeway traffic	70	
Man's voice (3 feet)	70	
Air-conditioning unit (20 feet)	60	Intrusive
Light auto traffic (100 feet)	50	Quiet
Living room	40	
Bedroom	40	
Quiet office	40	
Library	30	Very quiet
Soft whisper (15 feet)	30	
Broadcasting studio	20	
	10	Just audible
	0	Hearing begins

* Point at which noise begins to harm hearing.

Data in this table were collected from a variety of sources, including the American Academy of Otolaryngology and the American Medical Association, and it is meant to serve as a general, nonlegal guideline for the effect of sound on human hearing.

3.12 Wellness and Touch

There is a biological need for touch, an actual skin hunger, which can be met only in contact with another human being. When touching is denied, or severely restricted, infants die. During the nineteenth century, children who had been abandoned at birth and transferred to foundling homes died by the thousands. They literally wasted away, despite the fact that they were fed, kept clean, and protected from danger. The condition, known as marasmus (from the Greek, meaning "wasting away"), claimed the lives of nearly 100 percent of the infants under the age of one in U.S. foundling hospitals as late as 1920.[4] What these children lacked was physical contact. Other infants, raised in their own homes, were cradled and fed at their mothers' breasts. These foundlings weren't. When this connection between life and touch was realized, doctors and nurses in many institutions cooperated in a plan to supply "mothering" for these children. It consisted of holding, stroking, speaking to the infant, and allowing significant periods of cuddling the child, especially at mealtimes. The results were dramatic and immediate. Infant mortality rates dropped within one year of adopting these touching practices.

Despite the lessons we have learned about the necessity for touch, many child-rearing practices that discourage it endure today. So-called experts have encouraged mothers to feed children only on schedule, discouraged breast-feeding, and convinced us that independence is to be learned by exiling the little person to an oversized crib in a separate room. In many cultures, it is common practice for parents and children to share the same bed, yet in our society this is often considered unnatural.

The lack of sufficient touch has far-reaching effects on our development and shows itself in problematic ways when we reach maturity. Some people devise destructive means of compensation to satisfy the hunger for touch. These include the following:

- *Overeating,* which serves to gratify oral needs by stimulating the lips and mouth to fill us up with more of what we really don't need, to deaden the pain of emotional isolation

- *Self-destructive habits,* such as smoking, nail-biting, pulling out hair, rubbing the skin excessively, and even self-mutilation

- *Compulsive sex,* physical violence and aggressiveness, rape, and other forms of sexual abuse

The biggest problem that touch deprivation creates, however, is a sense of alienation from ourselves and isolation from others. We see this manifested in these behaviors:

- *Boredom with and lack of energy for life in general,* the experience of being out of touch with or disconnected from the world

- *Sexual dysfunction;* an unresponsiveness to the special electricity of the touch of another human body; overanxiousness, which can encourage both premature ejaculation and overall bodily tension; and fear of one's own body

- *Unsatisfying relationships,* unwillingness to attend to the needs of the other, self-preoccupation, excessive shyness, the fear of reaching out, and the fear of sustained intimacy

The need for psychological touch—attention, acknowledgment, love, praise—is as great as that for physical touch. As a primary input in the Wellness Energy System, it will be addressed further in chapter 6.

> **Researchers have found that the affectional touch climate in the subject's family of origin is the major psychosocial variable related to a person's current sexual attitude and behavior. Subjects who originated from physically affectionate families were more likely to enjoy pleasurable and more frequent experiences in the sexual-affectional aspects of their adult relationships. Adults who experienced rejection and touch deprivation in their childhood tend to treat their adult partners and their offspring in a similar manner.**
>
> —Mary Main

Why We Don't Touch

By now you should have a good idea of how important touch is for human growth and development, and how grave the consequences may be when it is lacking. The question now becomes—"Why don't we do more of it?" There are at least five possible answers.

First: Not everyone knows how essential touch is. Here, as in so many areas of life, we are often sadly lacking in information about what it takes to promote personal wellness. In an attempt to counter this ignorance, a popular bumper sticker appeared some years ago: "Have You Hugged Your Kid Today?"

Second: Much of our reluctance to touch and be touched stems from fear of our bodies—a fear we learned as children. To touch yourself and gain pleasure is still considered sinful by many segments of society. Children who masturbate frequently get their hands slapped. Many of us were told that masturbation is disgusting behavior. Messages like this communicate negativity about the body and create distrust of it.

Third: Societal attitudes increasingly connect touch with sexual advances and label as improper any public displays of affection. These attitudes show up in many ways:

- *A woman who breast-feeds her child outside the home receives disapproving looks.*

- *A preschool teacher tells her class that while it's permissible for girls, boys are not supposed to kiss each other.*

- *Two friends who recently met in the local bank after many years apart were asked to leave when their embrace lasted over twenty seconds.*

- *In some school systems, teachers are forbidden to touch children at all.*

Fear of the body in general and sexuality in particular are deeply embedded in the consciousness of the culture.

Fourth: We refrain from touching and allowing touch because we are depressed, anxious, or withdrawn. Living primarily in our heads, we are often simply unaware of our need for touch.

Finally: It is risky to touch. To be "touching" or "touchable" is to be vulnerable. If you reach out to another person, you might be rejected, and this would hurt. If you allow yourself to be touched by another, your defenses are down, and you might be hurt as well. Consequently, many of us have learned that it is easier to simply "keep our hands to ourselves."

When people lose touch with their inside world, when they fail to be sufficiently touched in a positive way by the world outside, they slowly die—sometimes physically, but more often socially, sexually, emotionally, and spiritually. We need to touch and be touched in order to learn, to communicate, to experience pleasure, to be healthy, and to grow. As you appreciate your needs for and fears of touch, you lay the groundwork for more creative ways to touch your world.

I Am Touched—Remembrances of Growing Up

We learn to touch by being touched. Some of us were raised in homes where physical contact was common-place. Others rarely received touching of any kind. A few remember only the hurtful incidents—the spankings. What do you recall about your early life relative to touching?

Settle back into a relaxed position. Put your feet up. Close your eyes. Take yourself back in time, as far as you can go. Don't feel that you have to progress logically or chronologically. Simply let your imagination suggest to you incidents that relate to your experiences of touching. Let them stay as long as they wish. Let them go when they are ready, especially if they are unhappy memories. Record your recollections.

_____

_____

_____

_____

_____

_____

_____

_____

_____

_____

_____

_____

_____

_____

_____

In writing, here or in your journal, ask yourself: What does this mean to me today? Does it help to explain some things for me? Does it highlight areas I would like to change?

_____

_____

_____

_____

_____

3.13 Wellness and Massage

Our everyday language is filled with references to the sense of touch. Besides the act of physical stimulation of the skin, we use the word "touch" to mean communication at a deep level—"Your words touched me"; correspondence or contact at a casual level—"Do keep in touch"; and the experience of just about every emotion—"How touching." We are fortunate to be living at a time in which some expressions of touch are being liberated. While certain walk-in massage parlors may still remain suspect, the offering of massage therapy at reputable health clubs, gyms, and hotels and the growing popularity of books on massage and new schools for the training of massage therapists indicate an increasing acceptance of this practice.[5] Massage is nonfattening, and if you do it yourself, it's free! Some of its benefits include:

- *Relief of pain and tension*

- *Improvement of muscle tone*

- *Maintenance of a healthy complexion*

- *Release of emotional blockages caused by trauma and repression*

- *Increased blood flow and electrical energy, to "wake up" deadened parts of the body*

- *Foreplay for sexual intercourse or sensual arousal*

- *General balancing of the right and left and the upper and lower parts of the body*

And it's so simple to do. You put your hands on and start moving them. Lotions, varied techniques,

ROSEMARY'S TEACHING

Rosemary was a student of mine for several courses, a remarkably talented woman—a counselor, a fine cook, and a weaver. Rosemary was born with a degenerative spinal condition that left her body twisted and hampered normal development.

One day in class we were working at the front of the room. One at a time, the students left their seats and came forward to take part. Rosemary remained at her place. When I asked her, "Shall I bring the equipment down to you, or clear some space so that you can get your wheelchair up to the front? Or," I hesitated, not sure that I really

wanted to make the offer, "shall I carry you?"

"I want you to carry me," she replied immediately. And so I did.

My reaction startled me. I was really afraid to touch her. Her body was no larger than that of a five-year-old child. I love to pick up children. But here was an adult. Here was a twisted body. Old voices filled my head. For one split second I was repulsed as if I might catch something. Catch her paralysis, her deformity? No, catch my own. . . . What was happening was that I was touching deep within myself—to the hidden, ugly places, which I don't usually let people see. I was reminded

of my own weakness, my vulnerability, my mortality. Tears streamed down my cheeks. Rosemary was crying too. I looked up and saw the entire class, as one pair of eyes, connected with us. Many others were crying too.

"I asked you to carry me," Rosemary reported, "because I needed to be touched."

As we left class that day, everybody touched. Hugs went all around—to me, to Rosemary. Men hugged men. Women hugged women. We had all learned an invaluable lesson.

—RSR

and training can certainly enhance the experience, but they can also lead you to believe that you need them to do it "right." This is just not true. The only rule that applies is to listen to the feedback from your own body, or ask your partner if he or she likes what you are doing. If it feels good—do it. The more you can quiet the chatter and judgment in your mind and allow your hands to move intuitively, the more creative, relaxed, and enjoyable the results will be.

Give yourself permission to receive and administer pleasure, if for no other reason than that it is a proven method of increasing overall health.

3.14 Communication Through Touch

As the infant takes its first breath, it reaches out to learn what this new world is all about. Sensory receptors located in the skin start picking up enormous quantities of information and sending them to the brain. Pressure, temperature, pain—each stimulation carries a message about the environment. Each one adds another dimension to the infant's accumulating experience.

As the largest organ of the body, the skin comprises almost one-fifth of the total body weight and engages a major percentage of the operation of the brain. The skin is constantly growing and changing in sensitivity as it performs its many functions: protection, sensation, regulation of temperature, excretion, respiration, and the metabolism and storage of fat.

The sense of touch communicates without the need for words. Gently stroking a child will induce sleep, soothe pain, and quiet rage. Physical contact informs the other of our presence, our caring, and our support. We hold the person who is grieving. We touch to say "Hello," "Good-bye," and "It's OK." A pat on the back signals approval, a slap on the hand says the opposite. And we rely upon the chemistry of touch in our sexual interactions.

Limiting ourselves to verbal expression cuts us off from the full range of communication. Since touching means closeness, it can help to bridge the distances that separate us from one another. Thus connected, you can communicate better. As you approach the other with your defenses down and your hand extended in a gesture of acceptance, you stand a better chance of reaching a mutual understanding.

In sexual relationships, touching becomes a special form of communication. Among the complaints most frequently voiced by women about sex is that their male partners do not use enough stroking and caressing prior to, during, and after intercourse. What these women are really asking for is the communication of presence, of acceptance, of tenderness, throughout. Sex therapists who work with couples encourage them to explore meaningful and pleasurable ways to touch each other, besides strictly genital involvement.[6] Experimenting with touch in sex sensitizes you to an awareness of the nonverbal messages that the body is expressing and opens up new options for intimacy.

3.15 Wellness and the Healing Powers of Touch

> **Now when the sun was setting, all they that had any sick with diverse diseases brought them unto him; and he laid his hand on every one of them, and healed them.**
>
> —Luke 4:40

Prophets and teachers in most of the world's great religions have been credited with the power to heal through touch. In our own time, reports of modes of healing that involve the "laying on of hands" are many.

Affectionate touch, whenever appropriate, in communicating with dying people and grieving family members, is recognized as an effective therapeutic measure. The dying experience extreme loneliness as they leave everything they have known and loved. Reassuring touch can reconnect them with the family, the community of support. Healing of this type is a healing of the spirit.

It is not the skin alone that is touched—it is a whole person. Touching brings with it a stimulation of the capillaries that increases blood flow to the area, a sharing of body heat, and a relaxation of muscular tension. Each of these factors will encourage the normal healing process. But more important, perhaps, is the way touching comforts a troubled mind, provides security for a lonely and scared victim, and communicates love, person to person. You probably know that pain is increased by anxiety, and that emotional imbalance feeds physical disease. Touch serves to ground a patient in the realization that he or she is not alone. That assurance brings healing. For ages, parents have used hugs and kisses to heal their children's hurts. Putting an arm around an asthma sufferer at the onset of an attack will frequently stop it.

When you are hurt, your hands will automatically move to the area of pain. Part of this is for protection. The other part is that we connect our hands with some ability to relieve or remove pain. A man will grasp his sprained ankle. A child curls up in a fetal position, hands covering her aching belly. A woman with a headache will frequently rub or hold her head. Watch a person with a severe toothache: you will almost always see a hand tightly pressed against the cheek and jaw. We attempt to heal ourselves through touch without much awareness. To use it more consciously can be a very powerful method of relaxation and pain reduction.

Therapeutic procedures, such as acupressure, that use touch for rebalancing and healing are growing in number and popularity. Some are based on ancient Chinese medicine, which describes a universal energy—called *chi* or *ki*—that circulates throughout the body. This energy can become blocked at any point, creating an imbalance in the system. Using massage and pressure at specified points is known to release the blockage.[7]

You can do a variation of acupressure for yourself with the guidance of a clear book and a little practice. Imagine being able to relieve a headache by pinching the skin below your nose and above your upper lip, or by pressing at a point on your hand between your thumb and forefinger! Strange as this may sound, these techniques sometimes work faster for many people than the leading brand of aspirin.

One of the most ancient of arts—the rubbing of tired feet—has been systematized into a science. Called *foot reflexology,* it correlates points on your feet with every part of your body—organs, glands, spinal column, and so on. Working on the feet is then comparable to massaging the entire body. Proponents believe that energy blocks broken up in the foot mean a recharging of the corresponding segment of the body. Many of these claims have yet to be clinically verified, but to anyone who has ever received one, the value of foot massage as a simple, loving, and healing tool is undisputed. See the following chart and instructions for a foot treatment on the next page.

Nurturing yourself through touch is a way of accepting and loving yourself—a form of preventive medicine, easy to do and immediately rewarding. Using touch with others is a primary way of opening communication and establishing intimacy with them. And intimacy is healing.

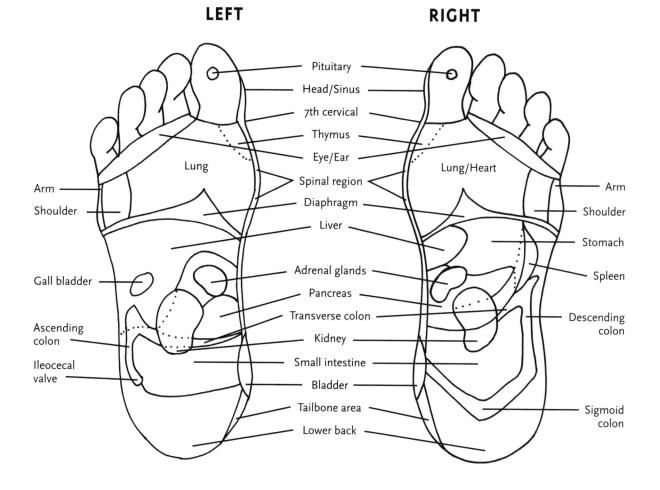

LEFT   RIGHT

Pituitary
Head/Sinus
7th cervical
Thymus
Eye/Ear
Spinal region
Diaphragm
Liver
Adrenal glands
Pancreas
Transverse colon
Kidney
Small intestine
Bladder
Tailbone area
Lower back

Lung
Arm
Shoulder
Gall bladder
Ascending colon
Ileocecal valve

Lung/Heart
Arm
Shoulder
Stomach
Spleen
Descending colon
Sigmoid colon

Give Yourself a Foot Treatment

In The Foot Book, *author Devaki Berkson writes:*

> *Otau was a wise, old, and wrinkled man. The whole village respected his healing abilities. One day a foreigner came to ask him many questions and write down the healing ways of Otau. However, all Otau would say was, "See to their feet and you have seen to their body."*
>
> *"I do not understand," insisted the foreigner.*
>
> *"Your understanding will never be enough," Otau chuckled. "See to their feet, and that will be enough."*

Foot reflexology, or zone therapy, is a type of pressure-point treatment applied to the feet. The theory behind reflexology is that the body is divided lengthwise into energy zones that end at the feet. The feet, therefore, contain reflex points that correspond to all major organs, glands, and body parts. Attention to your feet can thereby affect your whole body. Perhaps this is what Otau was referring to. Reflexologists attest to the overall therapeutic value of this type of treatment. It relaxes, stimulates energy flow, and often relieves pain.

1. *Position yourself so that you can comfortably hold one of your feet in both hands. This can be done more easily if you can sit in a chair. (You could also invite a friend to give you this foot treatment.)*

2. *Now, begin to massage this foot and ankle gently all over. Work between and around your toes. Give special attention to your ankles.*

3. *Using your thumb pads or the knuckle of your index finger, begin to explore your foot and ankle until you encounter a sore spot. Apply light pressure here and massage in a circular motion for no more than thirty seconds at a time. Then move on to find another spot that needs attention.*

4. *The chart on page 71 indicates the correspondence between places on your foot and the rest of your body.*

5. *When you are finished, stretch your toes. Bend, flex, and rotate your ankle. Gently rub your foot all over . . . and then go to work on the other foot.*

3.16 Acknowledgment and Recognition

In addition to the physical sensory energy we receive from our environment, humans need nonphysical energy from other humans, in the form of recognition or acknowledgment. To feel that we are seen, heard, and recognized by another is one of the most healing forms of sensory energy. Simply being present to another can have a profound impact on their wellbeing.

We are a social species and our connections with each other, the earth, and the numinous are crucial ingredients for our wellness. The earliest forms of acknowledgement we receive in infancy are related to input from our physical senses of touch, smell, and movement. Tragically, these three sources of sensory input are often severely limited for Western infants.

Modern child-rearing practices that support leaving infants alone for long periods of time scar our young ones, to whom words such as "I love you, I'll be back soon" mean nothing. These infants are left feeling abandoned and isolated. It is through touch, smell, and movement—the "near" somatic senses—that a newborn can continue to feel connected with her mother as she adapts to living outside the womb in an environment that is alien compared to the fetal environment. Of these somatic senses (in contrast to the cognitive senses of vision and hearing), the sense of movement is the most important, as it is the dominant sensory system in utero connecting the fetus with the mother. Similarly, postnatal movement from being carried on the mother's body creates an external "umbilical cord" that keeps mother and infant connected and bonded.

> These are our first real experiences of life—floating in a warm liquid, curling inside a total embrace, swaying to the undulations of the moving body, and hearing the beat of the pulsing heart.
>
> —Desmond Morris

Eye contact with the mother, as she holds the infant to her breast many times a day, begins to deepen the in utero connection previously established between the two and, more importantly, helps regulate the child's developing nervous system. Infants who are not held and carried most of the time, and who are not nursed while being held close to the mother's heart (the heart has been shown to radiate a strong electromagnetic field[8]) and gazing into the mother's eyes, develop more slowly and are more prone to depression, violence, and addiction.[9]

While this connection appears to be largely physical when we are young, as we develop first our vision and then language, we become able to experience connection by eye contact from afar and through the spoken language—both the words and the tone of voice. The ability to experience and express love is directly related to how connected we feel with those around us. Compliments, appreciation, and recognition are deeply embedded in the greeting rituals of most cultures. ("You're looking well today." "Thank you!") Clearly, the value of such rituals has been recognized for a long time. Unfortunately, many greetings have deteriorated into robotic generalizations that have far less meaning than a genuinely expressed, specific appreciation, such as "Thanks so much for your email the other day. I loved hearing your story about meeting my daughter at the game." Specific compliments or

As a fish is to water, we are so close to one of our fundamental sensory inputs that we rarely recognize that it exists. Ask someone what the "five senses" are and they will rarely mention our sense of motion. This sense resides in the inner ear (vestibular system) and, as it is the earliest sense to develop in the womb, should be labeled as our first sense. Generally we take this sense for granted except when it causes us trouble—feeling dizziness, vertigo, or motion sickness. But this sense is even more important when our brain first starts to grow.

From the work of James Prescott, Ph.D., of the National Institute of Child Health and Human Development (at the National Institute of Health) in the 1960s and 1970s, we know that input from our first sense is so important to the developing brain that without enough of it, actual brain damage occurs. Sensory input from the vestibular system travels to the cerebellum, the limbic system, and the prefrontal neocortex, which form the basis of the neurointegrative brain. Here, constant movement influences the development of neurotransmitter systems and "brain gestalts" in which the whole is greater than the sum of its parts. Most of us alive today did not get enough somatic stimulation and as a result suffer from some degree of somato-sensory affectional deprivation syndrome (S-SADS), which often leads to depression, violence, and/or addictions.[10]

Gentle rocking soothes infants, but if we didn't get enough, one way we can treat ourselves for this somatosensory deprivation is to self-stimulate our sensory system. Self-rocking and other stereotypical behaviors are well-known consequences of S-SADS.

Do you recall riding in the back of a car at night as a child and falling asleep? Was it upsetting to have this womblike state disrupted when the car stopped at a traffic light or, worse yet, you arrived home and had to walk to the house?

As young children we are drawn to naturally stimulate our vestibular system on playgrounds. This is probably the result of the various forms of sensory deprivation our bodies are otherwise enduring. Swings, slides, merry-go-rounds, and teeter-totters all happen to specifically stimulate the inner ear, which provides an important input to our nervous system. Due to liability fears, however, many of these devices have been removed from playgrounds—the teeter-totters and merry-go-rounds are usually the first to go, then the slides get shorter and the swings lower. In a few more years, what will be left besides static devices?

But older kids have found another solution—skateboards!

As adults, we pay money to have our vestibular system stimulated by carousels, Ferris wheels, and roller coasters, not to mention the upside-down terror machines of theme parks.

We crave it in the air, with sailplanes, hang gliders, parasailing, skydiving, bungee jumping, high diving, and so on; or on the water, with surfing, sailboats and sailboards, water-skiing, snorkeling, and scuba diving.

The correlation of the rise of interest in these sports and the increases in S-SADS among the very generations that create and pursue these sports is intriguing.

It must be a monumental shock to a newborn to come out of the womb, in which she was constantly in motion and being massaged by the movement of her mother's diaphragm and intestines, and be placed alone in a lifeless plastic container; yet this shock goes as unnoticed as our sixth sense itself. Carrying babies and sleeping with them mimics the experience of being in the womb; it has been the norm for millions of years of our ancestry. Cross-cultural studies have confirmed that tribes with high mother-infant bonding through movement are peaceful cultures. The lack of this mother-infant movement bonding produces violent cultures.[11] To think we can ignore such a basic need without severe consequences is probably arrogant and shortsighted.

recognition have much more value (energy) for their recipient than generalities like "Thanks." While this is probably related to the energy of the physical connection that we had (or didn't have) as infants, the energy that is passed between people in this kind of interaction defies physical measurement. It is significant, nonetheless, and it illustrates the power of symbols (words) in the flow of energy between people.

The beauty of this type of energy is that, when you give it, you usually receive as much energy back from the good feelings that arise in you when you allow yourself to really appreciate another person.

Love has been defined as being completely present to another (not a simple task). Acknowledgments, compliments, and appreciation are the building blocks of love—perhaps the most valuable form of energy on the planet.

3.17 Wellness and the Nonphysical Senses—Feng Shui

There are many forms of subtle energy that we cannot detect with our usual physical senses. The Chinese art and science of feng shui (prounounced "fung shway," meaning "wind-water"), which has gained enormous popularity throughout the West in recent years, is based on an understanding of the life force, or chi energy from the Chinese perspective, which is always moving throughout creation, as the wind is always moving. But at some points it can become blocked or trapped, even becoming stagnated, like unmoving water. By learning this art or consulting a feng shui practitioner, one gets to "see" and "feel" where this energy is trapped or has built up unnecessarily. One then must create balance between the light and the dark (the *yin* and the *yang*) of all the features in the environment—including the light, the color, the decorations, the placement of objects, the design of the room or the space, the sounds, the movements. A particular balance of these energies and features will maximize the environment's ability to foster health, wealth, and happiness: that is, for relaxation, for energetic accumulation, for healing, or for doing business.

Examine your home and workplace in this light. What moods does the lighting in various rooms create? Where is clutter building up, causing you to feel uneasy? If green plants can't thrive in your room, how do *you* expect to? Learn some valuable lessons from your green, growing friends. Experiment with lights of different colors and with altering the color scheme and furniture placement of a setting. You will discover that certain colors have a more relaxing effect on your nervous system; certain arrangements will open up something, giving you a sense that you can breathe more easily. Trust your intuition. Surround yourself with simple and beautiful things; dress yourself in colors that you really like. You are the judge of what feels good to you.

By developing this nonphysical sense that is built upon color, form, and location (but is more than a physical sensing of these elements), you will experience a systematized aspect of what we in the West might call *aesthetics*—an attunement to beauty and artistic expression that includes the sense of where and how energy is flowing, or feng shui.

3.18 Wellness, Silence, and Being Alone

Many of us experience great uneasiness when confronted with a lack of the types of input that we are used to, and particularly the types of distracting input we use to keep ourselves so occupied that we don't or can't attend to the subtleties of simply *being*—because silence may force us to think, to feel, to touch deep parts of ourselves. Learning to be comfortable with silence means learning to be comfortable alone with yourself. It is one of the healthiest habits one can cultivate. The teachings of many world religions speak of the necessity of silence to hear the voice of God or the voice of the inner wisdom. In the silence of the mind, the heart speaks. Watch yourself as you go through the course of a day, or several days.

- *When and for how long did you experience silence accidentally? Deliberately?*

- *How did you feel about these occasions? What, if anything, did it do for you?*

- *Would you like to cultivate a more loving relationship with silence? With yourself?*

> **When real silence is dared, we can come very close to ourselves and to the deep center of the world.**
>
> —James Carroll

A quieter external environment allows us to hear a level of sounds that are usually unobserved, like the wondrous sound of our own breathing or that of a loved one, the sound of a gentle breeze, the delicate sound of tea being poured into a waiting cup, the sounds of birds in the distant trees, the hum of insects. Try this: While outside, close your eyes and stand very still. Listen carefully. What is the most distant sound you can hear? How many different sounds can you hear?

As you move through the day, try to become aware of the sounds you make as you progress from one activity to another. "Listen" to yourself brushing your teeth, drinking a glass of water, dressing yourself, or walking up stairs. There are hundreds of experiences you can use to develop awareness and sensitivity about yourself and your environment. Becoming aware of your own "noise" can be an invitation to step more lightly in many ways. Try it.

Wonderful/Terrible Silence

Consider both the potential value of silence and the potential tyranny of silence with regard to your overall wellbeing. Use the space below to write a short poem or a brief reflection about either aspect—or both.

_____

_____

_____

SUGGESTED READING

Arvigo, R., and N. Epstein, *Spiritual Bathing: Healing Rituals and Traditions from Around the World* (Celestial Arts, 2003).

Beresford, S., et al., *Improve Your Vision Without Glasses or Contact Lenses: A New Program of Therapeutic Eye Exercises* (Fireside Books, 1996).

Campbell, D., *The Mozart Effect: Tapping the Power of Music to Heal the Body, Strengthen the Mind, and Unlock the Creative Spirit* (Quill, 2001).

Caplan, M., *To Touch Is to Live: The Need for Genuine Affection in an Impersonal World* (Hohm Press, 2003).

Childre, D., and H. Martin, *The HeartMath Solution* (Harper SanFrancisco, 1999).

Dodt, C., *The Essential Oils Book* (Storey Communications, 1996).

Downing, G., *The Massage Book* (Random House, 1998).

Fleiss, P., and F. Hodges, *Sweet Dreams: A Pediatrician's Secrets for Baby's Good Night's Sleep* (McGraw-Hill/Contemporary Books, 2000).

Graham, H., *Discover Color Therapy* (Ulysses Press, 1998).

Krieger, D., *The Therapeutic Touch: How to Use Your Hands to Help or Heal* (Fireside, 1992).

Liedloff, J., *The Continuum Concept* (Perseus Publishing, 1986).

Maxwell-Hudson, C., and S. Lousada, *The Complete Book of Massage* (Random House, 1988).

Montagu, A., *Touching: The Human Significance of the Skin* (Perennial, 1986).

Ryan, R., *After Surgery, Illness, or Trauma: 10 Practical Steps to Renewed Energy and Health* (Hohm Press, 2000).

Sang, L., *The Principles of Feng Shui* (American Institute of Feng Shui, 1995).

Wong, E., *A Master Course in Feng Shui* (Shambhala Publications, 2001).

Worwood, V., *The Complete Book of Aromatherapy and Essential Oils* (New World Library, 1991).

For an updated listing of resources and active links to the websites mentioned in this chapter, please see www.WellnessWorkbook.com.

NOTES

1. Montagu, A., *Touching: The Human Significance of the Skin* (Perennial, 1986), 31–37.

2. Autier, P., et al., "Sunscreen Use, Wearing Clothes, and Number of Nevi in 6- to 7-Year-Old European Children," *J. Nat. Cancer Inst.* (1998) 90:1873–1880.

3. Peters, R. R., et al., "Supplemental Lighting Stimulates Growth and Lactation in Cattle," *Science,* Vol. 99 (February 24, 1978): 911–12.

4. Montagu, 82–84.

5. For a list of schools, see www.amtamassage.org/schools/list.org, or write Robert K. King, National Education Director, American Massage Therapy Association, 820 Davis St., Evanston, IL 60201 (include a self-addressed stamped envelope).

6. Exercises for getting in touch with the skin, called "sensate focus," are recommended and explained in the *S.A.R. [Sexual Attitudes Restructuring] Programs.* For information, contact the Institute for the Advanced Study of Human Sexuality, 1523 Franklin St., San Francisco, CA 94109, (415) 928-1133, www.iashs.edu.

7. These techniques include acupuncture, acupressure, do-in, shiatsu, and others. See Carter, M., *Body Reflexology: Healing at Your Fingertips* (Parker Publishing Co., 1983); Namikashi, T., *The Complete Book of Shiatsu Therapy* (Japan Publications, 1981); and Teeguarden, I. M., *Acupressure Way of Health: Jin Shin Do* (Japan Publications, 1978).

8. Childre, D., and H. Martin, *The HeartMath Solution* (HarperSanFrancisco, 1999).

9. Prescott, J. W., "Breastfeeding: Brain Nutrients in Brain Development for Human Love and Peace" (1997), www.violence.de/prescott/ttf/article.html.

10. Prescott, J. W., "The Origins of Love" (2004), www.byronchild.com/arts21.htm.

11. Prescott, J. W., "How Culture Shapes the Developing Brain and the Future of Humanity" (2002), www.touchthefuture.org/services/bonding/02SpringNLJWP.pdf.

CHAPTER 4

Wellness and Eating

*The third energy input type in the Wellness Energy System is food. Eating (including diges-
tion and assimilation) is the process whereby nutrients are extracted from food, combusted
with the oxygen supplied by breathing, and transformed into electrochemical and heat energy.
The newly acquired organic molecules are also used in the production of raw materials
needed for building and repairing body parts.*

When all else fails, *eat!*

—Ashleigh Brilliant

Recent U.S. history has reflected a growing concern
with nutrition and its relationship to health. In February 1977, a select committee of the U.S. Senate
under the direction of Senator George McGovern
published the first *Dietary Goals for the United
States.* Its purpose, McGovern stated, was "to point
out that eating patterns of this century represent as
critical a public health concern as any now before
us."[1] Despite pressure from many special interest
groups and lobbies, especially in the meat and dairy
industry, the Committee's recommendations took a
radical departure from the nutritional dogma that
most Americans at that time had been raised on. We
were urged to increase consumption of fruits, vegetables, and whole grains and decrease our consumption of red meat, saturated fats, sugar, salt, and
foods high in cholesterol.

In 1992, the U.S. Department of Agriculture
(USDA) went further, issuing its Food Guide Pyramid as the beginning of a nationwide project to re-
educate Americans about the need for a healthy diet.
Dairy products and other protein foods like meat
and beans were relegated to a much less important
status than carbohydrates, fruits, and vegetables,
which formed the foundation of the pyramid. At the
narrowest part of the pyramid—indicative of the
minor role they should play in the diet—were placed

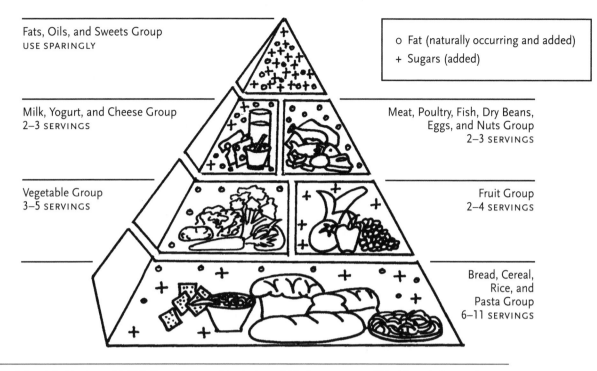

Fats, Oils, and Sweets Group
USE SPARINGLY

o Fat (naturally occurring and added)
+ Sugars (added)

Milk, Yogurt, and Cheese Group
2–3 SERVINGS

Meat, Poultry, Fish, Dry Beans,
Eggs, and Nuts Group
2–3 SERVINGS

Vegetable Group
3–5 SERVINGS

Fruit Group
2–4 SERVINGS

Bread, Cereal,
Rice, and
Pasta Group
6–11 SERVINGS

USDA Food Guide Pyramid. U.S. Department of Agriculture/U.S. Department of Health and Human Services, www.usda.gov/cnpp/pyramid.html.

"fats, oils, and sweets" with the disparaging recommendation, "Use Sparingly."

At about the same time as the USDA Food Guide Pyramid's introduction, studies from around the world began to pour in that correlated the consumption of fresh fruits and vegetables with a significantly lowered incidence of heart attack and many types of cancer. The U.S. National Cancer Institute instituted its "5 A Day" program throughout the United States in 1991, recommending five to nine *daily* servings of fresh fruits and vegetables. Research indicated that this change alone could reduce risk of both heart attack and cancer by as much as 55 percent.

These dietary guidelines were again updated in 2000 as the fifth edition of *Nutrition and Your Health: Dietary Guidelines for Americans,* a joint publication of the U.S. Department of Health and Human Services and the Department of Agriculture, and will continue to be updated every five years. The guidelines were expanded to include a number of vital distinctions—like the need for healthy fats (fatty

acids) versus the danger of unhealthy fats (saturated fats)—a recommendation for safety measures in storing and preparing foods, and a strong encouragement to exercise as a necessary part of a healthy lifestyle.

Some researchers, like Meir Stampfer, M.D., Dr.P.H., of the Harvard University School of Public Health (who served on the committee for the 2000 *Guidelines* update), and Walter Willett, M.D., Dr.P.H., chair of the Department of Nutrition at Harvard, think that additional changes should have been recommended. In fact, Willett's book *Eat, Drink, and Be Healthy* offers another pyramid model that makes more distinctions. Among the differences from the USDA model, the Harvard "Healthy Eating Pyramid" puts nuts and legumes in their own category instead of lumping them together with fish, poultry, and eggs. It de-emphasizes dairy products, placing them in a category with calcium supplements. It further recommends a daily multivitamin supplement and allows for moderate alcohol consumption, as appropriate.

Yet, even though we now have more healthy choices and can talk about nutrition with some sophistication, we need not look far to see that Americans in general are unhealthy. Most Americans' eating patterns represent a public health crisis. If a new disease erupted that was one-tenth as destructive as most people's diets, there would be a massive public outcry to find the cure. It isn't just the poor who die of malnutrition. The average diet in the United States is so full of empty calories, dangerous fats, and chemical additives that a whole new type of malnutrition is being established. We are overweight or dying in increasing numbers from conditions linked with dietary and related lifestyle patterns. Heart disease, cancer, diabetes, kidney disease, and stroke—these are the killers of today. The "minor" concerns, we would add, are that few of us really experience happiness, peace of mind, and good health. We suffer from:

- *Depression*

- *Tooth decay*

- *Indigestion*

- *Constipation*

- *Allergies, in ever growing numbers*

- *Headaches*

- *Learning disabilities*

- *Hyperactivity*

- *Lethargy*

- *Skin disorders*

- *Weak nails and brittle hair*

The list goes on and on. And each of these conditions is connected with what we eat, as well as how and why we eat it.

In 2003, Secretary of Health and Human Services Tommy Thompson reported that the United States was spending $1.4 trillion on "health" care annually. Thompson claimed that three-quarters of that amount was used to treat chronic illnesses that could be

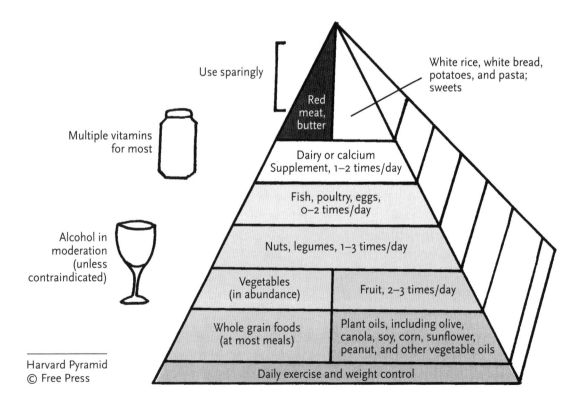

Harvard Pyramid
© Free Press

reduced through prevention. He further reported that 43 percent of the U.S. population had some type of chronic illness, 17 million people had diabetes (a diet-related disease), and 50 million adults (25 percent of the adult population) were obese. According to the U.S. Centers for Disease Control and Prevention, the prevalence of obesity among adults rose 60 percent nationally since 1991. "That is a dramatic increase in a relatively short period of time," said Donald Hensrud, a Mayo Clinic nutrition specialist.

Whether or not children eat proper foods, eat regularly, eat carefully, and eat politely has an effect on their health and their personalities.

—National Education Association, 1940

The basic problem, as we see it, is a lethal mix of dietary confusion with an increasingly sedentary yet stressed lifestyle. Our diets and eating habits are highly imbalanced. Our stress levels are increasing, thereby undermining our ability to digest and utilize our foods properly. Our overall level of physical exercise is generally not enough to keep pace with what we eat and with the stresses we bear. In some cases these imbalances exist because we lack information about nutrition, stress, and exercise; but the overall problem is more likely the result of changing lifestyle patterns and the choices that result from these. For instance, as people take more sedentary jobs, increase their home TV viewing, and decrease their exercise, obesity is creeping across the nation's high-rises and office parks, accounting for about 300,000 U.S. deaths each year.

Today, "convenience" and "comfort" are the primary drivers of consumer food choices. We can now buy our "fresh" vegetables already peeled and cut up; our frozen or deli dinners ready to "pop in the microwave." The growing popularity of fast-food and restaurant fare has added to our diminishing control over our diets; many fast foods are excessively high in the things we don't need—like salt and saturated and trans fats—and low in the things we do—like vitamins and minerals. Because food preferences are generally learned, food companies using modern advertising can fuel our cravings for snack foods and fast foods and teach our children that the only fun is had in eating saturated fats (potato chips, french fries, and ice cream), sugars (cookies, candy, and soft drinks), and high-protein "meals" (burgers and milkshakes).

The confusion around food shows up in the ways we have learned to use food to relieve emotional and physical pain. Moreover, in addition to the issue of what we eat or don't eat in the way of nutrients, many of us are addicted to various drugs in foods, beverages, or food-like substitutes: caffeine, alcohol, nicotine, and a wide variety of pharmaceuticals.

It's a vicious circle in which each unbalancing factor leads to another and then turns back to reinforce itself. The more stressed you are, the more you may eat in an attempt to relieve your pain. The more you eat, the more pain you may create through increased weight or compounded guilt. The more pain you create, the more you may want to eat to relieve it. Round and round you go. It makes no difference at what point on the circle you jump in. Anywhere you turn, you lose. Winning requires breaking this cycle—moving into another circle altogether.

While some of your choices—like job availability and certain stressors—are often beyond your control, many other choices are still yours to make. The message of this book is that we *can* take responsibility for overall food selection. We *can* choose to limit much of the stress in our lives and learn ways to manage unavoidable stress. We *can* choose to exercise. In this chapter, we will present some basic data about nutrition, examine the reasons behind our imbalanced use of food, and highlight ways of growing in awareness and love through our diet and eating habits. These suggestions will help us define a whole new circle within which to live.

4.1 The Food Story—Back to Basics

All foods are made of one or more of seven types of essential nutrients—so called because they are necessary to sustain life in the body. These types of nutrients are:

- *Carbohydrates*
- *Fats*
- *Proteins*
- *Phytochemicals (the hundreds of vital substances in plants)*
- *Vitamins*
- *Minerals*
- *Water*

Nutrition is the study of how to provide these nutrients in the right amount for good health. Changing these nutrients into smaller, simpler substances for ready use within the body is the process of digestion. Its main activity is breaking down and extracting. Digestion entails:

- *Breaking down carbohydrates into simple sugars (glucose)*
- *Breaking down fats into fatty acids and glycerol*
- *Breaking down proteins into amino acids*
- *Extracting phytochemicals from plant-based foods*

Carbohydrates, fats, and proteins are the only three nutrients that contain heat-producing energy. They are the fuels that the body burns in order to provide it with the heat energy it needs. The amount of heat generated when food is oxidized is measured in units of heat called *calories.* One calorie represents the quantity necessary to raise the temperature of a kilogram (roughly one quart) of water by 1°C (1.8°F).

These three nutrients burn at a different rates—some providing instant but short-lived "flames," others burning slowly and efficiently for the warmth needed on a cold winter's night. Fats contain about 225 calories per ounce and are the slowest-burning fuel—the coal. Proteins contain about 115 calories per ounce and burn almost twice as fast as fats—they are the hardwood. Carbohydrates (including sugars) contain 115 calories or less per ounce and burn quickly—they are the softwood and kindling. However, since carbohydrates should be eaten in greater proportion than fats or proteins, they can provide consistent, efficient service.

Carbohydrates

Carbohydrates are the most common source of food energy. Our grandparents lived quite well on diets high in unrefined or natural carbohydrates—vegetables, fruits, and whole grains. These foods supplied starches, natural sugars, vitamins, minerals, plant chemicals, and adequate fiber to keep everything in good working order. So why do some people (especially dieters) fear and avoid carbohydrates today?

The question has many sides to it, and lack of understanding is rampant—the old "potatoes are fattening" myth, for example. The most important point to remember about carbohydrates is that there is a significant biochemical difference between *unrefined* carbohydrates (like potatoes and other vegetables, for instance) and *refined* carbohydrates, such as bleached-flour bread or pasta, white rice, and sugar.

Refined carbohydrates, like kindling in the fireplace, provide a burst of flame that is soon gone. They are immediately absorbed into the bloodstream, creating the short-lived "rush" that you experience after eating a chocolate bar or drinking a soft drink for a quick pick-me-up. What the advertisers neglect to tell you, however, is that refined carbohydrates provide just as quick a letdown. Refined sugar (sucrose) is not digested in the mouth or the stomach but passes directly to the lower intestines and thence to the bloodstream. The extra speed with which sucrose enters the bloodstream does more harm than good. As the body swings back and forth from stimulation to depletion, sometimes all day long, this puts a huge stress on the adrenal glands and other glands and organs responsible for keeping a happy state of balance within. When our glandular system is stressed, our immune system is also compromised.

Today we find refined sugars in just about all processed foods—cold cereals, pies, and snack foods, as well as in canned vegetables, fruits, meats, and many prepared baby foods. Since 1942, when the American Medical Association expressed concern about sweetened carbonated beverages, candy, and other foods rich in sugar but poor in nutrients, consumption of soft drinks (or "liquid candy") has increased about sevenfold (excluding diet soft drinks), and overall sugar consumption has increased by one-third. In 1975, average sugar consumption in America was 120 pounds per year. In 1999, it had jumped nearly 40 pounds to 158 pounds per year. This equals 170 grams of sugar (nearly three-quarters of a cup) per day. In 1970, Americans drank an average of one soft drink per day. Today, the average U.S. teenager drinks 868 cans of soft drink in one year.

Unrefined, natural carbohydrates (vegetables, fruits, whole grains, potatoes) burn like softwoods in your fireplace. In addition to being rich sources of vitamins, phytochemicals, and minerals, these foods provide a steady burning fire that will last many hours.

According to the diet recommended by *Nutrition and Your Health: Dietary Guidelines for Americans* (fifth edition, 2000), more than 60 percent of our foods should be in the form of complex carbohydrates. Lots of salads, fresh or lightly cooked vegetables, and raw fruits are primary in this approach. Whole-grain cereals and breads, brown rice and other whole grains, beans, nuts, and seeds—these foods will adequately supply necessary fiber as well as fuel reserves.

While these dietary guidelines may not be the ideal for everyone (see module 4.10), in general they offer a sane starting point, an alternative to the highly saturated fats and the sugars that are so rapidly damaging health and leading to obesity.

Fats

Few people would deny that fat is a big problem in our society. It is also big business! How easily our TV-motivated culture is bandwagoned into eating gigantic hamburgers and buckets of deep-fat fries, then shamed into joining a health club, eating diet bread, or buying control-top pantyhose. Is it any wonder our lives are not happier and our bodies not healthier?

Let's clear up a few common misconceptions. First, there is fat, and then there are *fats*. The latter need not be singled out as the cause of the former. You can become *fat* as a result of eating excessive amounts of protein or carbohydrates, too. Second, healthy fats (essential fatty acids) are a necessary ingredient in a well-balanced diet. You *must* consume fats, period! The point is not to eliminate fats, but to supply the body with fats of a certain type and in a certain amount.

Essential fatty acids can be found in their healthy form in high-quality, cold-pressed, less-processed, nonhydrogenated oils. These may include extra-virgin olive oil, flax oil, sesame oil, and fish oils such as from canned sardines or wild (not farmed) salmon—but read the labels on bulk oils to be sure they meet the above criteria and are not hydrogenated or even partially hydrogenated. These fats supply us with cancer-fighting vitamins A and E, aid in the production of healthy hair and skin, and give the liver the necessary building blocks for a vast number of chemical processes, including the production of hormones and brain neurotransmitters, and energy production within the cells themselves. For extraordinary mental and physical health, most of the components in the biochemical cascade of fat metabolism absolutely depend upon the regular (almost daily) intake of balanced varieties and proper quantities of essential fatty acids from healthy fats and oils. This is nonnegotiable.

Fruits like avocados, fresh coconuts, and olives supply these healthy fats in a pure form that is both easy to take and delicious. And fish and poultry (especially if raised in unpolluted environments) are also a much healthier source of naturally healthy fat than is red meat.

There are also very unhealthy fats—saturated fats and trans fatty acids. These fats are extremely difficult to break up in the process of digestion. Consequently, they tend to clump together and form droplets of fat that accumulate as a part of plaque in our arteries. Saturated fats are found in meat and dairy products, including the cheese that we are eating in astronomical amounts these days; and trans fatty acids are found in highly processed hydrogenated oils—those inexpensive "vegetable oils" that we pour on our once-healthy salads and in which we deep-fry our potatoes and other foods.

Fats, in the fireplace analogy, burn like coal, the hardest and slowest-burning fossil fuel. They contain twice as much energy per gram as the other fuels—proteins and carbohydrates. With significant physical exercise, which requires a large turnover of energy, our bodies can use fats to great advantage. Without activity, however, we would do well to remember the old adage "A moment on the lips and forever on the hips," and limit our intake of foods that are high in saturated fat.

Protein

The word *protein* comes from the Greek *proteios,* meaning "primary." Your body is composed chiefly of proteins (18 to 20 percent by weight), and consequently needs to be supplied with them in order to build new cells, replacing those that are constantly dying. If the protein intake is so high that some are burned for energy, they are slow to digest. Thus, while they may be likened to hardwoods in our heat-generating analogy, their slow breakdown rate may cause them to remain long in the digestive tract, which is especially dangerous where meat and dairy products are concerned. Every naturally occurring food contains some protein, so the sources are abundant.

THE CASE FOR FIBER

The bran of cereals constitutes more than half of their vitamin and mineral value, but in order to make cereals more palatable, food manufacturers remove this part and feed it to livestock. Cereals are then "enriched" by putting back four of the twenty-two nutrients that were removed. The whole situation is ironic in the wasteful pattern it encourages. Moreover, by the time most of these foods reach our plates they are soft, smooth, and almost entirely lacking the fiber necessary to keep the colon adequately stimulated. Diverticulosis starts showing up in people over fifty, whose "unstimulating" diet has been the pattern of a lifetime. In this condition the colon wall is stretched into blind pockets that accumulate fecal matter and may become sealed off from the main cavity. Other related problems include constipation, obesity, and even cancer.

Proteins are like words, and the amino acids that comprise them are like letters. When a protein is digested, it is taken apart and the "letters" made available to spell whatever new words the body needs. Proteins (the "words") are used to build and repair the body. In order to perform all the necessary functions, an adequate supply of all the amino acids is imperative. Twenty-two different amino acids are required to build all the proteins needed by humans. Fourteen of these can be manufactured within the body. They are called the *nonessential* amino acids, not because they aren't necessary but because we don't have to do anything to supply them. The other eight cannot be easily synthesized by the body; they must be supplied with regularity and in certain proportions. They are called the eight *essential* amino acids. Some foods contain all eight of these essential amino acids; others contain varying amounts. It is important to know that you don't need to consume them all within the same meal.

High amounts of protein are found in meat, fish, eggs, milk, nuts, and soybeans, as well as in lesser-known food sources such as the grains amaranth and quinoa. Even fruits and vegetables contain amino acids that can be combined to form proteins. The idea that you must have superprotein foods like meat or dairy products in order to have adequate protein in the body is a myth, as many vibrantly healthy vegetarians will testify.

Phytochemicals

While most of us know that foods supply us with vitamins and minerals, fewer are up to date on the hundreds—in fact, thousands—of other chemical components in our foods, particularly those found in plant foods. These substances are referred to as *phytochemicals,* from the Greek word *phyto,* meaning "plant." Phytochemicals are the compounds that give plant foods their color, odor, and flavor; they also serve as the plant's own self-defense system. Some may be familiar to you, such as chlorophyll, that incomparable green power in plants. Others are less well known, although the plants they live in are recognized as disease fighters—like kale and broccoli,

RESTRICTING CALORIES: FOUNTAIN OF YOUTH?

There is a consensus among health professionals that avoiding obesity can help us live a long and healthy life. There is now evidence that it's possible to live longer and healthier by restricting calories. Previous studies have found that rats placed on a very low-calorie diet lived up to 30 percent longer, and scientists have been working to see if that translates to humans. In a similar study with monkeys, published in the *American Journal of Physiology,* George Roth and colleagues at the National Institutes on Aging and the Arizona Center on Aging found that a 30 percent reduction in calories led to higher levels of HDL—the "good" cholesterol that decreases the risk of heart disease. "In addition to enhanced HDL and lower triglyceride levels, we also see a small drop in blood pressure," Roth said. "My own personal belief is . . . these beneficial effects that we see in calorically restricted monkeys could be translated into people." He noted that his research could serve as a model for human studies.[2] In addition to extending longevity in many animals, studies show that caloric restriction slows age-related deficits in learning, immune response, and causes changes in the genetic expression of DNA. And, in related cancer research, calorically restricted rats and mice get fewer and/or smaller tumors than do animals that can gobble all they want, according to David Kritchevsky, the Caspar Wistar scholar at the Wistar Institute in Philadelphia.[3]

which contain phytochemicals known as *indoles,* which have been shown to protect against a variety of cancers by making dangerous toxins in the body easier to excrete. The phytochemical allium, present in garlic, lowers cholesterol.

Phytochemicals are found in micro amounts, which is why one vegetable can contain so many. Yet, despite these micro quantities, they are highly advantageous to the body. Eating one carrot, for instance, can supply the full day's dosage of the important phytochemical beta-carotene, a precursor to vitamin A. Among other things, beta-carotene helps to counterbalance the harmful effects of pollution, like cigarette smoke and other air-borne pollutants, on the body.

The moral of the phytochemical story is that your health is greatly enhanced by consuming a wide range of fruits and vegetables in a variety of colors— and the fresher and less processed, the better. That means that a raw apple is prized over processed applesauce (especially the kind with sugar added!). One of the benefits of eating fresh salads is that in one bowl you can have a banquet of gorgeous and life-saving phytochemicals. Think green (leafy vegetables, including the dark greens) . . . and red (tomatoes contain coumarins, which prevent blood clots, and lycopene—important for prostate health) . . . and orange/yellow (carrots, of course, as well as yams and squash, contain lutein, a carotenoid, which is important for the eyes) . . . and purple (purple cabbage, grapes, black raspberries) . . . and every other color! Eating a rainbow of color, you'll be enriching your body with the best medicine known to humans.

Vitamins and Minerals

Our concern about vitamins and minerals is relatively recent in human history, and new discoveries are being made all the time. If we lived more in harmony with the earth and sea, the foods we'd eat would probably supply us with all the vitamins and minerals necessary for good healthy bodies. But since we have robbed our soils of these nutrients, polluted our waters, and overprocessed our food, we must compensate for the empty calories, missing nutrients, and toxic residues of most commercial foods.

Many people therefore have learned to supplement their diets in other ways—through buying so-called "vitamin-enriched" foods, or by taking vitamins and minerals in tablet form. Paradoxically, many people prefer to eat polished (white) rice instead of brown rice, then buy bottles of B vitamins that are made from the parts removed from brown rice in the processing! You need vitamins and minerals so that your body can properly regulate its metabolic processes. In and of themselves, vitamins and minerals are not sources of energy, but they do determine and direct the ways in which ingested foods are assimilated and distributed. Minerals also provide building materials for teeth and bones.

Because each of us is different, it is impossible to set absolute standards for all. The charts in this section list the essential vitamins and minerals and tell what they are needed for and where to find them. It is important to note, however, that the minimum daily requirements (MDR) and recommended doses are merely averages. They are based on minimal amounts needed to prevent serious disease, not the amount that those seeking high-level wellness may wish to use. Also, keep in mind that while the meats, fish, grains, fruits, and vegetables listed in this table supply certain vitamins and minerals, you should always seek out foods that are organically grown or farmed, to avoid toxicity.

VITAMIN AND MINERAL SUMMARY

The following listings present information about vitamins and important minerals, including their sources in foods, details of toxicity, consequences of deficiency in each substance, and recommended daily allowances (RDA) for adults (and some for children). Since the need for vitamins and minerals varies tremendously from individual to individual and from day to day, these figures are only approximations and statistical averages. An RDA for one person may be too much or too little for another.

Water-Soluble Vitamins

All B vitamins: B_1, B_2, B_3, B_5, B_6, B_{12}, biotin, folic acid
Vitamin C

Fat-Soluble Vitamins

Vitamin A
Vitamin D
Vitamin E
Vitamin K

Antioxidant Vitamins

Vitamin A
Vitamin C
Vitamin E
Beta-carotene

WATER-SOLUBLE VITAMINS

Vitamin B_1 (thiamine)

NONTOXIC

DEFICIENCY
Causes a disease called beriberi, which affects the function of the nervous system and the heart; found in cultures that eat a lot of polished rice.

RDA
Adult: 0.5 mg/1000 kcal per day
Elderly: 1.0 mg/1000 kcal per day
Pregnancy/lactation: 1.5 mg/1000 kcal per day

SOURCES
lean pork, wheat germ, liver, poultry, egg yolks, fish, dry beans, cereals, whole-grain breads

Vitamin B_2 (riboflavin)

NONTOXIC

DEFICIENCY
Causes angular stomatitis—dry cracking of the corners of the mouth—along with skin lesions (sores).

RDA
All ages: 0.6 mg/1000 kcal
Pregnancy: 0.3 mg extra
Lactation: 0.5 mg extra

SOURCES
Widely distributed in small amounts:
Excellent: organ meats, milk, cheese, eggs, green leafy vegetables
Good: whole grains, legumes, nutritional yeast

NOTE
Ratio of B_1:B_2 should be close to 1:1

Vitamin B_3 (niacin)

NONTOXIC

DEFICIENCY
Causes a disease called pellagra that affects the skin, nervous system, and intestinal tract; occurs primarily when a diet consists largely of corn (maize).

RDA
Based on a unit called the Niacin Equivalent (NE)
Average person eating approx. 2000 kcal requires:
Males: 13–14 NE/day
Females: 14–18 NE/day
Pregnancy: 20 NE/day

SOURCES
Best: organ meats, nutritional yeast, peanut butter
Good: meat, poultry, fish

(continued)

Vitamin B$_5$ (pantothenic acid)

NONTOXIC
Aids in the production of adrenal hormones.

DEFICIENCY
Causes stomachache and burning feet.

RDA
Adults: 4–7 mg/kg
Pregnancy/lactation: no evidence that more is needed

SOURCES
Present in all plant and animal tissues
Best: eggs, liver, salmon, whole-grain cereals

Vitamin B$_6$ (pyridoxine)

NONTOXIC
Involved in more bodily functions than any other single nutrient.

DEFICIENCY
Rare, because B$_6$ is found in most foods.

RDA
Related to protein intake
Males: 2.2 mg/day
Females: 2.0 mg/day
Children: 35–50% above adult needs
Increased requirements in pregnancy, oral contraceptive users, elderly, cardiac failure patients, chronic alcoholics

SOURCES
Best: nutritional yeast, wheat germ, pork, glandular meats, cereals, legumes
Poor: milk, eggs, fruits, vegetables

Vitamin B$_{12}$ (cobolamin)

NONTOXIC

DEFICIENCY
Causes anemia—*vegetarians are particularly susceptible to B$_{12}$ deficiency and must therefore either make an effort to eat foods that contain it or take supplements.*

RDA
Adults: 2.0 μg/day
Pregnancy/lactation: 2.6 μg/day

SOURCES
Excellent: liver, kidney, lean meats
Good: raw (unpasteurized) milk, eggs, fish, cheese
Poor: pasteurized or evaporated milk

Biotin (a B vitamin)

NONTOXIC
Helps metabolize fats and carbohydrates.

DEFICIENCY
Causes decreased immunity but this is rare, because it can be manufactured in the intestinal tract from food.

RDA
30–100 μg/day

SOURCES
cooked egg yolks, kidney, liver, mushrooms, nuts, nutritional yeast

Folic acid

NONTOXIC

DEFICIENCY
Causes megaloblastic anemia, in which red blood cells are oversized and do not transport oxygen properly.

RDA
Adults: 180–200 μg/day
Pregnancy: 400 μg/day

SOURCES
Excellent: dark green leafy vegetables, spinach, broccoli, liver, kidney, lima beans
Good: lean beef, potatoes, whole-wheat bread
Poorer: most meats, milk, eggs, most fruits

Vitamin C (ascorbic acid)

NONTOXIC
Used in the formation of collagen, which is required for wound healing, ligament repair, and so on.

DEFICIENCY
Causes scurvy—internal bleeding, weak bones and teeth.

RDA
Adult: 60 mg/day
Infant: 35 mg/day for first year
Children under 11 years: 45 mg/day
Older children: up to 60 mg/day
Pregnancy: 80 mg/day
Lactation: 110 mg/day

SOURCES
citrus fruits, raw green vegetables, tomatoes, kiwi

FAT-SOLUBLE VITAMINS

Vitamin A (retinol)

TOXIC
Causes spleen enlargement, headache, peeling skin.

DEFICIENCY
Causes night blindness.

RDA
Men: 1000 RE*/day
Women: 800 RE/day
Children: 400–700 RE/day
Pregnancy: 1300 RE/day
Lactation: 1100–1200 RE/day
*NOTE: 1 Retinol Equivalent (RE) = 1 µg retinol or 6 µg beta-carotene

SOURCES
Retinol: storage organs (liver, kidney), fish oils, animal fats
Beta-Carotene (which most people can convert to retinol): dark green leafy vegetables, yellow vegetables, yellow and orange fruit (other than oranges)

Vitamin E (tocopherol)

NOT LIKELY TO BE TOXIC

DEFICIENCY
Causes many conditions, including decreased circulation, slow tissue healing, and leg cramps.

RDA
Males: 10 mg alpha TE/day
Females: 8 mg alpha TE/day

SOURCES
wheat germ oil, soybean oil, corn oil, leafy green vegetables

Vitamin D (D_2 and D_3)

TOXIC

DEFICIENCY
Causes rickets in children and osteomalacia in adults. Both are bone-softening disorders that cause bones to be malformed. Vitamin D helps bring calcium into bones to make them strong.

RDA
Adults: 5 µg/day (200 IU) 1 IU = .025 µg
Children: 10 µg/day
Pregnancy/lactation: 10 µg/day

SOURCES
The skin is a major source, as a compound in the skin is converted by sunlight into vitamin D. Sources also include nutritional yeast, fish liver oils, and fortified milk.

(continued)

Vitamin K

TOXIC

Used to make blood-clotting factors.

DEFICIENCY

Causes defective coagulation (clotting) of blood.

RDA

Males: approx. 80 µg/day
Females: approx. 65 µg/day
Infant formulas should contain 4 µg/100 kcal

SOURCES

Up to 50% comes from bacterial synthesis in the gut. Food sources include cabbage, spinach, broccoli, lettuce, cheese, egg yolks

IMPORTANT MINERALS

Calcium

NONTOXIC

Only 25%–35% absorbed from diet.

DEFICIENCY

Causes weak bones, bad teeth, muscle spasms.

RDA

Age	Male	Female
8–11	800 mg	900 mg
12–24	1200 mg	1200 mg
>24	800 mg	800 mg
Postmenopause		1200 mg

SOURCES

milk, cheese, yogurt, broccoli, spinach, turnips, beans, almonds

Phosphorus

WELL ABSORBED

(60%–65%)

DEFICIENCY

Causes irritability, weakness, blood-cell disorders.

RDA

Same as for calcium.

SOURCES

Occurs naturally in dairy and meat products; also found in processed food and as a preservative in soft drinks.

NOTE

It is important to understand that phosphorus binds with calcium in the blood and is excreted as a waste product. This causes more calcium to be drawn out of the bones to keep blood levels of calcium at normal levels. Excess phosphorus in the blood can therefore lead to weakened bones. The average North American diet has four times the required phosphorus! This is largely due to the amount of phosphorus found in processed foods and soft drinks, which are overconsumed in our society. It is also worth noting that some experts debate whether or not the calcium found in dairy products is of any use to the body because the naturally occurring phosphorus in these products may simply bind with the calcium, leaving it inactive.

Iron

TOXIC

DEFICIENCY

Causes anemia due to decreased red blood cells and hemoglobin.

RDA

Males: 10 mg/day
Females: 15–18 mg/day
Infants: 10–15 mg/day
Children: 15–18 mg/day

SOURCES

Best: liver
Next Best: oysters, shellfish, kidney, meat, poultry

Magnesium

Important because it is used in all living cells.

DEFICIENCY
Causes neuromuscular irritability.

RDA
Males: 350 mg/day
Females: 300 mg/day
Pregnancy/lactation: 450 mg/day

SOURCES
widely distributed, part of chlorophyll in green vegetables, found in cocoa, nuts, cereals, grains, meat (best source), milk, seafood

Zinc

Aids in collagen formation and therefore wound healing, as well as enhancing the immune system to help fight infections. Excess causes intestinal upset.

DEFICIENCY
Causes growth retardation.

RDA
Males: 15 mg/day
Females: 12 mg/day
Pregnancy: extra 5 mg
Lactation: extra 10 mg

SOURCES
Better: wheat germ, lima beans
Good: meat, liver, eggs, seafood (oysters)

Sodium

Necessary for many cellular metabolic functions; excess causes water retention, high blood pressure in susceptible individuals only.

RDA
Adults: 1100–2400 mg/day
Children: lower

SOURCES
seasoning used in cooking and processing, protein foods, some antacids

Potassium

Necessary for many cellular metabolic functions.

DEFICIENCY
Causes cardiac disturbances.

RDA
none; safe/average level is 0.8–1.5 g/1000 kcal
(or 2000 mg/day)

SOURCES
Best: apricots, cantaloupes, honeydew melons
Good: bananas, fruit juices, dried beans, legumes, nuts
Adequate: milk, meat, cereals

4.2 **Food Supplements**

What vitamin or mineral supplements should you take? Granted, it can seem confusing, even overwhelming at first. Yet, with a little time and effort you can find out what you need and supply it. Start by consulting your healthcare professional, especially if you have a condition that requires careful monitoring. Speak to those who work in the field. With health-food stores and huge whole-food supermarkets continuing to spread in towns and cities all over North America and in Europe, there are many knowledgeable individuals available to assist you in your quest for the right products. Books on the subject are numerous, and Internet sources can be most valuable, as long as you are careful to sort out the sales pitches from the information. Rather than trying to supply yourself with each element individually, which can be dangerous, look for a balanced multivitamin and mineral complex supplement, or *superfood* complex, to give you the support that may be missing from your diet. In the last few years, Regina has replaced nearly all her vitamin and mineral pills with one powdered green superfood mixture added to fruit juice once a day. This product alone supplies her with a unique blend of vitamins, minerals, and other phytochemicals, specially formulated for women of her age range.

Don't forget that foods should be your main source of phytochemicals, vitamins, and minerals. An important factor in getting vitamins from your vegetables is the preparation method you choose. The heat of boiling destroys most vitamins; the rest are dissolved in the water, which is usually just thrown away. Eating your vegetables raw would ensure that you get maximum value from them. But since most of us are used to having our string beans cooked, we suggest lightly steaming or stir-frying to preserve as many essential vitamins as possible.

As for minerals, many of us are unaware of how essential they are. Even fewer people know that we need not only the familiar major minerals, like calcium, phosphorus, and zinc, but trace minerals as well. In recent years, trace minerals (like selenium) have been cited for their powerful cancer-fighting abilities, as well as in their role as facilitators of other minerals (calcium's absorption and usability multiplies in the presence of the trace mineral boron). Both major minerals and trace minerals are available in fresh fruits and vegetables; in this form they are highly available to the body, although when cooked they become less so.

It is possible to get too much of a good thing, however. Salt (sodium chloride), for instance, is an essential mineral. It occurs naturally in vegetables, grains, and meats—in nearly all the foods we eat. Because of its flavor-enhancing qualities, and because we have dulled our taste buds through misuse, we have been adding more and more salt to our foods—and thereby consuming ever-increasing quantities. This abuse has been found to cause an increase in blood pressure and hypertension in some people, and is thought to encourage heart disease and migraine headache in others. In general, the path of wellness is one of balance, so megadosing with some vitamin or mineral is rarely wise unless you are under the care of a health professional. Even then, trust your intuition about what feels good to you and keep your doctor or caregiver informed of your reactions.

4.3 Antioxidants

Certain vitamins and minerals, along with numerous phytochemicals, are often given another fancy name—antioxidant—based in their ability to prevent certain types of harmful oxidation (such as peroxidation; see module 4.15) in the body. Excessive peroxidation results in premature aging as well as an overall weakening of the body, leading to disease. Antioxidants are receiving a lot of attention for their cancer-fighting ability, but equally because our youth-obsessed culture wants to keep looking good.

At present, the big three antioxidants are vitamins A, C, and E, but hundreds of lesser-known phytochemical substances also have strong antioxidant properties. Antioxidants are needed to balance out the wild activity of "free radicals"—not some holdover from the 1960s, but a molecule containing an oxygen atom with an unpaired electron inside it. As it tries to find a mate for its lonely electron, that particular oxygen molecule will often behave in a violent fashion, bashing around among other molecules looking for Mr. (or Ms.) Right. (This drive for relationship can make people *and* electrons act in strange and unpredictable ways.) Antioxidants neutralize free radicals, which is why they are known affectionately as "free radical scavengers."

In an ideal world, you wouldn't need to be concerned about free radicals getting out of control. Your body would handle them naturally, and you would age "normally." But today we are literally bombarded with arsenals of free radicals generated by air pollution, cigarette smoke, ultraviolet light from the sun through the damaged ozone layer, and pesticides and other contaminants in our food. Other sneak attacks of free radicals occur if we eat foods fried in fats and junk foods of all types.

We can supplement our diet with antioxidant substances (vitamins A, C, and E) or increase our consumption of fresh foods that are particularly high in antioxidant phytochemicals, especially fresh fruits and vegetables—or do both.

ANTIOXIDANTS TO THE RESCUE

The first scientific discovery of the link between the antioxidant vitamin C and the condition of scurvy was made by the Scottish physician James Lind in 1753. In those days, when sailors set out to sea their rations comprised salted beef, biscuits, and water. Frequently they would develop weakness, swollen and bleeding gums, their teeth would drop out, joints would swell, old wounds would reopen and eventually many died. "Scurvy," as this condition was called, became the major cause of death at sea. Lind maintained that the cure for this disease was lime juice and, following his recommendations, sailors began to take provisions of limes on their long voyages. The British Navy finally issued general orders to provide lime juice (as well as rum) to its sailors in 1795, hence the generic term for the English as "Limeys." Sailors of other nations only gained parity by the mid-nineteenth century.

Hasnain Walji, *Live Longer, Live Healthier: The Practical Handbook of Antioxidants* (Hohm Press, 1996).

PRESERVING THE MAXIMAL ANTIOXIDANT CONTENT OF FOODS

In *The Antioxidant Revolution,* Kenneth Cooper, M.D., tells exactly how to preserve as many of the vital antioxidants (and, therefore, most other vital functional components) as possible by keeping the following points in mind in food preparation. Food expert Lalitha Thomas summarizes his suggestions and adds a bit more:

- Avoid wilted produce and *do not buy* precut produce.

- Don't trim off or discard the highly useful and edible skins, outer leaves, and so on. Eat them as part of the dish you are preparing. Exceptions to this are nonorganic produce that cannot be cleaned of offending chemical coatings, such as the skins of waxed apples and cucumbers. For nonorganic produce, make a case-by-case judgment on this "to trim or not to trim" question, depending on how effective you think the cleaning methods have been and how offending some of the coatings are. Waxed coatings should be trimmed off.

- Don't cook foods with the "swimming in water" methods. Use as little water as needed, or use a steamer basket that holds foods up out of the water, thereby keeping the nutrition in the food instead of in the cooking water, which is often thrown away. Add any leftover cooking water back to the food whenever possible— it contains antioxidants!

- Avoid excessive heat in cooking. Long boiling or other extended cooking, and exposure of foods to flame or smoke can damage antioxidants. Do not fry foods.

- Use the syrups or liquids that result from thawing frozen foods.

- Do not refrigerate once-cooked foods for more than a day, and always store them in airtight containers.

- Try not to reheat once-cooked fruit or vegetable dishes.

- Avoid keeping foods warm for more than thirty minutes before you serve them, as antioxidants are being lost increasingly with this passage of time.

- Do not hold fresh produce in your refrigerator for more than a few days, and certainly not longer than a week. Buying frozen fruits and vegetables is a better choice if you think you won't consume the fresh produce within a few days of purchase.

Lalitha Thomas, *10 Essential Foods* (Hohm Press, 1997). Used with permission.

4.4 Water

Sometimes the water in my house can taste weird, so it makes me wonder if there isn't something else in it that shouldn't be there.

—Pittsburgh-area high school student

The need for water in the human body is absolutely critical. The human body is 70 percent water, and the brain alone is 75 percent water. We rely upon water for digestion, cooling the body, elimination, and, of course, the circulation of nutrients to every cell. Failure to replenish the supply will mean death. Your need for water is clear.

The exact amounts of water required daily will vary depending upon the foods you eat, the temperature and humidity of the air, the amount of exercise you do, and your individual rate of metabolism. (Some of us just sweat more than others!) As a general recommendation, drinking six to eight glasses of water a day is a good habit to acquire. We also get water by eating solid foods (some of which, like lettuce, tomatoes, and watermelons, are more than 90 percent water), and some from body cells as a by-product of metabolism.

In general, however, most people don't drink enough pure water, relying instead on other liquids—especially coffee, tea, and soft drinks, many of which contain sugar and caffeine, which actually have a dehydrating effect. After drinking these beverages, the body requires more water to aid in their metabolism. Many common health problems would be eased or remedied if we kept ourselves better hydrated. Headaches, irritability, and constipation are just a few of the conditions that point to the need for more water. Sports enthusiasts know the necessity of keeping hydrated as they exercise, and travel pros will tell you that drinking lots of water is one of the primary means of preventing jet lag as you fly across time zones.

Water *quality*, however, is another problem. Most of our waterways and much of our groundwater is now contaminated from thoughtless practices. Safety standards for tap water focus on bacterial contamination, which is controlled by adding chlorine. These standards were set decades ago, before the massive discharge of toxic heavy metals and organic industrial or agricultural byproducts into the environment. We now find toxic pollutants such as lead, asbestos, and mercury in the water. As a result, urban tap water is unfit to drink in many communities across North America, Europe, and other parts of the world as well. Because large amounts of water are filtered through our bodies, even small traces of these toxins will accumulate over time. There are now private companies that will test your water quality for a reasonable fee.

Even many bottled waters are not as pure as the bottlers would have you believe, and if the waters were pure when bottled, the plastic solvents that leach from the bottle into the water are seldom measured. A high-quality water filter is probably the most reliable source of pure water, but read the manufacturer's specifications closely, as there are many types. Reverse osmosis (RO) processing seems to be the water-safety system of choice among discriminating water connoisseurs. Since water is the most important substance you take into your body, it's doubly important that you pay close attention to what else is in the water available to you and select accordingly.

4.5 **Our First Food**

We learned about food long before we ever started feeding ourselves. In fact, our concern with food began even before we were born. So let's go back to the beginning—to that tiny mass of protoplasm within the uterus, sustained by the nutrients in the mother's blood, awaiting its entry into the big world outside.

Until its birth, the fetus is warm, secure, and totally dependent for all its needs, which nature so generously fills. This is not to say, however, that it is *completely* safe. Mother's diet and mental state are subtly exerting their influence upon the unborn child. The mother's food needs to be rich in the vitamins, minerals, and phytochemicals essential to growth, and unadulterated by harmful substances and contaminants that may retard the normal development of the vulnerable fetus.

Once it arrives on the scene at birth, the child spends the first months of life in two basic activities—sleeping and eating. The quality of its food is of great importance, not only in keeping it alive and well *now,* but in setting the stage for later eating habits. Equally important is the way food is supplied. Traumatic or unsatisfying feeding experiences may color the infant's view of the world and have far-reaching effects upon its physical and mental health.

We know that breast-fed babies evidence strong advantages over bottle-fed infants. Breast-fed children have significantly fewer respiratory infections, conditions such as asthma and hay fever, gastrointestinal problems, and skin disorders such as eczema.[4] Joseph Chilton Pearce, in *The Magical Child Matures,* reports that chemicals found in mother's milk are actually necessary to stimulate midbrain functions that regulate certain aspects of intelligence. At the National Institutes of Health, researchers followed 855 children from birth to school age and found that the longer a child had been breast-fed, the smarter and more coordinated he or she was.[5] This may be due as much to the touch and nurturance involved in breast-feeding as to the nutritional value of mother's milk. More than milk is needed to satisfy hunger.

What you are *really* looking for is not in here.

—Sign on a refrigerator door

As we learned in the last chapter, the intimate association between being fed and being cared for is realized very early in life. Need satisfaction and food are joined so strongly that the union endures throughout our development and into adulthood. And so, at age eighteen, or thirty-two, or fifty-five, sitting in your chair reading this book, you are a complex network of needs and assets. Your hunger may be for security, for companionship, or for self-worth, but the easiest and quickest source of satisfaction will probably be food.

4.6 Food as a Pain Reliever

Many of us have learned to use food to alleviate physical pain. Recall for a moment a typical scene. Jenny is riding her tricycle on the sidewalk; the wheel hits a bump and she topples to the ground, crying. Dad rushes from the house and gathers her up in his arms, kissing her baby tears and consoling, "There, there now, don't cry, you're all right. Come inside and I'll give you a piece of candy."

For a long time, big people have been trying to convince children that vaccinations, vitamins, spinach, and lots of other things will not hurt or taste bad, provided that they are quickly accompanied by a lollipop or chocolate bar. We have been programmed from our earliest years to use food to deal with pain.

While some adults who experience migraine headaches lose their appetites during an episode, Regina found that she actually ate more. "Eating may have been simply a good distraction," she explained, "but I really felt an alleviation of pain when I was eating." In fact, there seems to be a physiological basis to this. The addiction to food appears to be linked with the release of a brain substance called *beta-endorphin,* which is governed by the pituitary gland and serves as a natural opiate that may temporarily relieve pain and stress, creating a biologically comforting effect.

4.7 Filling Up the Emptiness

Food fills up the empty spaces in the body, but not those in the mind and soul. Learning to tell the difference between "mouth hunger" and "stomach hunger" is important if you have a weight problem.

Eating out of boredom—a form of emotional pain—is one of the chief reasons for compulsive eating and poor nutrition. The work ethic and need for achievement that characterize life in contemporary culture can lead you to the conclusion that you must be "doing something" or keep busy to be of value to yourself and society. When the motivation for work or involvement wanes—due to physical exhaustion, an emotional setback, or an inability to find meaning in life—we commonly experience a sense of guilt for not being productive. Many people attempt to resolve this condition by eating.

Time and again in the classes and workshops that we conducted, we would hear stories like these:

"My problems with overeating started when my last child went off to school."

"I'm eating a lot of junk food lately, but I'm under a lot of emotional stress. Since I lost my job, I'm bored."

Deborah, who conducts weight-awareness seminars for women, has found that many people eat to gain weight so that they will have something tangible to work at—that is, trying to *lose* weight. No one makes this a conscious plan—but the pattern is common enough that she believes it is a real one. She personalizes it this way: "If I wasn't on a diet, what else would I have to do?" or "If I ever reached my ideal weight and found that I still wasn't happy—what would I do then?"

I was bulimic for fourteen years. Today I am free of this destructive binge-purge cycle and have been for over twenty years. My recovery began when I made a commitment to myself—to do whatever it took to stop this obsession that kept me hating myself and feeling powerless.

In 1981, treatment centers for this eating disorder were unknown to me, so it was a lot harder to get help than it is today. I created a support system by deciding to write my master's thesis on the recovery from bulimia. I interviewed therapists and recovering bulimics. Talking to women who were farther along the path of recovery inspired me to keep going even when I felt scared and hopeless. One person in particular I'll never forget—a woman who had hidden her binge-purge behavior from her husband and children for twenty-five years. She shared so openly, as did many others, and helped me to open to the strong part in me that knew I could and would overcome this destructive behavior.

Here are the major steps I took:

• I became ruthlessly honest with myself and everyone in my life. Basically, I stopped hiding my behavior and my feelings.

• I learned to ask for what I really wanted, and to say no to what I didn't—in my relationships and all other areas of my life.

• I realized that food and weight issues were not really about food and weight, so I attended groups and workshops to work through the underlying emotional issues— like low self-esteem, perfectionism, and a need to be in control.

• I gave up the need to be thin, and decided I'd rather be happy. (Paradoxically, after a temporary weight gain, I lost weight and have maintained it with ease.)

• I stopped looking for an external authority to tell me how to live my life (that is, what I should eat, what I should weigh, how I should act or feel) and began to look inside and trust that I had those answers for myself.

• I stopped beating up on myself when I had made a mistake.

Instead, I used my energy to learn about myself, rather than feeling wrong or guilty about my mistakes.

• I stopped being a victim, blaming circumstances and people in my life, and took responsibility for myself and my bulimia. Once I accepted that I had chosen to be bulimic, I freed myself to choose otherwise.

My life isn't problem free now by any means. But knowing that I conquered bulimia gives me courage to face any problems in my life.

If you are currently struggling to overcome any eating disorder, you need to know that *recovery is possible*. Today, most hospitals have special programs for dealing with your particular needs, and there are therapists who are trained to work with you. Please don't be ashamed to seek help. I did it. You can too.

—Jo Sherrill

4.8 Food as Emotional Insulation

Many people use food as emotional insulation to protect themselves from further hurt, or as a drug to dull the pain of a meaningless existence, a broken marriage, or the death of a loved one. When the U.S. government started giving tax breaks for insulating homes to conserve energy, it made environmentalists very happy. Many chronically overweight people have been giving themselves a "feeling" break for a long time as they pile on layer after layer of fat in an attempt to insulate their hearts, and guts, and sexual organs from emotional energy loss. But the break is only temporary and eventually leads to something worse. The real needs aren't being addressed. Cindy's story illustrates this.

Cindy gave birth to a beautiful eight-pound boy, only to learn that her child was deaf. Distraught with grief, she began to eat excessively and consequently to gain weight. Fifteen years and an extra eighty pounds or so later, she realized that she hadn't cried since "I can't remember when," her desire for sex had long since died, and her world was shaded in gray. Cindy's body had become her refuge. She had attempted to shield herself from being disappointed and hurt again, but she was far from happy. It had been an unsuccessful and costly strategy that produced new and different problems and had really not alleviated the pain.

It isn't hard to understand the lessons in Cindy's case. At some time in our lives most of us have used food to mask or alleviate pain, or as an unconscious means of punishment and self-destruction. Or we may have denied ourselves food and so diverted our attention to a new pain.

Conditions such as anorexia and bulimia are a serious health issue in Western cultures. Alarming numbers of young people, especially women, are jeopardizing their health by using food in self-destructive ways (for example, by gorging on food, then vomiting or taking laxatives) or by denying food to themselves altogether. For some, it is a misguided attempt to gain control over their lives. For others, it is an obsession with weight gain, which is considered the greatest of all evils. In nearly all cases, low self-esteem is strongly evident. The table becomes the battleground, and food, whether it is the enemy or the only trusted ally, is the one thing that matters. Needless to say, when this kind of emotional war is being waged, considerations such as nutrition or real nourishment are rarely addressed.

Still another type of eating disorder is evidenced by "nutrition addicts," who devote the greater part of their day's work to worrying about and planning the balancing of their foods. They can be found wandering the aisles of the health-food stores, diligently studying vitamin bottles; they then hurry home to administer to themselves some new intestinal cleanser. They are obsessed with "toxins" and fascinated by the consistency of their feces. This excessive concern may be temporarily necessary during certain critical periods, especially in treating serious illness, but as a way of life, it more likely indicates another obsession with food that fills time and may serve to discourage the cultivation of relationships with others and the creation of more dynamic and rewarding forms of self-expression.

4.9 Eating and Stress

In a remarkable series of books describing his training by the Yaqui sorcerer Don Juan, Carlos Castaneda describes the characteristics of the warrior, the person of power. Far from being a creature of habit at the mercy of societal convenience, the warrior is attuned to both intuition and the body's natural rhythms. Consequently, the warrior will sleep when tired, rise when rested, and eat when hungry. Certainly not dramatic prescriptions, but difficult for most of us to follow nonetheless.

In contrast, we generally eat from 12 to 1 because that's when lunch hour on the job is scheduled , or eat dinner at 6:30 because that's when the *News at Six* is over—paying little attention to whether we are hungry or not at those times. The whole scene is strongly reminiscent of Pavlov's dogs, who were conditioned to salivate at the sound of a bell.

The demands of a job, a school schedule, or child-rearing frequently necessitate altering our mealtimes accordingly. In order to get our kids to their soccer practice on time or get ourselves to work on time, we may eat too quickly. Have you ever seen a pie-eating contest? Definitely not an aesthetic experience! While most of us will probably never qualify for the national teams, the speed with which we empty our plates or finish off our lunches might indicate that we are in training for some degree of fast-eating competition.

Never eat more than you can lift.

—Miss Piggy

When you eat rapidly so as not to miss your plane, your history class, or your favorite TV program, you put yourself under time pressure, which creates stress throughout your body. The body, in its natural wisdom, will generate a variety of hormonal secretions, as well as increase both heart rate and respiration, to attempt to cope with the situation. Eating in this condition will result in any number of sorry effects, including indigestion and acid reflux. The remedy for this, offered by high-pressure advertising, is to consume a candy or liquid preparation that "reduces excess stomach acid." Thus relieved, you can continue the practice that got you into trouble in the first place. The American way really does support "a pill for every ill."

Speed-eating further subjects us to the risk of choking on our food, since we don't take the time to chew it properly. Choking is currently the sixth highest cause of accidental death in the United States

Regina grew up in a large family and remembers well the humorous grace before meals in which she prayed: "Father, Son, and Holy Ghost; the one who eats fastest gets the most." While we are on the subject of childhood memories, picture, for a moment, the family gathered around the dinner table. The TV sitcoms and romantic novels suggest that they are discussing what the children learned in school today, the literary merits of a current best seller, or plans for the summer vacation. More realistically, if they eat together at all, they may spend mealtimes watching high-speed car chases on the television, arguing over whose turn it is to do the dishes, or worrying about whether the money will hold out long enough to get the car repaired or the phone bill paid. Sound familiar? It certainly doesn't make for relaxed, aware eating.

Since mealtimes provide some of the rare occasions for getting together with loved ones, and can be tax write-offs for business, they are often used as opportunities to discuss "big deals" or to deal with problems. Handling hassles over lunch is an effective way to increase stress and give yourself an upset stomach.

Where you eat can also contribute to stress. The availability of fast food has made it possible to buy and consume a meal without ever leaving your car. Simply driving your car through the city, or on freeways, in so many places in the United States today can be a very taxing experience. Eating your meals while doing so rings the bell at the top of the stress scale. The food served at fast-food establishments are usually highly refined, filled with sugar and chemical preservatives, and loaded with unnecessary fat, which makes it even worse.

CHANGES IN U.S. DIETARY PATTERNS

Figures provided by the University of California and the USDA give a startling overview of the changes in the amounts of items commonly consumed by Americans between 1970 and 1996:

- 35 percent less coffee
- 23 percent less eggs
- 22 percent less beverage milk
- 15 percent less red meat
- 17 percent more alcoholic beverages
- 21 percent more fats and oils
- 23 percent more fruits and vegetables
- 24 percent more caloric sweeteners (includes caloric sweeteners used in soft drinks)

- 26 percent more fish
- 46 percent more flour and cereal products
- 90 percent more poultry
- 114 percent more carbonated soft drinks
- 143 percent more cheese

Keep in mind that these figures may be deceiving. They do not indicate the form in which the fruits and vegetables are consumed. If "vegetables" are consumed as tomato sauce that is topped by thick slices of high-fat, high-protein cheese, or as potato chips or fries washed down with carbonated soft drinks, although they may provide some benefit, the detrimental effect is far greater. The same disclaimer applies to the consumption of poultry. Eating more chicken rather than red meat is one thing, but eating more batter-covered, deep-fried chicken may defeat the purpose of cutting down on red meat.

As a population we seem to be in a period of profound media-driven dietary confusion. While some statistics would indicate that we are making positive choices, the growing rates of chronic illness and obesity cannot be denied.

U.S. Department of Agriculture, *Agriculture Fact Book 1998*, www.usda.gov/news/pubs/fbook98/afb98.pdf.

4.10 We Forget Our Uniqueness

We have relinquished self-responsibility and awareness in our eating habits as we have in so many other areas of our lives. Few people are in touch with themselves and knowledgeable enough about their own metabolism to design their own nutritional programs. We therefore follow patterns we learned as children, or the recommendations of "experts," or the lead assumed by the advertising media. Because nutritional education is filled with talk of "norms," "minimum daily requirements," "average weights," and "ideal diets," it is easy to become confused and forget our uniqueness.

If you watch what people eat and observe their resulting bodies, you soon realize that what works for one may be the downfall of the other. One friend consumes huge quantities, has tremendous energy, rarely gets sick, and never gains weight. Another generally eats sparingly and yet constantly battles overweight. A chronically overweight woman complains that she merely has to drive past a bakery shop and she puts on a few extra pounds!

The realization that differences exist in the ways our bodies metabolize food was offered by Dr. George Watson of the University of Southern California in the 1960s, when he observed the different effects that foods had on people's emotions.[6] Around the same time, Roger J. Williams, Ph.D., was developing his similar theories expressed in his book *Biochemical Individuality*. Williams remarks: "If normal facial features varied as much as gastric juices do, some of our noses would be about the size of navy beans while others would be the size of twenty-pound watermelons."

Williams believes that we all come into life with unique biochemical needs that can be met only with a proper balance of nutrients. Failure to supply these nutrients in the right amounts results in disease.

Furthermore, what is excessive for one may be insufficient for another. According to Williams, there is no such thing as the "average" man or woman.

Our metabolic needs are all subject to periodic fluctuations as well. The change from summer to winter, falling in love, preparing for a crucial exam, the death of a dear one—each of these factors will alter the body's chemistry and motivate a change in eating habits. Yet these factors are rarely appreciated and honored. Our diets are imbalanced because we often don't know *what* we really need. The paradox is that few of us give our automobiles as little preventive care as we give our bodies.

Every age and culture has had its ways of classifying bodies and personalities: the ecto-, endo-, and mesomorphs . . . the phlegmatics and sanguines . . . the type As and the type Bs . . . Metabolism Type 1 through Metabolism Type 10. True to form, this interest in "types" found expression in various approaches to diet throughout the 1990s, and the movement continues today. Following upon the popularity of books by pioneer Vasant Lad, M.D., and Deepak Chopra, M.D., the ancient Indian science of Ayurveda has been receiving widespread public interest. According to this system, individuals are designated according to one of three principles—*vata, pitta,* and *kapha*—and advised to eat foods that support that principle. In 1996, Peter D'Adamo, M.D., author of *Eat Right 4 Your Type,* presented a somewhat revolutionary approach to dieting determined by blood type. He made a persuasive argument that your blood type is an evolutionary marker that tells you which foods you'll process best and which will be useless calories. The book became an overnight sensation. While there are many serious critics of his program and the research that supports it, there are also numerous testimonies to its lifesaving values.

Another response to this need for individualization has been the introduction of the personalized health plan, the personally designed diet, the nutritional analysis, the metabolic profile. Far from being satisfied with recommending calorie limits based on sex and weight, many of these methods use in-depth surveys to determine lifestyle factors that affect nutritional needs. Others test pulse rate, saliva, blood, hair, and urine.[7]

These trends, aside from confirming that we humans are fascinated with technology and with putting ourselves into categories, indicate a positive and growing appreciation for the needs of individuals. Any viable system, including those advanced in this book, must offer a wide range of tolerance. No matter how much an approach to nutrition may have served me personally, my dietary successes are based on my own needs and experiences and *will not* work for everybody.

4.11 Eating "Junk"

The problems with what we eat are many. As a population, we eat a lot of "junk," or empty calories. We eat highly processed foods, chemical additives, irradiated and genetically altered foods, "bad" fats . . . and more. This module, and modules 4.12 through 4.16, will elaborate on these issues.

Snacking and eating out, particularly at fast-food restaurants, have become great American pastimes, indicative not only of our love for burgers, tacos, and pizza, but also of a lifestyle shift in the population at large. Just take a trip to your local shopping mall and watch how many people walk along with food or drinks in hand. Many malls also have food courts in which one can purchase a slice of pizza, a deep-fried egg roll, a corn dog, and a sugar-filled frozen yogurt cone and consider that a "meal." In addition, modern food processing methods, such as milling, lead to nutritionally empty foods. While we may be eating more grain-based foods today than we did in 1975—which sounds positive at first hearing—many of these "grains" are actually white-flour breads, pastas, and pizza crusts, or tortillas and corn chips. When these highly-processed foods are covered with melted cheese, moreover, they fill us up but don't necessarily do us a lot of good. As to fat consumption, we have cut our consumption of red meat significantly since the 1970s, but we have turned to another high-fat source as our substitute. During the 1970s, the average American consumed ten pounds of cheese per year. Today, the average American consumes more than thirty pounds of cheese per year. Twenty more pounds and a 200 percent increase! In general, even though vast segments of the population are always "on a diet," we are eating slightly more food—around three hundred additional calories per day—than we did in 1975. While that may not sound like a big increase, it is compounded by the fact that we are exercising less.

4.12 Chemical Additives

Highly processed foods typically abound in chemical additives, preservatives, and sugar—and over the years some researchers have claimed a link between food additives and hyperactivity in children. The average adult in America eats approximately ten pounds of these chemicals each year. Currently, more than 1,300 of these substances are approved by the FDA for use as colors, flavors, preservatives, and thickeners. Some have been rigorously tested, others far less. Almost daily, the observant reader can find reference to studies linking one or another of these additives with cancer of some sort.

As long as we demand a convenience-store diet of pink cupcakes with yellow cream filling, there will be little chance of curtailing the use of these substances in our food. Necessity is one thing, as in the use of small amounts of nitrates to control bacterial growth in meat. But commercial gimmickry is another. Stroll down the breakfast cereal aisle of your local food store and observe that you can now feed yourself and your children chocolate cereals and purple and pink puffs that taste like blueberry muffins or strawberry shortcake, while the fine print reads, "artificially flavored."

Match the "Food" with Its Ingredients

1. Fruit drink mix _____

2. Instant tomato soup _____

3. Instant mashed potatoes _____

4. Diet soft drink _____

5. Non-dairy coffee creamer _____

6. Canned dog food _____

7. Canned cake frosting _____

A. Corn syrup solids, hydrogenated coconut oil, lactose, sodium caseinate, dipotassium phosphate, mono- and diglycerides, sodium silico aluminate, artificial colors, lecithin, artificial flavor.

B. Potato flakes, mono- and diglycerides, sodium acid pyrophosphate, sodium sulphites, citric acid, BHA, BHT.

C. Sugar, dried tomato, modified corn starch, salt, hydrogenated cottonseed and soy oils, natural flavors, dried onion, lactose, dried garlic, artificial flavor, sodium caseinate, monosodium glutamate, dipotassium phosphate, soy flour, artificial color, chicken fat, dried chicken meat, thiamine hydrochloride, disodium inosinate and disodium guanylate, turmeric, spices.

D. Citric acid, monocalcium phosphate, artificial flavor, vitamin C, artificial color, BHA.

E. Sugar, hydrogenated vegetable oils, BHA, BHT, water, corn syrup, cocoa processed with alkali, salt, natural and artificial flavors, wheat starch, polysorbate 60, citric acid, potassium sorbate, lecithin, cellulose gum.

F. Carbonated water, caramel color, phosphoric acid, sodium saccharin, sodium citrate, caffeine, natural flavor, citric acid.

G. Meat by-products, chicken parts, poultry by-products, wheat flour, soy flour, whole egg, salt, dried yeast.

Answers: 1D, 2C, 3B, 4F, 5A, 6G, 7E

4.13 Chemically Contaminated, Irradiated, Genetically Modified Food

Since fresh, unprocessed foods spoil more quickly than processed, preserved foods, high nutritional value is at cross-purposes with the goals of today's food industry. Our present economic system of food production, transportation, and distribution makes ease of shipping and long shelf life its most important considerations. Not only are foods grown in depleted soils enriched with chemical fertilizers, they are heavily sprayed to avoid insect attack and spoilage from molds. In preparing foods for the grocery produce department, moreover, the industry again sprays, waxes, and sometimes irradiates our fruits and vegetables, all in an attempt to retard spoilage and increase eye appeal. Consumers would rather have a bright orange–colored "orange" that has been dyed orange, rather than eat a lighter-colored orange with more true orange taste that is free of additives and preservatives. People are turned off by the sight of a non–chemically treated apple with a tiny brown spot, preferring instead to buy a picture-perfect fruit that has been waxed and polished—and tastes it. These waxes on our apples and cucumbers are actually *plastics,* which cannot be removed and can never be digested. You must peel them to remove them. But even peeling them doesn't remove the toxins that have seeped through the skin into the fruits or vegetables themselves.

According to the U.S. Environmental Protection Agency (EPA), continued exposure to the pesticides and insecticides commonly used in commercial farming today causes cancer, birth defects, nerve damage, and genetic mutations. Also according to the EPA, 60 percent of all herbicides, 90 percent of all fungicides, and 30 percent of all insecticides used in nonorganic food are carcinogenic. As the USDA

offers plans to irradiate more types of foods, the debate over the potential for mutagenic effects caused by radiation of meat, seafood, and vegetables continues to rage. Large food industries tend to favor such processes, because radiation increases shelf life. But many citizen action groups and consumer protection agencies in both the United States and Europe have protested, claiming that irradiated foods pose a serious health hazard for both humans and animals.[8]

Genetically modified foods are those altered with the purpose of improving them by the introduction of specific genes, rather than by the more lengthy process of selective breeding. While some forms may be relatively harmless, others sound downright scary! The Monsanto Company, for example, makes an herbicide called Roundup that kills any plant it touches. This would create a problem in farming, however. So, Monsanto has genetically modified many crop plants, including soybeans, to make them "immune" to Roundup. These are called "Roundup Ready" strains. Now, the farmer can spray Roundup on everything—the genetically modified plants are unaffected.

Needless to say, this has become a highly desirable form of agriculture, as it reduces production costs and increases yield. But the long-term effects of such modifications are still unknown. The controversy continues.

Organic foods, on the other hand, are grown without pesticides or chemical fertilizers and constitute the fastest growing segment of commercial food production. Once an oddity, now organically produced foods can be found, at least in a small selection, in most supermarkets. Ounce for ounce, organic fruits and vegetables are twice as rich in certain nutrients compared to nonorganic produce, according to a recent study reported in the *Journal of Applied Nutrition*. Starting in 2002, a USDA Organic label began appearing on foods offered in markets. Choosing this label is a vote against genetically modified foods and toxic pesticides and a vote for reducing environmental pollution and supporting healthy farms, farm workers, and our own and our children's health.

The difference in taste between organically and chemically produced food can be extraordinary. If you don't believe it, test it for yourself.

4.14 Caffeine Addicts

Caffeinated beverages and foods cause erratic blood sugar levels, and their addictive properties are well known to the user. Many people are treated for sleep disorders, anxiety, high blood pressure, and other symptoms, when a simple reduction in their caffeine intake would solve their problems. Coffee, black teas, colas, and chocolate, which are all high in caffeine, should therefore be approached with caution.

You know you are a caffeine addict if your doctor measures your heartbeat on the Richter scale.

—Anonymous

A switch to decaffeinated teas and coffees is a big improvement, but be aware that even these contain low levels of caffeine and other chemicals—so restrict your intake. The cycle of stress, leading to exhaustion, propped up by stimulants, leading to deeper levels of exhaustion is indeed a vicious one, condoned and even glorified by our culture.

The chemical brews that make soft drinks so popular can also wreak havoc with our health. These drinks are either high in sugar—offering empty calories that displace hunger for more nutritious foods—or they are laced with chemical sugar substitutes that may cause even more harm after years of consumption. And, of course, many contain caffeine as well.

---

de·caf·a·lon *n.*
The grueling event of getting through the day consuming only things that are good for you.

Many caffeine lovers today are making the switch to green tea, which supplies a much lower amount of caffeine while offering the benefits of being one of the most potent herbal antioxidants available. As already mentioned, antioxidants "eat" free radicals, thus counterbalancing their damage to the immune system.

Caffeine has been cited as a contributing factor in breast tumors and has been linked with ulcers, some birth defects, osteoporosis, and fertility problems. William Uy, Ph.D., in his book *Curing Airborne Allergies,* has found increased caffeine use to be directly connected with the increase in airborne allergies that growing numbers of the U.S. population, including children, suffer today.

4.15 We Eat Too Much "Bad" Fat

Most of us have too many of the wrong kind of fats and oils in our diet—the heavy salad dressings, the fatty hamburgers, the cheese sauces. A diet of natural whole foods would ideally contain sufficient natural fats to meet the nutritional needs of healthy individuals (from fruits and vegetables, like the oil-rich avocados and olives; grains, nuts, and seeds; and for some, fish from unpolluted waters). Even so, most of us will profit from supplemental use of the right kinds of fats and oils that are necessary for proper brain chemistry and hundreds of other essential metabolic functions.

It is therefore important to choose organic nuts, seeds, oils, and butter whenever possible because most toxins are fat-soluble and find their way into your body via dietary fats and oils. Likewise, it is important to avoid hydrogenated fats in commercial shortenings and packaged foods, which are high in trans fatty acids, as much as possible. Rancid fats and oils, including nuts and seeds—alone or mixed in cereal products, trail mixes, and treat bars—can also pose problems. Rancidity in commercially sold products like these is quite common. When extreme, rancidity produces a bitter taste, but it is often undetectable by taste.

A good source of the essential fatty acids is fresh, organic, unprocessed vegetable oils (such as flax, olive, sesame, canola and safflower oil) when used in salads and other room-temperature (or lower) recipes. But beware that these oils are fragile, go rancid quickly, and are rapidly oxidized at cooking temperatures. Despite the food industry's large marketing campaign to the contrary, at cooking temperatures the more heat-stable saturated fats—butter, coconut oil, and palm oil—produce fewer free radicals than do the vegetable oils.

One of the biggest problems with lipids (fats, oils, cholesterol, and so on), especially the unsaturated lipids, is that the fatty acids in them become oxidized very quickly on contact with oxygen, creating free radicals, as described earlier. Free radicals are molecules that lack an electron, so they will take one from whatever source they come near. Ingested free radicals will, as they circulate in your body, steal electrons from healthy cell walls, damaging them in a process called *lipid peroxidation.*

Severely peroxidized lipids reveal the smell and taste of rancidity, but at much lower levels than are detectable by our senses, the free radicals present can be destructive to tissues, accelerating the aging process.

Since many of the foods we eat are prepared long before they are purchased and consumed, the amount of free radicals potentially available in your food is significant considering the time that has elapsed since the oils were pressed, the butter churned, and so on. But it is also likely that you will increase the amount of free radicals when you cook your foods. Even if you use oils that are low in free radicals, when you put them in the frying pan, where they are exposed to both heat and oxygen, you bring on massive oxidation and free-radical production.

It's not the lipids themselves that are dangerous, but the way they have been processed. For a long time eggs were linked with a high blood cholesterol count—an erroneous connection between dietary cholesterol and the body's independent natural production of cholesterol. Soft-boiling an egg in its shell is very different from frying or scrambling it with oils in a hot skillet; during boiling, the proteins are cooked gently without ever reaching the high temperatures of a skillet's surface, where they would be exposed to hot oils and oxygen.

4.16 Problems with Protein Foods

As we approach the subject of the potential problems created by meat and the high consumption of other protein foods, we enter an area of extreme controversy. The beef, egg, and dairy industries (our main suppliers of protein foods) exercise powerful lobbies and advertising programs to keep us eating their products.

It is no secret that growth-producing hormones, chemical foods, and grains sprayed with pesticides are the daily fare of beef cattle, and that these toxic residues build up in the bodies of those of us who consume the beef. We note further that among populations whose meat consumption is high, mortality rates from a variety of cancers are correspondingly high.[9]

In the United States, the Seventh Day Adventists, a religious group whose members do not eat meat, offer living proof of the health benefits of vegetarianism. Studies in this group indicate their general health is far superior to that of the rest of the U.S. population. Obviously, meat protein is not essential.

There are other problems with the typical meat-centered diet. For one, it is heavy—that is, filling—so it discourages children and adults from eating more vegetables. It also necessitates the use of large land areas for grazing and growing food for cattle. One-half of the harvested agricultural land in the United States is planted with feed crops; 78 percent of all our grain is fed to animals. Grain fed to cattle is not being fed to people. And the world is starving. Once again, it is a question of balance.

It is paradoxical that we, who may be so cautious about taking risks in other aspects of our lives, would be willing to run such high ones when it comes to the foods we eat and feed our children. In teaching and conducting workshops, we are continually amazed at how much our students and participants know about what they shouldn't do. What is lacking is the motivation to attack the problem.

Knowing all this, we offer in module 4.17 the recommendations of the 2000 Dietary Guidelines for Americans and the Harvard Food Pyramid, a few important recommendations for pursuing personal nutritional awareness, and some encouragement to help you in your wellness process.

LOST: 22,000 SEATS IN YANKEE STADIUM!

One of the most graphic examples of increasing obesity in the United States is the disappearing seats of a famous baseball park. Yankee Stadium was built during the 1920s. It had about 82,000 seats. After remodeling during the 1970s, the seating was only 59,000. During that fifty-year period, between Babe Ruth and such baseball greats as Thurman Munson, Ron Guidry, and Reggie Jackson, the average American "bottom" had widened from fourteen inches to nineteen inches. Today, patrons at the Mickey Mantle Restaurant in New York, where a few of the original seats were installed, have found them to be a tight fit.

Charles Atwood, M.D., *A Vegetarian Doctor Speaks Out* (Hohm Press, 1998).

Americans probably eat more dairy products than any other food items except meat and refined sugar products. Millions of dollars are spent each year extolling the virtues of milk. It ranks right up there with Mom and apple pie. In some instances, though, milk itself can be harmful, and in others, problems arise from excessive intake or from the way in which it is processed.

For infants, cow's milk is a poor substitute for mother's milk. It has the wrong fat-to-protein ratio and lacks hundreds of key nutrients, enzymes, and antibodies that infants need for development. Many adults, especially those of Asian or African origin, lack the enzyme used to digest the lactose present in milk, so milk ferments in their intestines rather than being absorbed as a nutrient. The amount of phosphorus present in milk is so great that it may prevent the absorption of other minerals, such as magnesium, zinc, and copper. The milk protein casein binds up much of the iron in other foods that may be in the digestive tract (milk itself has little iron), causing iron deficiencies.

Beyond these problems inherent in the use of cow's milk, let's look at what happens when we alter the milk. First, we pasteurize it, destroying vitamins and helpful bacteria in order to enable it to sit longer on the shelf without spoiling and to ensure that no harmful bacteria have infected it. Then, it is usually homogenized, a process whereby the large fat molecules of the cream are smashed up into a smaller size so they will stay in the solution rather than rising to the top. This causes biochemical changes in milk that are poorly understood. Also, the fluid is bombarded with ultraviolet radiation, which converts some of the naturally-occurring ergosterol into vitamin D to make up for the vitamin D we don't get from the sun. This source of vitamin D has been a very useful crutch for our indoor society in recent years.

We process much of our milk into cheese, butter, ice cream, or yogurt. In its natural form, yogurt is one of the best dairy products we can eat because the lactose is predigested in the yogurt culture. However, what is actually chemically added as it is processed we can only begin to tell from reading the labels, because the dairy industry has special exemptions from many of the labeling disclosure laws. The yogurt you eat may contain so much gelatin, sugar, cornstarch, and preservatives that they cancel out any of the beneficial effects of the acidophilus culture. As for ice cream, do you know what's in it besides petrochemicals and air? Certainly little ice and no cream! (with a few notable exceptions becoming available).

I realize that challenging the dairy industry and the sacred institution of milk drinking—contradicting those wholesome, milk-mustached lads and lassies who extol the virtues of this "wonder" food—will be considered un-American by some, but the facts don't support their claims.

—JWT

4.17 Eating for High-Level Wellness

This book won't prescribe systems everyone can or should follow; this would undermine the concept of self-trust that has been its underlying thesis. However, some consideration of the components of basic nutrition is needed to develop an intelligent, broad-based awareness of the role that food plays in your wellbeing. Moreover, in the midst of the confusing data surrounding this subject, some common recommendations continually surface from almost every source consulted. While it would be foolish to latch onto this or any other plan as the final word, we do believe that the overall guidelines offered by the 2000 Dietary Guidelines for Americans and supplemented by the Harvard Medical School guidelines represent a balanced approach. To view and download a copy of *Nutrition and Your Health: Dietary Guidelines for Americans* (fifth edition, 2000), visit www.usda.gov/cnpp/Pubs/DG2000. Single copies of the guidelines can also be purchased from the Federal Consumer Information Center, (888) 878-3256.

For the Harvard recommendations, see www.hsph.harvard.edu/nutritionsource/pyramids.html or *Eat, Drink, and Be Healthy.*

In brief, combining these guidelines, we suggest the following:

1. *Let the pyramids guide your food choices. (The pyramid diagrams are shown on pages 79 and 80.) Primarily, let plant foods serve as the foundation of your diet.*

   A. *Choose a variety of grains daily, especially whole grains. Keep white rice, pasta, starches, and sweets to a minimum.*

   B. *Choose a variety of fruits and vegetables daily.*

2. *Keep food safe to eat by avoiding contamination or improper storage.*

3. *Aim for a healthy weight.*

   A. *Evaluate your body weight.*

   B. *Find out your risk factors for disease.*

   C. *Choose sensible portion sizes.*

   D. *If you need to lose weight, do so gradually.*

   F. *Encourage healthy weight in children.*

4. *Be physically active each day.*

5. *Choose a diet that is low in saturated fat and cholesterol and moderate in total fat. Use plant oils (like olive, canola, sunflower, etc.) regularly.*

6. *Choose beverages and foods to moderate your intake of sugars.*

7. *Choose and prepare foods with less salt.*

8. *If you drink alcoholic beverages, do so in moderation.*

9. *Use a multivitamin and multimineral supplement, or a type of plant-based superfood, daily.*

As with all general recommendations, don't expect to make massive changes overnight. Focus on one or two small changes at a time. Take three or four weeks to allow your new habits to become firmly established, even natural to you. Keep them going while you then choose another recommendation to work on. Take your time. These are the habits of a lifetime that you are addressing. Be gentle but consistent.

4.18 Check Those Labels

If you don't already do so, start reading the labels on cans and packages of food products. You may be in for a real shock. Ingredients are listed in order by amount; that is, the main ingredient is listed first, on down to the smallest. Comparative shopping often reveals that while one product contains sugar and/or strange-sounding chemicals, another brand may not. Keep in mind, however, that ingredient labeling has some limitations. There are many additives that the U.S. Food and Drug Administration (FDA) does not require to be listed on labels. Some ingredients must be listed on some products but not on others. Incomplete or inadequate labeling is also evident; for example, certified food coloring may be listed, but the specific type is not indicated. Ingredient labeling is not required at all on some products. For instance, due to powerful lobbying, the dairy industry has been exempted from listing most additives.

Also realize that the processed food industry may use wording on the labels and techniques in their advertising that can make you feel confused, deceived, and downright pressured. To give you a few examples:

- *"Enriched" or "wheat" flour means white flour. White flour is made from wheat, except that the bran and wheat germ have been removed. To be sure you're getting a true whole-grain product, look for the words "stone-ground whole wheat" (or rye, or other grain). "Natural sweetener" usually means sugar (as opposed to artificial sweetener).*

- *Supposedly knowledgeable professionals or celebrities may be paid to recommend a product.*

- *Labels may list the vitamins and minerals with which a product has been enriched. This usually means that a minimal amount of vitamins has been added to a deficient (that is, junk) food product to make the label look good. The product is often high in sugar, white flour, and/or fat.*

As products of our environment, most of us are strongly influenced by food ads and consequently are lacking in both nutrition education and nutritious food.

Food producers boast an annual advertising budget as big as the portion sizes they advertise. McDonald's alone spends about $1 billion a year promoting its products, and soft-drink companies spend about $600 million. All told, the food industry spends about $25 billion on advertising and other forms of promotion. Only 2 percent of the ads are for fruits, vegetables, grains, and beans—the foods that should make up the bulk of a healthy diet.

—Michael F. Jacobson, Ph.D., executive director of the Center for Science in the Public Interest

---

4.19 Awareness and Self-Trust

Nutrition is a subject as highly charged as politics or religion. For just about any set of facts substantiated by one group of studies, you will find a comparable number of articles and "experts" to refute it:

Sugar is poison *vs.* Sugar is a quick energy food

Meats are the best source of protein *vs.* Meat is harmful

Vitamin and mineral supplements are a rip-off *vs.* Commercial croplands are so depleted, supplementing is essential

Distilled water is best; it prevents kidney stones *vs.* Hard waters are associated with a lower incidence of heart disease

Confusing? Well, before you abandon your search, remember that there is one expert who does have answers for you—and that authority is you. Learning to listen to your own body will help you piece together the parts of your own nutritional puzzle. The appreciation of biochemical individuality demands that, above all else, we develop awareness of and trust in our own bodies. Ultimately, you are the one who is responsible for the health and wellbeing of your own body—not a chemist, a computer, or a physician.

To "listen" in this context means to be aware, and to be effective this requires honesty and thoroughness. You may crave sweets because they have been your sustenance and reward throughout life. If you listen only to this craving and set about satisfying it in all circumstances, then you will end up in more trouble. A craving may be an indication of metabolic need, or it may be the result of an addiction. There are lots of other signs you must attend to if you are to practice self-trust correctly. Let's consider some of these.

The condition of your teeth and gums are strong indicators of just how well you are eating. Frequent cavities and bleeding gums are not normal—and changing your brand of toothpaste will do little to alleviate them.

Look at your tongue. Is it discolored and coated? Do you have a sour taste in your mouth and consistently bad breath? Your mouth is trying to tell you something.

The strength of your fingernails and the overall condition of your skin are strong indicators of your diet-related health.

Despite what the TV advertisements may lead you to believe, chronic headaches are not something to treat with aspirins and dismiss. Headaches are loud-and-clear messages that something about the organism is amiss. They commonly indicate general stress. But that level of stress would be a lot less if not compounded by a host of diet-related conditions. Most people don't realize the connection between constipation and headaches, but the two are strongly related. Headaches are also commonly the result of imbalances such as hypoglycemia (low blood sugar) and alcohol consumption. In any case, those long-lasting, fast-acting, extra-strength pain relievers can only muffle the warning sounds temporarily.

It doesn't take too much nutritional sophistication to appreciate the connection between overeating, indulging in spicy, rich food, and drinking alcohol and acid indigestion, acid reflux, and upset stomach. Listen to your body on "the morning after"—it can provide you with lots of valuable information about what doesn't work for you. It can also be a great motivator for change.

4.20 Signs of a Balanced Diet

The regularity of bowel movements is strong indicator of dietary balance. Constipation is a huge chronic problem for many. So many factors contribute to a lack of regularity. Diets with adequate fiber produce large quantities of bulky stools that usually float in the toilet, an excellent indicator of whether you are getting enough bulk in the diet.

Physical strength, endurance, and flexibility are other factors to consider in developing awareness of the relationship between the food you eat and the foods you need. While it is difficult to quantify the changes in strength level that happen as a result of eating different foods, most people notice that some foods make them feel heavy, bloated, bogged down, or sleepy, while others induce a feeling of lightness. Eating for lightness is an excellent criterion to use in changing your dietary patterns for the promotion of high-level wellness. Christina sums up her approach to nutrition by saying, "I eat what makes me feel light and what makes me feel strong."

The list of signs and clues goes on and on. They include mood swings; frequency of colds, flu, and other contagious diseases; and difficulty in sleeping. By now, you are probably getting a clearer picture of what it means to be your own food expert. Sure, go on reading and learning what others have to share, but balance this with quiet reflection in which you courageously face the question: "How do I feel?" In addition, you may wish to set up experiments with certain foods or ways of eating. Allow enough time in each experiment to really experience the effects. Add a food or abstain from a food for awhile and keep a nutritional journal, recording each day what you have done and how you feel. Above all, as your own food awareness grows, resist the temptation to criticize other people's diets. Redirect this energy as loving acceptance of your fellow beings, and offer a hug instead of a lecture.

WHERE IS FIBER FOUND?

Whole-grain cereals are a major source of dietary fiber. Bran has 9 to 12 percent crude fiber; dry beans, lentils, and soybeans have over 4 percent (equivalent to 1.2 to 1.5 percent after cooking with added water); roasted nuts have 2.3 to 2.6 percent; and most fruits and vegetables contain 0.5 to 1 percent, although there is some loss during cooking.

4.21 Slowing Down

If you are intent upon developing a more generalized sensitivity and awareness for a richer and more fulfilling life, there is no better place to start than at your table. The key to awareness about eating is to slow down. Eating fast is a disservice to the cook who prepared the food, to your companions at the table, and primarily to your own body. Ask any weight-control expert and you will learn that slowing down your eating speed will cause you to eat less. It makes sense. When you allow time for the food to reach your stomach and for the digestive juices to begin the breakdown process, hunger sensations will begin to diminish. It will take a smaller amount of food to satisfy you, and that is a help not only in maintaining your ideal weight, but also in sustaining a longer life.

To appreciate food requires the varied use of many senses and organs besides the mouth, tongue, teeth, and taste buds. Many cooks will complain that they have little hunger left after looking at and smelling food for hours in the preparation. While this condition is far from desirable to most of us, it illustrates the important role that sight and smell play in the whole drama. And that is just what eating can become—a drama. Imagine your disappointment, even anger, if you had spent $80 or $100 for front-and-center theater seats to witness a famous production, only to have the actors and actresses race through their lines, as if they were reciting grocery lists or multiplication tables, on a stage devoid of sets with no complementary lighting. To eat purely out of habit or in a race against the clock is to participate in a similar travesty.

Food has aroma, and texture, and color, and form, and temperature, and weight, both on the plate and in your mouth. How often have you allowed these characteristics to enter your awareness? To do so, you simply have to slow down.

A CONTEMPORARY MEAL PRAYER

Countless beings have contributed their precious life energies to supply this food that we are about to eat. Let us remember them, with gratitude. Let us eat with reverence for all life.

In many cultures and religious traditions it is common to offer a prayer before a meal. Whatever your particular spiritual orientation may be, you can undoubtedly appreciate the wisdom of this practice. The body is given a few moments to rest, to orient itself in preparation for the task of eating. The eyes are temporarily closed, shutting out distractions and allowing one to focus awareness on breathing. A few deep breaths will facilitate general relaxation of the entire organism. Reflection may be made about the love and caring that went into the preparation of the meal, the richness of life in general as symbolized in the richness and abundance of the food, and the resolution made to eat with reverence and awareness. Not a bad habit to start, if this is not already a part of your mealtime practice.

The healthiest way to slow down speed-eating is to start chewing—a long-forgotten activity in the repertoire of most moderns, adults as well as children. If for no other reason, the prevention of death by choking should serve to motivate us to start masticating. There's a saying, "Drink your solids and chew your liquids." To "drink" your solids means to chew them so well that they pass like liquids down your throat. To "chew" your liquids means to enjoy the sensation of them throughout your mouth. Good advice for the gulpers among us.

Besides the physical effect (the aid to digestion through the breakdown of complex carbohydrates by the enzymes in saliva), the advantages of chewing include a ready outlet for stress, a strengthening of the will, and patience and peace enhanced by conscious eating.

Finally, while there is little evidence to prove claims for foods as aphrodisiacs (substances that increase the sexual urge), it is general knowledge that seduction is more readily accomplished in a quiet candle-lit atmosphere than at the corner taco stand. Few would argue that the sensual pleasures of food can be heightened by the proper setting, the mode of preparation and presentation, and the service. There is more to eating than satisfying hunger pains. Why not slow down and allow yourself a greater share of life's pleasures by appreciating food for its sacramental and multisensual qualities?

4.22 Love and Compassion

The saying goes, "There is nothing more obnoxious than a reformed [fill in any appropriate word]." While this may be a cruel and unjust generalization, you have probably experienced a real-life case. Take the food faddist, for instance: three weeks of eating nothing but nuts and figs, a condescending smile, and an unasked-for lecture directed at a companion across the table who has made the sorry mistake of ordering a cup of coffee. (Or even a bowl of yogurt— "mucus-producing, you know.") What good will it do you to put perfect food in your body if you use your knowledge to alienate yourself from the love of others?

While this may be an extreme example, it helps to make some important points on the subject of moderation and balance in the area of foods, diets, and nutrition in general. Here, as in many other areas, the key words are *patience* and *compassion*. Making radical changes in a very short period of time will more often set you up for failure and disappointment, and it can also upset your system enough that you temporarily feel worse instead of better. So take slow steps, reward yourself for your satisfying changes, and love yourself for being noncompulsive when you choose to break your regimen.

Realize that because something works for you now, it may not always. Neither is it necessarily the remedy for someone else.

Keep in mind that your body has an amazing resiliency; it can tolerate just about any foods or beverages for a limited time or in small amounts. So try to restrain your tendency to set unrealistic demands on yourself, like "I'll never eat candy again."

Whatever you do, attempt to do it with awareness. As long as you've chosen to eat that apple or that piece of cake, please enjoy it in the process. The reward for a well-balanced and more conscious lifestyle is the realization of high-level wellness.

A Nutrition Journal

A nutrition journal can be used as your personal record of the ways your body responds to the foods you eat; a balance sheet to observe the kinds of raw materials or fuels with which you supply your body; a place to keep special recipes; a diet notebook for weight gain or loss; and a record of emotions felt, resolutions, etc. Here is a sample entry, using breakfast as the subject under consideration:

Day/Time	Foods	Effects
Monday 3/22 9:00 A.M.	2 eggs, 2 strips bacon, 2 pieces toast, butter and jam, 2 cups coffee	Left the table feeling stuffed. Too much food. Generally good day. Not hungry until 3 P.M.

Record your observations for a one- to two-day period here:

Day/Time	Foods	Effects

Record your reflections and resolutions here:

_____

_____

_____

_____

_____

4.23 Growing Your Own

Growing your own food can be a very pleasurable and satisfying experience. Not only will you have tastier fruits and vegetables, you'll save money and get a little exercise and sunshine at the same time. An added benefit is that you can eliminate or control the chemicals used—the fertilizers, pesticides, and herbicides.

Even the smallest plot of land can yield a fair crop. You might consider tearing out your lawn and replacing it with a vegetable garden. There is probably enough space devoted to lawns in the United States to feed the entire population!

4.24 Feeding Our Planet

On this day, 24,000 of our brothers and sisters throughout the world will die of starvation while we pursue the luxury of deciding between steak or pork chops, health food or junk food, a high-protein or a high-carbohydrate diet.

The reasons given for mass malnutrition range from the simplistic and crass to the frightening and complex:

- *It's nature's way of population control.*

- *People are lazy and ignorant.*

- *The rich will demand what they have come to enjoy.*

- *We have upset the ecological balance.*

- *Food costs have risen with the rising costs of oil.*

- *Food corporations control the world.*

And the situation continues to worsen.

Any decision for high-level wellness as a way of life must take this reality into account. The choices and demands we make will impact all the people who share our small planet. They affect the conditions of our soil, the prices we have to pay for food, and its availability to others.

Our responsibility is a heavy one. It means that we must:

- *Become informed.*

- *Resist waste and greed.*

- *Possibly change our diets and eating habits.*

- *Work for equitable distribution of food and rightful control of the land.*

- *Do everything within our power to end starvation.*

Nature's way is the way of balance. High-level wellness for any must mean a balanced diet for all.

See The Hunger Project website, www.thp.org, for more ideas.

SUGGESTED READING

Attwood, C., *A Vegetarian Doctor Speaks Out* (Hohm Press, 1998).

Chopra, D., *The Chopra Center Cookbook* (John Wiley and Sons, 2003).

Cousens, G., *Conscious Eating* (North Atlantic Books, 2000).

D'Adamo, R., *Eat Right 4 Your Type* (Putnam, 1996).

Dufty, W., *Sugar Blues* (Warner Books, 1993).

Jeavons, J., *How to Grow More Vegetables* (Ten Speed Press, 2002).

Katzen, M., *The New Moosewood Cookbook* (Ten Speed Press, 2002).

——, *The Enchanted Broccoli Forest* (Ten Speed Press, 2002).

Kristal, H., and J. Haig, *The Nutrition Solution: A Guide to Your Metabolic Type* (North Atlantic Books, 2002).

Ladd, U., and V. Ladd, *Ayurvedic Cooking for Self Healing,* 2nd edition (Ayurvedic Press, 1997).

Lappé, F. M., *Diet for a Small Planet* (Ballantine Books, 1992).

Robertson, L., C. Flinders, and B. Godfrey, *The New Laurel's Kitchen: A Handbook for Vegetarian Cookery and Nutrition* (Ten Speed Press, 1986).

Roth, G., *Feeding the Hungry Heart* (Plume, 1982).

Santillo, H., *Intuitive Eating* (Hohm Press, 1993).

Schwartz, B., *Diets Don't Work!* (Breakthru Publishing, 2002).

Smith, E. K., *The Quick and Easy Ayurvedic Cookbook* (Charles Tuttle, 2000).

Thomas, L., *10 Essential Foods* (Hohm Press, 1997).

Willett, W., and P. J. Skerrett, *Eat, Drink, and Be Healthy: The Harvard Medical School Guide to Healthy Eating* (Free Press, 2002).

Williams, R., *Biochemical Individuality* (McGraw-Hill, 1998).

For an updated listing of resources and active links to the websites mentioned in this chapter, please see www.WellnessWorkbook.com.

NOTES

1. *Dietary Goals for the United States,* Select Committee on Nutrition and Human Needs, U.S. Government Printing Office, Washington, D.C. (February 1977), v.

2. The original study was condensed in "Biomarkers of Caloric Restriction May Predict Longevity in Humans," *Science,* Vol. 297 (2 August 2002), 811.

3. Established in 1892, the Wistar Institute was the first independent medical research facility in the United States. Wistar's mission is to pursue basic scientific research in medicine, to develop treatment and prevention of chronic and acute disease. Wistar is a National Cancer Institute Cancer Center, funded by endowments, the National Institutes of Health, and private foundation grants.

4. Excellent resources and research are provided at www.breastfeeding.com; and Saarinen U. M., and M. Kajosaari, "Breastfeeding as prophylaxis against atopic disease: prospective follow-up study until 17 years old," *Lancet* 346 (1995):1065–69.

5. Reported in "Breastfeeding and Intelligence," *Pediatrics for Parents* (July/August 1993), 12.

6. *Journal of the Nutritional Academy,* Vol. II, No. II (August 1979).

7. Among many different types of personal health evaluation, the hair mineral analysis offers a clear understanding of the body's mineral and trace element levels. It can usually identify inorganic toxic materials that may be present, so that appropriate treatments can be begun to eliminate them naturally from the body. Search the Internet for hair/mineral analysis.

8. Public Citizen, "The Top 10 Problems with Irradiated Food," www.citizen.org/documents/Top10.pdf. Public Citizen is a national, nonprofit consumer advocacy organization founded by Ralph Nader in 1971 to represent consumer interests in Congress, the executive branch, and the courts.

9. *Dietary Goals,* 33.

CHAPTER 5

Wellness and Moving

Movement is one of the most basic expressions of energy output in the Wellness Energy System. When nourished and stimulated with oxygen, sensory data, and food (fuel), the body responds with internal movement (lungs expanding, heart pumping, and so on) and external movement (walking, smiling, and so on). The ability to move is the basis for more complex bodily activities such as working and playing, creative expression, communicating, and sexual activity.

**It's no fun . . . it's for athletes . . .
I'm too busy, etc. . . .**

—Anonymous couch potato

Everything in us is moving. Our heart pumps, blood flows, lungs expand and contract, eyes scan, eardrums vibrate. To be alive is to be moving. Inhibit the movement and you create illness. Stop it and you are dead. Allow it fully and you realize wellness.

In his wonderful book *Stalking the Wild Pendulum,* Itzhak Bentov takes us on a journey inside the human body. We find ourselves immersed in a sea of atoms ". . . weaving back and forth like a field of ripe wheat blown by the wind. They move in unison and

in beautiful rhythm." Moving inside an atom, we discover there also that ". . . everything is in a constant, very rapid, but very orderly motion."

Because of this movement, everything is changing from moment to moment. To block movement, therefore, is to block change. The moving river cleanses itself. The unmoving water becomes the stagnant pool. The moving body freely channels the energy of life. The unmoving body becomes a home for infection and depression.

Think about it. Close your eyes for a moment and create a mental picture of an unhealthy person. Your image may include a colorless and drooping face, an overweight body—possibly seated in a chair—or a tired form sluggishly climbing a flight of stairs, puffing at every step. Or perhaps an anorexic, emaciated body, moving along the path at a rapid pace, muscles and nerves strained with tension. . . . Now, imagine the opposite. See a person at the peak of health. Chances are you have pictured a healthy complexion and a well-toned, beautiful body in motion—running, or jumping with arms reaching out, or making love, or dancing. Dancing is a great metaphor for living—for being—in harmony, since the whole universe, the sum total of energy, moves as in a dance. The person dancing is the person at one with the universe. The person dancing is fully alive.

If you have a body with physical challenges, don't let that stop you. The National Center on Physical Activity and Disability (www.ncpad.org) has links to fact sheets, monographs, bibliographies, slide shows, and abstracts of current research on physical activity and disability.

Without movement you have no dance, no work, and no play either. It's that elementary. Movement changes both the inner world and the outer world. Moving encourages movement. The more you move, the better you move. Energy creates energy—in a continuous, circling process—in a constant dance.

5.1 The Need for Movement

Many sedentary-type people have had such negative experiences from childhood sports, physical education classes, or the dance class our mother forced us to attend, or are so habituated to spending hours in front of the TV or computer screen, that we have completely suppressed any sensations from our body about its need for movement. By paying attention to subtle but constant messages—such as tense muscles, a restricted range of movement, shallow breathing, or lethargy—with some practice we can begin to notice that muscles were made to be used.

You may be tempted to feel guilty if you aren't exercising regularly. The reasons why we don't move more are as many and varied as the people who ask the question. Take Jerry, for example.

He doesn't hate exercise—he just hates boredom. He's often experienced them as one and the same. Left to himself, he would rather spend the morning listening to music, reading a good book, or doing a crossword puzzle. But his whole world brightens when an energetic friend appears at the door inviting him to go swim, to play tennis, to take a hike up a nearby mountain.

For Jerry to berate himself for his lack of self-motivation would be a great energy waste. For him to consciously program situations in which he will have others to accompany him while he works out will meet his needs for both emotional stroking and physical exercise.

Roselyn, on the other hand, loves to run alone along the flat country roads near her home. Every morning she does yoga for one hour. Every evening she does tai chi, a slow, dancing form of martial art.

For Roselyn to dictate what Jerry needs would be foolish and frustrating. For Jerry to expect Roselyn to react as he does would be unrealistic. They are unique and extraordinary individuals. Each will be happy only if they trust their own internal messages and design their environments so they can best meet their own needs for exercise. The options are almost limitless. Remember that the *one way* to wellness is *your way*.

**but if the dance of the run
isn't fun
then discover another dance
because without fun
the good of the run
is undone
and a suffering runner
always quits
sooner or later.**

—Fred Rohe

5.2 Stair Climbing

With few exceptions (such as farm work, or running from the neighbor's dog), our needs to move with vigor are usually few. Our cars, trains, and planes, plus the countless laborsaving devices that surround us, do the work for us.

While these conveniences may lighten the load, they also discourage us from moving. The words of John F. Kennedy, spoken in the early 1960s, still apply today: ". . . the labor of the human body is rapidly being engineered out of working life." To counteract this continuing trend, we need to focus on integrating movement into our daily lifestyle. Unless we consciously seek out ways to engineer exercise back into our daily life—such as taking the stairs, parking at the far end of the parking lot, or riding a bike for short errands—we will unconsciously continue to follow the herd and remain sedentary.

5.3 Exploring and Caring for Yourself through Movement

Since the Industrial Revolution, the need for human activity has changed dramatically. Most of us no longer chop wood and carry water. Our work more likely involves sitting for long hours at a desk or in an automobile, or standing behind a counter or at an assembly line. Much of our business, moreover, is tedious and stressful. Even if we enjoy the opportunity of working in the out-of-doors, our range of movement is probably limited. Joyce, for instance, stands on the highway all day changing a sign from SLOW to STOP and back again. She has learned to exercise while standing in place, using isometrics (two opposite muscle groups tensing against each other, giving both a workout). Through practice, she can now individually locate and contract many separate muscle groups as she stands there doing her job. When there are no cars in sight, she practices her dance moves, or just abandons herself to what her muscles feel called to express.

Movement is life, and we're always in motion, even while asleep. You can bring consciousness and add a touch of creativity to some of your everyday movements—hand someone a glass of water with a little flourish, skip down the sidewalk or stairs (when no one's looking), or invent a new "silly walk" for Monty Python's Ministry of Silly Walks.

Don't Get Out of Bed (Before You Start Moving!)

How you start the day can set the tone for how you live the rest of it. These exercises are designed to get you moving easily, first thing in the morning. Releasing the kinks that you may have built up will energize you and may even make the transition from bed to floor a less traumatic one. Choose among the movements below and develop your own routine.

On Your Back

- *The rack stretch—Extend your legs as far as they will go; point your toes and stretch your arms out to either side, extending your fingers. Hold for a few seconds. Release. Repeat two or three times.*

- *Reach for the ceiling. Extend and then contract your fingers. Tense, relax, and shake your arms.*

- *Extend your right leg over your left leg at a 90-degree angle from the trunk, if possible (go as far as is comfortable). Repeat several times. Then do the same with your left leg. Rest.*

- *Bring your knees up toward your chest. Grasp them with your arms. In this position, roll to your left, then back to center, then roll to your right. Repeat as often as is fun. Release your knees. Extend your legs.*

- *To the count of 1-2-3, arch your lower back. Hold. Repeat the count and lower it to the bed again. Rotate your pelvis clockwise three times. Rotate counterclockwise three times.*

- *Bend your knees and place your feet flat on the bed. Raise your buttocks off the bed. Hold for a count of 1-2-3. Lower your buttocks back onto the bed. Repeat three or four times.*

- *Inhale as you turn your head to the right slowly, lowering your right ear to the bed. Exhale as you return to the center. Repeat, turning your head to the left. Do this three or four times. Relax.*

On Your Belly

- *Bend your knees and bring your heels back toward your buttocks. Hold. Lower your feet to the bed again. Repeat twice.*

- *Bring your knees up under your chest, then reach back and hold your feet. Tuck your head down toward your chest. Feel your neck and back stretch with this one. Release your feet; raise your head and straighten your back, sitting back on your legs and feet.*

When you're done, look in the direction of the sunrise. Smile and greet the day. Get out of bed.

5.4 Vigorous Physical Effort

In many areas of wellness, simply allowing the body's natural processes to be unfettered will tend to keep it in balance. With respect to moving however, minimal maintenance will not be enough. If you want to be well, you are going to have to do something more—exercise.

There are many excuses for neglecting exercise:

- *It's no fun.*
- *It's for kids.*
- *I'm too busy.*
- *I'm too tired.*
- *I'm too fat.*
- *I look awful in tennis outfits.*
- *I can't afford the equipment.*
- *I don't have anyone to play with.*
- *I tried it once and it didn't work; I can't keep up the pace.*
- *I don't know how.*
- *I'm afraid!*
- *Who knows what might happen if I did!*
- *I'm still afraid . . .*

We can look at our resistance with compassion and deal with it. When we realize that these excuses, combined with our poor diet habits and stressful lifestyles, have resulted in overweight, dire heart conditions, high blood pressure, and energy-robbed lives, we can decide to join the millions of Americans who are choosing to get moving!

Interest in exercise is becoming greater, in part because of our growing concern about our appearance. Fat is the enemy. The models of success and happiness that the media present to us are young, energetic, slim, and good-looking. A possible upside to the long hours of TV many Americans watch is that this may well contribute to the interest in exercise. The interconnection between self-image, physical appearance, and exercise is very strong.

Fitness centers, spas, running clubs, and dance classes are places to meet people, to gain a sense of community, to receive the encouragement and support we all need. Besides, exercise makes us feel good—not just physically, but emotionally and spiritually.

There is clearly a relationship between the growing interest in exercise and the public recognition that coronary heart disease is the number one cause of death in the United States. When a friend suffers a heart attack, you take notice. Such an event may shock many people into running, swimming, or some other vigorous, heart-healthy activity.

Heart disease is the subject of much research, and there is no one explanation for why some people get it and others don't (unless you support the notion that we choose our illnesses). We do know the leading risk factors in heart disease:

- *High blood fats*
- *High blood pressure*
- *Obesity*
- *Smoking*
- *High blood sugar*
- *Family history of heart disease*
- *Diabetes*
- *Lack of exercise*
- *Hostility*

Perhaps most enticing and rewarding of all outcomes, exercise increases the levels of endorphins (the "feel good" hormones) levels in the bloodstream. Feeling better further encourages you to continue your exercise program for all those other benefits it affords you—a safety valve for stress, help in shedding unwanted pounds, and lowering of blood sugar levels. Many smokers are able to cut down significantly or stop smoking altogether when they start a regular program of exercise.

Exercise is beneficial in treating some backaches, ulcers, arthritis, insomnia, nervous tension, indigestion, asthma, diabetes, plus anxiety and low-level depression. It truly is a wonder "drug."

5.5 Breathing, Movement, and Body Awareness

As if the physical advantages of exercise were not enough, its connection to the ways we think and feel about ourselves is remarkable. As shown in chapter 2, the crucial link between the mind and body is the breath—the life force. Encouraging fuller breathing through exercise is one of the most dynamic ways of increasing overall vitality. Many disciplines, such as yoga or the martial arts, focus on the breath—especially abdominal or diaphragmatic breathing—as a core factor in reconnecting the mind, body, and spirit.

The key to diaphragmatic breathing is simple: as you inhale, expand your abdomen; as you exhale, contract your abdomen.

- *Lie on your back with your legs bent, feet close to your buttocks, and eyes closed. Inhale, expanding the abdomen while keeping the chest still.*

- *Exhale, pulling in the abdomen and drawing it back to the spine.*

- *Repeat five times, following this ratio:*

- *Inhale: five seconds (expand abdomen)*

- *Exhale: ten seconds (contract abdomen)*

Finding a regular discipline that reinforces this type of breathing is a vital part of a wellness program.

An Exercise Journal

Exercising is a form of play—we encourage you to use it that way. If you want results of any kind, however, you will need to apply yourself to your practice with some consistency. One way to keep yourself motivated is to use a record or journal to chart your progress. You don't need to do the same type of exercise every day, unless you want to. Regina often varies her morning workouts. She may start with stretching, yet some days do race-walking, other days play tennis, and on still others ride her bike. Here is a sample journal entry:

Date	Time	Type of Exercise	Comments
7/25	6:30–7:15	Tennis with Jere	Clumsy; we laughed
7/27	7:30–8:30	Bike ride (five miles)	Magnificent day; good push

Use this page as your journal for one week:

Date	Time	Type of Exercise	Comments

At the end of the week, record your overall impressions, insights, and accomplishment of goals here:

_____

_____

_____

Record your resolutions here:

_____

_____

_____

5.6 Aerobic Exercise

Aerobics include any exercises that increase the heart rate and breathing rate for a sustained period of time, greatly increasing the flow of oxygen and blood to all parts of the body. Aerobic exercise, or cardiovascular exercise, provides all these benefits:

- *Increased lean muscle*

- *Decreased intramuscular and subcutaneous fat*

- *Improved circulation*

- *Elevated metabolism*

- *Increased energy and stamina*

- *More restful sleep*

- *Reduction of mild depression, anxiety, and muscle tension*

- *Improved appearance*

- *More positive self-image and outlook on life*

- *Reduced use of coffee, tea, alcohol, tobacco, sugar, and refined carbohydrates*

- *Increased immune function by increasing the white blood cell count*

- *Increased HDL and decreased LDL*

To be most effective, the exercise must raise your pulse rate to the range indicated in the formula on page 129, and keep it at that level for not less than twenty minutes. (Note: People who are not in good cardiovascular condition should begin at a lower level and can break their exercise time into five-minute periods with rests in between.) Try to exercise three times a week.

Examples of aerobic exercises are bicycling, aerobic dance and step classes, running, swimming, jumping rope, and vigorous walking. Stop-and-go exercises (such as golf, downhill skiing, housework,

and gardening) and those of short duration (like sprinting, square dancing, and calisthenics) do not produce the desired cardiovascular benefit.

As soon as you start moving, your heart starts working harder, pumping more blood with each beat. The blood then rushes with greater speed and force through the vessels, which expand to allow for this increased volume. The working muscles call out for more oxygen. The body responds by breathing more deeply. In moving to arms and legs, the blood is diverted from the digestive organs. Blood vessels in the exercising muscles expand tremendously, allowing a greater influx of oxygen. The process returns to its starting point as the blood goes back to the heart, faster and in greater volume, filling it to capacity and keeping the whole operation working smoothly. Stressing the whole system in this way improves its function and increases its capacity to handle more stress.

Circulation is not the only process affected during aerobic exercise. The body's energy supply shifts from glucose to fat usage. Fat stored in body tissues is released, moving first to the liver for breakdown, then out to the needy muscles to fuel them. Hormones and enzymes jump in to keep the system in balance, and the chemistry of the brain itself is altered.

Other Types of Exercise

It is important to understand that the exercise most effective in preventing heart disease is cardiovascular exercise (see pages 128 and 129), but there are also two other types of exercise, each categorized by the body systems most influenced:

- *Cardiovascular exercise (aerobics) stimulates heart and lungs and builds endurance.*

- **Flexibility exercise** *lengthens and stretches muscles to enhance balance and overall grace and agility.*

- **Strength-developing exercise** *(such as weight training) increases muscle mass, potentially creating a leaner appearance.*

For basic fitness, all three are essential. Flexibility and strength-developing exercises will be covered in modules 5.9 (although yoga does more than just increase flexibility) and 5.10 respectively.

CREATING AN AEROBIC EXERCISE PROGRAM

Aerobic exercise is much more than an antidisease, antiaging tool. Whether you're working, playing, or dancing, moving your body is a wonderful gift, and experiencing its movement will give you much joy.

You must still be careful when doing aerobic exercise, especially when starting a new exercise program. Get a physical and ECG (especially if you are over age forty) first, and if you have medical problems, seek professional advice to help you create a routine that fits your needs.

How to Exercise?

Aerobic exercise doesn't mean just running. Many people find running boring or too hard on the ankles, feet, and knees. Luckily, we now have a wide range of lower-impact aerobic exercises from which to choose, including step aerobics, in-line skating, "spinning," and some martial arts. Swimming is a wonderful aerobic exercise, too. Try one, or try them all to find a form of aerobic exercise that suits you.

When to Exercise?

The time of day should fit your individual schedule. You may prefer to exercise after work, because it is an extremely effective way of revitalizing yourself and eliminating tensions. The morning holds other advantages: In the hot summer months it is a cool time of day. Also, some people find their morning schedule more controllable and less likely to vary than their evenings. Others just find morning exercise a great way to start the day.

How Long and How Often?

Regular exercise is imperative. As mentioned in module 5.6, twenty minutes, three times per week is good for a maintenance program. Four or five times a week is ideal for increasing your fitness or aerobic capacity. Weekend exercisers—or only-now-and-then exercisers—place themselves in potential danger because the heart and body are not strengthened sufficiently to withstand a really vigorous workout.

Note: While regular exercise is important, you should temporarily suspend it when ill or excessively fatigued.

Warm up. About five minutes is all you need. Calisthenics (such as sit-ups and push-ups) or any forms of movement that elevate your heart rate are particularly good for warming up. These exercises serve to get blood into the muscles and raise their temperature so they're not operating cold. They also get the heart going gradually, rather than in one quick burst, which could potentially be dangerous.

Cool down. After a period of vigorous exercise, cooling down is just as important as warming up. A gradual transition is good for the heart. During exercise such as running or cycling, there's a greater volume of blood in the large leg muscles. While the activity continues, the muscles are squeezing the blood back to the heart and rest of the body. When the exercise is stopped suddenly and completely, the increased volume of blood is still in the legs, but now there is no contraction of the leg muscles to return it to the heart and brain, so the blood pools there. Dizziness, fainting, or even more serious consequences can occur. A gradual (three- to five-minute) cool-down allows the heart rate to gradually return to resting and eases the transition between vigorous exercise and rest. Walking after running is a good example.

How Much Is Enough?

To gain the desired effect, you should not overexert yourself, nor should you go too slowly. Using the following formula to determine your minimum and maximum pulse rates will help guide you in determining that in-between, optimum level.

Minimum pulse rate =
   (220 – your age) times 0.55
Maximum pulse rate =
   (220 – your age) times 0.9
For future reference, we suggest that you record your range here:
Minimum _____; Maximum _____

A person who is terribly out of shape may be able to raise the pulse to the desired level by walking in place or doing seated arm circles, while another person, who is conditioned, may have to run quite hard to reach the same heart rate. Don't try to keep up with someone else— use the formula above to find your own pace.

The first few times you exercise, stop after a minute or two and take your pulse. If it is less than the recommended exercise rate for your age as determined by the formula above, you aren't pushing yourself hard enough. If it is too high, ease up a bit.

Take your pulse regularly. With the palm of your hand facing you, locate the place in your wrist where you can feel a good pulse. Place your index and middle fingers side by side in the groove just inside the bone that leads to the base of your thumb—about two inches below the bump at the end of that bone.

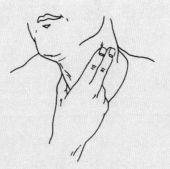

Many people (and vampires) prefer to locate the carotid artery pulse in the neck. First locate your Adam's Apple with your index and middle finger. Slide the fingers over to the side of the windpipe and feel deep into the neck for your pulse.

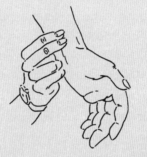

While looking at a clock, begin counting your pulse, beginning with the number zero (not one). After fifteen seconds, stop, and multiply your results by four to get the number of beats per minute. This is your pulse rate.

How Much Is Too Much?

There are several good ways to determine if you are exercising too hard:

- **Breath test.** If you can still talk comfortably as you are exercising, you are probably not overexerting yourself. If not, you are training too hard and need to slow down.

- If you experience **health problems** like faintness, dizziness, nausea, tightness or pain in the chest, severe shortness of breath, or loss of muscle control, **stop exercising immediately** and seek medical attention.

- **Heart-rate recovery.** Count your pulse five minutes after exercise. It should have returned to 120 beats per minute or below. If it hasn't, you're pushing yourself too hard. Count your pulse again after ten minutes. If it isn't back below 100, ease up a little on your exercise program.

- **Breathing recovery rate.** If you still find yourself short of breath ten minutes after exercising, your exercise is too strenuous.

- **Fatigue.** Ordinarily, exercise should be stimulating and invigorating. If you find yourself worn out and tired all the time, it may be a sign that you are overdoing and should slow down on your exercise program. An elevated resting heart rate (taken before rising in the morning) is a good gauge of overtraining. If it is higher than what is normal for you, this indicates the need for a milder workout or more recovery time.

Don't be in a hurry! You need time to condition your heart and muscles to the new demands. Begin slowly, then gradually increase intensity, duration, and frequency. Always be gentle, and enjoy yourself.

Adapted from B. Franklin, *ACSM's Guidelines for Exercise Testing and Prescription* (American College of Sports Medicine, 2000), and an out-of-print publication by Susan Stewart, R.N., and Richelle Aschenbrener, R.P.T., produced by the Calabasas Park (California) Center for Cervical and TMJ/Craniomandibular Orthopedics.

5.7 Exercise for the Heart and Soul

At some point during an extended aerobic workout, many exercisers describe moving into an altered state of consciousness—a place in which the rational mind is temporarily quiet, when the sense of separate self is overpowered by the sense of connectedness with everything that exists. It is a feeling and a deep "knowing" of peace and balance. Similar descriptions are found in religious literature. Many of the techniques used for meditation are present in a good run or an extended swim, for example. Both exercise and meditation contain a point of focus—a word or chant, the breath, or the repetitious act of simply putting one foot, or one arm, in front of the other again and again and again. A rhythm is set. Often the rhythm takes over. The runner becomes the movement. The meditator becomes the sound. For centuries, repetitious movement has been the basis of religious ritual in many traditions. The Sacred Dance again! The American Indian, the African tribesman, the whirling dervish, the yogi—all have made use of the moving body in spiritual practice or communal celebration. The Hindus' Nataraj is a dancing god. China's Taoism is based upon the flow of the moving universe; the art of tai chi, which developed from Taoism, is a representation, a dance, of this flow.

Many who have grown up in Jewish or Christian homes never learned that dance and movement could be a form of worship or prayer. Church was a place for sitting still and listening or reading. Singing may have been OK, but moving certainly wasn't. Maybe we heard about Shakers and "Holy Rollers"—more than likely as the subject of jokes. At best we were uninformed about what they did and why. The mind alone will never grasp the fullness of creation. Mind, heart, and body moving in harmony may begin to approximate the totality that is "God."

A body that moves is a body "taking shape." Regular exercise can firm muscles, shed pounds, and add a healthy glow to your complexion. Liking how you feel and how you look are among the rewards. When you think of yourself in more glowing terms, you "enlighten" those around you and can approach them with greater confidence. You are less dependent on other people for approval because *you know yourself,* and *you approve of* what you know.

Keeping to a regular program of exercise is a statement of personal power. It says that you are in control of your own life; that you have endurance, strength, and flexibility. You witness yourself as the chooser, the mover, the changer. *You* are doing it! What you do in your body, you can do in your work, your relationships, your dreams, your world at large.

The moving body is the body releasing stress, letting go of pent-up emotions, and unblocking channels for energy. In the chapter on breathing, we noted that the breath is the life force. Encouraging fuller breathing through exercise is one of the most dynamic ways of increasing overall vitality.

Time spent in exercising, moreover, is time away from your books, your budgets, and your boss. It is time for your body. Time for a break. As you allow the busy, problem-solving brain a chance to take a backseat, you give an opportunity for the sensual, creative brain to direct you for a while. Many runners testify to the inspiration that often occurs as they exercise. The change of pace that movement brings can refresh you. Back at work, you are better able to address the challenges of the task at hand.

Pride in the appreciation of a job well done; happiness at being alive; the chance to release frustrations; inspiration, clear thinking—these are the powers that heal. These are the joys of high-level wellness.

5.8 Guidelines for Stretching, Moving, and Exerting Your Body

Here are eleven easy steps to keep in mind as you learn how to enjoy moving your body:

1. *If it's not fun, avoid it. Many of us begin exercise programs with vigor, only to drop them abruptly. We set ourselves up for failure and guilt when we push ourselves, demanding that we do something we do not really enjoy. There are so many different ways to exercise. Be creative in finding one that is both challenging and enjoyable for you.*

2. **When pain starts, stop.** *Pain is the body's protective feedback system. Use it responsibly to gauge how much to do, how far to go. While it is OK to push our usual limits when we are in excellent condition, beginners should be respectful of the body's warnings and learn the difference between discomfort and pain.*

3. **Whatever you're doing, dance it.** *Whether you are running or playing handball, all of your movements can be smooth and flowing. From the study of martial arts we learn that movement directed from the center—the place of balance below the diaphragm, in the middle of the body—intensifies strength and enhances overall form. Finding this center and moving from it makes everything you do a dance.*

4. **Avoid imitation.** *As beginners we have much to learn from the pros. Many of them, however, became great because they tried something different, and it worked well for them. But beware of modeling yourself too closely upon someone else. What works for them may only serve to frustrate you. If it works for you, do it. If it doesn't, find your own way.*

5. **Deal cautiously with competition.** *The challenge of competition can be a great motivation for growth and development in any discipline. It can also lead to excess stress, cheating, and bad feelings. Become your own competitor. Use opportunities of playing with others as chances to better your last performance. Lose graciously or win graciously, knowing that the only lasting reward will be your sense of accomplishment and your own integrity.*

6. **Reward every effort.** *The more often you try, the more likely you are to succeed. Realize that it is never too late to begin, and that there are no limits to the number of times for starting over. Congratulate yourself for two minutes of exercise well done. Avoid being hard on yourself for the eighteen minutes not done. Set realistic times for yourself and give yourself lots of acknowledgment and perhaps, on occasion, a treat (a new bathing suit, a night out, an overdue massage) for accomplishing it. Remember that guilt is an enormous waste of precious energy.*

7. **Follow spontaneous impulses.** *When the urge to move arises, use it! Head toward the door and take a walk around the block (breathing every step of the way). If you feel like dancing, get on your feet. Close your office door and jump rope. Hang up the phone and run around the house. These impulses are jewels— don't pass them by.*

8. **Use every means to stay inspired.** Especially in the initial stages of an exercise program, it is easy to forget why you started it in the first place. You need to create inspiration for yourself. Start by scheduling your exercise time as if it were a high-priority meeting—which it is. Mark it on your calendar. Find a partner or a group to exercise with. You will keep each other inspired. No friend? Invite your dog to be your exercise companion. Set short-term goals for yourself. "Short-term" means no more than two weeks ahead. If you are walking for fifteen minutes a day, four days a week, what can you expect of yourself fourteen days from now? Be realistic, and challenge yourself, too. Keep a daily log and a weekly summary of what you did and how you felt when you did it. Reevaluate your goals often.

9. **Respect the earth you move on.** If your exercise takes place outdoors, capitalize on the opportunity to breathe and celebrate the sun, the sky, the fresh air. Don't miss the flowers as you run along the path, and leave the environment unharmed in your travels.

10. **Breathe.** As you move and exercise, you may notice that you are holding your breath. This is a sure sign of unnecessary straining. Inhale as your movements expand. Exhale as they contract or move back to center. Allow the breath to flow naturally.

11. **Love yourself.** Acknowledge what you like about your body and what it does for you. Compose a little song or lyric for yourself and sing or recite it as you exercise. "I am moving with grace and beauty." "I love myself as I grow in strength and agility." "Look at me, I'm beautiful."

This approach to exercise may not win you a place on an Olympic team, but it may help you build body-wise habits that will last a lifetime.

EXERCISING IN WATER

Here are some simple and enjoyable ways to use swimming pool time effectively for heart-stimulating exercise, as well as for firming and trimming of the body.

- **Jogging/cycling.** Keep yourself afloat with arm motions while you tread water, using your legs to "jog" or "ride a bicycle." Time yourself. Rest when tired.

- **Milk jug movements.** Secure two empty plastic gallon-size milk jugs with caps and handles. Screw on the caps tightly so water can't seep in. Hold one in each hand. Use them to support you as you kick, do leg lifts, "jog," and so on. To exercise your arms, play with trying to push them under the surface—you'll be amazed at the resistance. Extend your arms in front of you in chest-deep water and drag the jugs in large circular motions out to your sides and behind you. Have fun being creative with many different movements.

- **Ballet practice.** Stand in chest-deep water, holding on to the side of the pool on your right side. Do leg lifts to front, side, and back. Bend your knee and bring it up toward your chest. Reverse your position and do exercises with the other leg.

- **Dancing.** Bring along your radio or portable music player. Play active dancing music. Do water dancing, standing up or floating. Choreograph a water ballet. Be creative.

- **Swim-a-thon.** Challenge yourself to learn how many different ways you can get from one side of the pool to the other without standing up.

Joining the Dance—An Experience

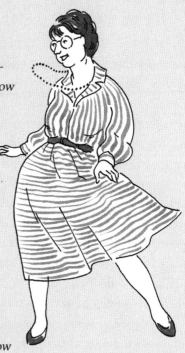

While some of us need no invitation to start exercising, others are less inclined. This exercise is designed to ease you into an enjoyable and energetic dance experience—something you can do without worrying about how you look. Try it and see how simple and joyful movement can be.

In the privacy of your room, put on a favorite piece of energetic music. Close your eyes and simply listen for a few minutes. Let yourself feel the music entering your body with your breath or vibrating the cells of your skin. Now direct your attention to your right hand. Begin to tap or stretch your fingers in any way that the music suggests. Allow the movement to extend itself, to encompass your wrist as well. Stay with this simple experience for a while.

Now direct attention to your left hand and do the same. Imagine that you are shaking off tension, or splashing in water, or kneading a piece of clay—whatever the movement inspires. Next, engage your right arm, and then your left, allowing yourself to move from shoulders to tips of fingers. How many different ways can you find to dance with your arms alone? How many different ways can you move your arms in unison or in opposition?

Keep your arms and hands going, doing whatever they want to, as you give attention to your head. Let the music direct it. Imagine conducting a symphony with a baton that extends from the center of your forehead, or from the crown of your head, or from your chin.

Your upper body now wants to get into the act. Concentrate on your middle section. Allow yourself to move from the waist in any ways that feel good. Pretend that your whole body exists from waist to head— forget the rest. Let the hips and pelvis come along whenever you are ready for them. Careful here—they will want to take over.

Imagine yourself as a tree in the wind. Roots are firm. Only the branches and upper trunk move. Be a fettered bird, wanting to escape, but restrained by a silver thread. Unlock your knees and allow your legs to move without lifting your feet. Challenge yourself with how many ways you can direct them—ways that you have never tried before. Pretend that you are scientifically cataloguing all the possible combinations of movement that legs can make. Keep your feet still until you can't stand it a minute longer. Go inside yourself and take note of what your body feels like all over. Imagine your blood cells dancing in your veins, oxygen dancing in your lungs, energy dancing everywhere.

Now let go completely and allow yourself to move totally—head, arms, belly, pelvis, legs, feet. Surprise! Want another one? This time simply try a different, dramatically more- or less-active, piece of music.

5.9 A Different Way to Exercise

Many of us are reluctant to start exercising regularly because it involves pain, or strain, or special equipment, or others to work out with, or traveling to get to the playing field. If this is true for you, then yoga may be just the approach you need to start you on the road to overall fitness. Anusara (AHN-u-sahr-a) yoga, one of many yoga systems being taught worldwide, not only focuses on the alignment of your outer body but also encourages awareness of your spiritual essence. This type of yoga is as much an art as a science, and those who study it seek to embody qualities of the heart through the movements—not just to stretch or strengthen the body.

The word *yoga* means "union." It is a discipline that seeks to unite the body, mind, heart, and spirit. It is an ideal practice for those in search of high-level wellness.

Anusara yoga, like the other forms, consists of a series of physical postures or poses (*asanas*) and breathing exercises (*pranayama*) that are easily learned and yet may have dramatic effects. Regular practice increases flexibility, strength, balance, grace, breath control, endurance, and overall health and integration. The exercises provide special stimulation of the endocrine glands and thus promote a rebalancing of vital energy throughout the body. Many people experience a greater serenity about life in general, improved circulation, a firmer, trimmer figure, and less illness.

In doing most forms of yoga, you are advised to move slowly and with concentrated awareness, to avoid strain or pain, and to coordinate your breath with your movements. Yoga exercises can be done almost anywhere. It helps to wear loose clothing to make stretching easier, and to have a mat or cloth under you, something that marks this spot as your yoga practice space. You can teach it to yourself simply by following a book or set of instructions, although a trained teacher is highly recommended, especially as you advance into more difficult postures. You can begin this very minute without leaving your chair. Interested? Try this one, it's called the Lion.

Inhale deeply; then forcefully exhale through your mouth. While exhaling with mouth wide open and eyes wide and staring, thrust out your tongue and stretch your arms down with fingers stiff and spread tautly apart. Hold the breath for a few seconds. Then close your mouth and inhale deeply through the nostrils (expanding the abdomen). Exhale again slowly through your nostrils and relax. Repeat three times.

Congratulations—you have done a yoga posture! How do you feel? On pages 135 through 138, you'll find a few more you may want to try. Remember—do not strain, move slowly, and follow instructions for breathing.

These descriptions are supplied by anusara yoga instructor Christina Sell, author of *Yoga from the Inside Out: Making Peace with the Body Through Yoga.* We chose this method because it reflects our wellness approach, and because it takes the emphasis off perfect bodies and puts it on enthusiastic hearts.

Centering

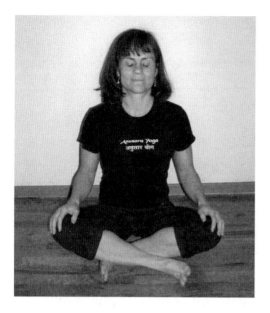

Anusara means "to flow with grace." At the beginning of your yoga practice, take a few moments to center yourself, to connect with your sense of the sacred, and to reflect on your reasons for practicing yoga. When you are ready, move into the Easy Pose, which in Sanskrit is called *Sukhasana. Sukha* means "easy," or "happy." This simple seated posture sets the tone for a happy, easeful relationship with your body and yourself as you practice yoga.

1. *Cross your legs comfortably in front of you.*

2. *Keep your pelvis heavy as you sit up as straight and tall as you can.*

3. *Fold your hands in front of your heart. This is* anjali mudra, *a gesture of prayer and offering that reminds us that every pose begins as an offering from our heart.*

4. *Breathe deeply, slowly, for two to three minutes.*

Standing Reach

Since yoga is about union, in every pose we seek to create a union between opposing forces. In this pose the legs root down into the earth and the torso and arms reach up to the heavens. The yogi or yogini (a female yogi) is balanced and aware in the middle of these opposing forces.

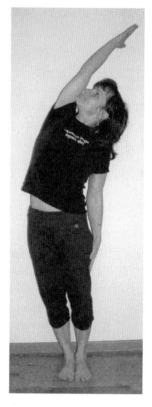

1. *Place your feet hip-width apart.*

2. *Inhale and draw the energy of the earth up into your legs and pelvis.*

3. *Exhale and send that energy back down through your legs into the ground.*

4. *Keeping your legs steady, inhale and stretch your arms over your head.*

5. *Exhale and reach joyfully up to the sky. Imagine even your fingernails stretching upward.*

As you practice this pose, see if you can stretch up through the upper half of your body at the same time that you root down through the lower half of your body.

Tree

This is an excellent way to improve your balance. Remember, even huge trees sway in the wind. There is no need to be perfectly still. Look for a place of balance inside of you that will stay steady no matter what winds may come.

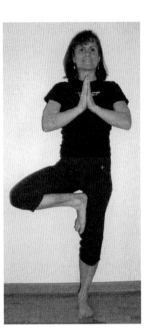

1. *Standing first on two feet, infuse your legs with the strength of a tree trunk.*

2. *Imagine your left foot growing roots deep down into the earth.*

3. *With your left foot rooted, and your left leg strong like a tree trunk, slowly lift your right foot toward your left inner thigh. (Note: It is perfectly acceptable to modify this pose by placing your foot on the inside of your ankle, calf, or knee. You can also practice this pose next to a wall or using a chair to assist your balance.)*

4. *Stretch your arms up to the sky like the branches of a tree.*

5. *Breathe deeply.*

6. *Return to standing on two feet and repeat, this time rooting your right foot and lifting your left foot.*

Warrior

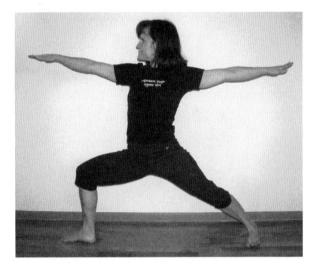

A true warrior fights with dedication for causes that have heart and meaning. In this challenging pose, the heart stays lifted and expanded while the legs remain strong and steadfast.

1. *Step your feet wide apart.*

2. *Inhale, filling your heart with the thought of the causes you believe are worth fighting for, and raise your arms out to the sides, palms facing down.*

3. *Exhale and lunge into your right leg until your calf forms a right angle with the ground. Make sure your right knee stays lined up with your right hipbone and keep your back leg straight and strong. (You can modify this pose by not bending so deeply into your front leg.)*

4. *Look out over your right arm and breathe deeply into your heart. With your torso vertical, reach your arms out to express the vision of your heart.*

5. *Inhale, return to standing center, and repeat on the other side.*

Side Angle

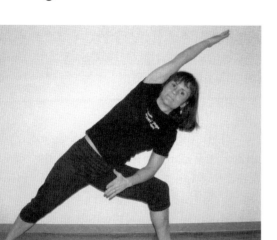

In this pose, the side of the body gets an excellent stretch.

1. *Step your feet wide apart.*

2. *Lunge into your right leg, keeping your back leg straight and strong.*

3. *Place your right forearm on your right thigh.*

4. *Stretch your left arm over your head.*

5. *Breathe deeply and on exhale, extend your energy from the center of your pelvis out all of your limbs so that the pose is even and all parts of you are active and stretching.*

6. *Inhale, return to standing center, and repeat on the other side.*

Bound Angle

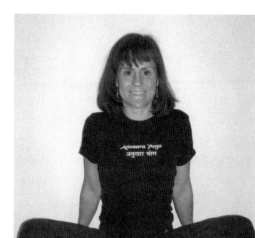

This pose is sometimes called the Cobbler's Pose. In India, cobblers place a shoe between their feet when they work. This pose is excellent for stretching the inner thighs, opening the hips, and maintaining the health of the internal organs.

1. *Sitting on the floor, join the soles of your feet together.*

2. *Inhale and make your legs strong; even draw your knees slightly up toward the sky in order to really feel your legs working.*

3. *Exhale and, keeping your legs strong, reach your knees out to the side. You may notice that your knees will begin to lower; this is good, but do not force them to lower. Instead, keep concentrating on your knees extending out to the side.*

4. *Breathe deeply.*

5. *Inhale, relax your legs, and return to standing.*

Conclusion

Finish your yoga exercise, or any exercise for that matter, by doing a total body relaxation. Lie on your back on your mat or cloth, on the floor, with arms at your sides and legs uncrossed. You can keep your legs straight, flat on the floor, or place your feet flat on the floor, thus allowing the knees to be bent, to relieve undue stress on the lower back. Starting with attention on your feet, slowly progress up the body like this:

1. *Become aware of the space occupied by each body part.*

2. *Attend to how it feels in relation to the ground.*

3. *Allow all tension, pain, and memories of pain to flow out and into the floor.*

4. *Surrender your weight, totally, in every part, letting the floor support you.*

5. *In this state of rest and balance, remember to breathe, and reaffirm your basic goodness.*

6. *Remain at rest, yet aware, for several minutes.*

7. *Slowly stretch, and carefully turn to your side before attempting to sit up.*

8. *Proceed on your way.*

These yoga asanas are only a sampling of hundreds of variations that are used. To learn more about yoga, see the suggested readings, videos, and websites at the end of this chapter.

In addition to yoga, there are many other forms of stretching from which to choose. What is most important is to stretch for twenty to thirty minutes at least three times a week, with emphasis on the lower back and upper legs. Don't stretch past the point of minor discomfort.

BALLOON WALK

Because there is entirely too much seriousness attached to many forms of exercise, most exercise ceases to be play. The following piece was created by our friend Kenneth Maue and is used here with permission. We offer it to you as a playful reminder, an alternative.

Go on a balloon walk. Start anywhere, with a sturdy balloon and some extras. Blow up the balloon, then release it, letting it scoot wherever it goes. After the balloon lands, walk to that place. Then do the process again—blow up the balloon, release it, walk to where it lands.

You may also add something specific to do at each place the balloon lands, such as touching your toes or jumping into the air.

If you are a musician, you may take your instrument and play for a bit at each spot.

Continue until you are finished, then end.

Kenneth Maue, *Water in the Lake: Real Events for the Imagination* (Harper & Row, 1979). Used with permission.

5.10 Strength or Weight Training

Strong muscles are needed for even the most mundane activities, such as getting up from a chair or lifting groceries and children. Strength training can make a big difference in pain control with conditions such as low-back pain and arthritis, and with maintaining and increasing bone density, a big factor in dealing with osteoporosis. The flexibility and strength of your muscles are crucial to remaining independent as you age. Research suggests that the muscle loss occurring in many older people is not from aging itself, but rather from lack of activity. Even a young person who does not get regular exercise loses muscle mass and strength.

In recent years, strength or weight training, also known as strength-developing exercise, has been more widely recognized as an important third component of a personal fitness program, along with cardiovascular and flexibility exercise. Strength training is done through multiple repetitions of several sets of exercises, often using moderate weights or other means to challenge the muscles by creating additional resistance. Besides using weights, excellent strength training can also be accomplished by rowing, climbing stairs, and doing exercises like push-ups. This type of exercise is designed to strengthen and condition the musculoskeletal system, not primarily to build huge muscles. Such training can result in improved muscle tone and endurance, increased bone mass, increased metabolism, and overall toning of the body.

The Department of Kinesiology and Health at Georgia State University summarizes the widely accepted benefits of strength training:

- *Increased muscular strength*
- *Increased strength of tendons and ligaments*
- *Potentially improved flexibility (range of motion of joints)*
- *Reduced body fat and increased lean body mass (muscle mass)*
- *Potentially decreased resting systolic and diastolic blood pressure*
- *Positive changes in blood cholesterol*
- *Improved glucose tolerance and insulin sensitivity*
- *Improved strength, balance, and functional ability in older adults*

It was shown that adding three pounds of muscle increases resting metabolic rate by 7 percent, and daily calorie requirements by 15 percent. At rest, a pound of muscle requires about 35 calories per day for tissue maintenance, and dramatically more during exercise. Replacing fat with muscle uses more calories all day and reduces fat accumulation. Campbell found that strength training produced four pounds of fat loss after three months of training, even though the subjects were eating 15 percent more calories per day.[1]

While "no pain, no gain" may be a catchy advertising slogan, it is false and dangerous advice when applied to strength training. Always take care and listen to your body when you start any new exercise program. Start slowly, move slowly, and increase weights and repetitions only gradually. You will be amazed at how quickly a few repetitions with lighter weights or small resistance will have a cumulative effect as your muscles strengthen.

Take a little time to warm up with breathing and stretching (even some enjoyable dancing!), especially when you are working out early in the day. In the early stages keep your focus on the technique and precision of your exercise, rather than the number of repetitions, and practice breathing thoroughly. Don't exercise for more than one hour, but if you feel "spent" don't go on, even if you've only been exercising a short time. Stop and rest.

Beginners will do well to abide by the American College of Sports Medicine's recommendation for eight to ten repetitions of eight to ten exercises, at a moderate intensity, two days a week. Allow your body to rest and rebuild for one to two days between workouts.

Get some guidance. Especially when using weights and other forms of resistance equipment, it is important to learn a few things before you plunge ahead and overdo it, a common way to invite injury. Your local YMCA or fitness center probably offers classes or the advice of a professional trainer. Your coach or trainer can advise you about how and when to intensify any workout by first adding sets of repetitions then increasing the size of weights.

You should also combine your strength-training routine with regular aerobic exercise (see module 5.6).

5.11 Exercise with a Destination

If you have ever been caught in a traffic jam on a hot summer day, you know firsthand about the stress and pollution created by dependence on the automobile. The situation will continue to deteriorate unless we each decide to do something about it. If you start using your body to take you places instead of your car, you will be rewarded many times over. Running, bicycling, walking, skateboarding and in-line skating do not pollute the air. They increase your own sense of power and also conserve valuable energy resources.

As responsible citizens of planet Earth, we can do much to encourage ecological and healthful alternatives to gas-guzzling and fume-spewing automobile use. We can support efforts to increase public transportation and car pools, especially in our cities. In many places, bicycling paths are being designated for both urban and rural use. As a taxpayer and a voter you can promote these actions. This may entail both higher taxes and lifestyle changes—but so will letting things progress the way they are going now.

. . . the waves are really dancing the measure of a tune.

—Havelock Ellis

SUGGESTED READING

Anderson, B., *Stretching* (Shelter, 2000).

Anderson, S., and R. Sovik, *Yoga: Mastering the Basics* (Himalayan Institute, 2000).

Cooper, K., *The Aerobics Program for Total Well-Being* (Bantam, 1985).

Dychtwald, K., *Bodymind* (J. P. Tarcher, 1986).

Gallwey, W. T., *The Inner Game of Tennis* (Random House, 1997).

Hittleman, R., *Yoga: 28 Day Exercise Plan* (Workman, 1980).

Huang, A. H., *Embrace Tiger, Return to Mountain* (Celestial Arts, 1988).

Johnson, D., *The Body in Psychotherapy* (North Atlantic, 1998).

Katz, J., *Swimming for Total Fitness* (Mainstreet Books, 1993).

Kuntzleman, C., *Maximum Personal Energy* (Rodale Press, 1981).

Lasater, J., *Relax and Renew* (Rodmell Press, 1995).

Leonard, G., *The Ultimate Athlete* (Avon, 1977).

Lusk, J., *Desktop Yoga* (Perigee, 1998).

Rosato, F., *Jogging and Walking for Health and Fitness* (Morton, 1995).

Sell, C., *Yoga from the Inside Out: Making Peace with Your Body Through Yoga* (Hohm, 2003).

Sheehan, G., *Running and Being: The Total Experience* (Second Wind II, 1998).

Stevens, J., *The Secrets of Aikido* (Shambhala, 1997).

Yanker, G., *Walking Medicine* (McGraw-Hill, 1990).

Videos

Beginning: Yoga for the Young at Heart. Susan Winter Ward, Living Arts, (800) 558-9642.

Yoga Journal has a series of excellent yoga videos for beginners, relaxation, strength, flexibility, energy, and meditation; contact at (877) 364-2935, www.yogajournal.com.

Anusara Yoga information, including books, videos, CDs, and how to find a teacher near you, is at (800) 436-9642, www.anusara.com.

For an updated listing of resources and active links to the websites mentioned in this chapter, please see www.WellnessWorkbook.com.

NOTES

1. Campbell, W., et al., "Increased Energy Requirements and Changes in Body Composition with Resistance Training in Older Adults," *American Journal of Clinical Nutrition* 60 (1994): 167–175.

CHAPTER 6

Wellness and Feeling

The expression of emotions—the primary ones being anger, fear, sadness, and joy—is an important form of human energy output. Feelings are generated from within the limbic system of the brain, and serve to motivate both thought and action.

The only thing that is required for healing is lack of fear.

—*A Course in Miracles*

From the moment of birth, with our very first breath, we experience feelings and emotions. They can be intense, or frightening, or wonderful. They can also be the most misunderstood—and, consequently, mistreated—gifts we receive as human beings. We judge them, repress them, drug them, worship them, and run from them. Yet, what a bore to be without them! Life fully lived is life filled with feeling! Life fully lived is high-level wellness.

Sensing . . . Feeling . . . Thinking

The first distinction we need to make is that *feelings,* as the word is used in this chapter, means "emotions." The physical experiences of heat or cold or hunger are *sensations*—the subject of a previous chapter.

Secondly, feelings are not the same as thoughts, even though we commonly hear them spoken of that way. Actually, thoughts and feelings are experienced in very different areas of the brain. The limbic system, deep within the brain, is the source of emotions, while thoughts occur in the neocortex, or gray matter, which is the surface of the brain and a rather recent development in the evolution of mammals.

We respond to any given event with both thoughts and feelings. Yet most of us give priority to our thoughts about a subject and sometimes ignore the feelings. If you ask a person how he feels about a controversial political figure, and he responds by saying, "I feel he should be recalled," he is really expressing an opinion (a thought), not a feeling. Recalling is not a feeling. Anger, fear, sadness, and joy are feelings. A more accurate answer, then, might be, "I feel angry with him and afraid of what he might do; I think he should be voted out of office."

Sometimes we are confused about what we are feeling. It is possible to feel both angry and sad at the same time, and one feeling may predominate only slightly over the other. It is possible to be both angry and fearful, or happy and sad about different aspects of the same situation. Also, when we are shocked by a traumatic event, the body-mind may temporarily shut down feelings that are too painful to experience all at once. In such a case, "numb" may best describe how we feel.

In most cases we have a feeling instantaneously, even though we may have learned to suppress it. Then, a fraction of a second later, the intellectual processes have time to compute, and we decide what position we will take and what we will do. This movement from feeling to thinking or from feeling to acting is described in many different ways by learning theorists and psychologists. Having some awareness of this important transition in our minds is a key wellness skill. When we know the interrelationship of feeling and thinking we can then decide what, if anything, we want to *do* about our feelings or our thoughts.

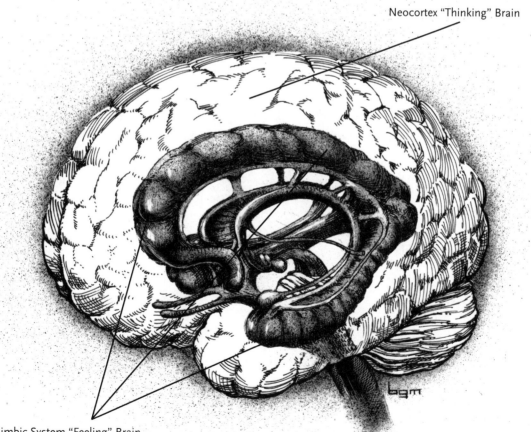

Neocortex "Thinking" Brain

Limbic System "Feeling" Brain

1978 (Looking Back)

It is midnight in April of 1972. Two-month-old Hannelore is sleeping in the nursery in the cherry cradle I built for her from plans out of the *Ladies' Home Journal* (if only I had known what I know now about the importance of children sleeping with parents). In the next room her mother and I are in bed having an argument. An observer would think it rather a strange argument because my wife is shouting angrily at me and I'm saying nothing, looking very martyred and wondering what the neighbors will think. The subject of her anger is my lack of emotional expression. I feel hurt inside, but am speechless when I try to express any of my feelings. I feel a growing pressure and sense of unreality and suddenly I sit up, yell loudly, and ram my head into the plasterboard at the head of the bed (I happen to be a Capricorn—the goat—but the symbolism eluded me at that point). Stunned, I look at the smashed hole conforming to the size of my head, mentally express gratitude that I missed the studs in the wall—or it would have *really* hurt—and collapse, sobbing. She puts on her overcoat and runs to the next-door neighbor, a former campus minister, who returns alone to our apartment. Through my tears I tell him I don't know what's come over me since Hanne's birth. My depressions are getting worse and my wife is spending so much time nurturing Hanne that she hardly has any time for me. David suggests I talk with our mutual friend Ann, who knows several pastoral counselors.

This event marked a major milestone in my personal and professional development as I began one-to-one counseling the next week and started reading the first psychological book that seemed like more than gobbledygook to me (*Born to Win*). I discovered a wholly different world of feelings and my own responsibility to deal with them effectively. The implications for my own health and for others were profound, yet nowhere in my previous medical training had I learned to be open to the concept of self-expression and self-responsibility.

—JWT

VARIATIONS ON A THEME—CLUES AND GAMES

On the opposite page is a list of feeling states that people often have but fail to identify. It can be used or played with in a number of ways:

- Use it when you're not sure if you're feeling anything, or if you have so many feelings that you are confused and frustrated. Read over the list quickly and check any words that come close to identifying your present state.

After you have noted them, ask yourself why you have them, or what has triggered them. For instance, if you identify with "stupefied," record for yourself: "I feel stupefied when all my plans fall apart; I feel stupefied by my inability to make a decision; I feel stupefied . . ." Challenge yourself to come up with as many as possible explanations as you can.

- Use the list with a friend. Ask one another: "Tell me about a time when you felt melancholy."

- Use it to inspire journal writing. Take one feeling, write it in the middle of a blank page, circle it, and record all your associations with it. After you've done this for ten minutes or less, write a little story, or poem, or letter for yourself about this experience. The main thing is to have fun.

I feel . . .

I am . . .

abandoned
adequate
adamant
affectionate
agony
almighty
ambivalent
angry
annoyed
anxious
apathetic
astounded
awed
awkward
bad
beautiful
betrayed
bitter
blissful
bold
bored
bothered
burdened
calm
capable
captivated
challenged
charmed
cheated
cheerful
childish
childlike
clever
combative
competitive

condemned
confused
conspicuous
contented
contrite
crazy
cruel
crushed
culpable
deceitful
defeated
delighted
desirous
despair
destructive
determined
different
diffident
diminished
discontented
distracted
distraught
disturbed
divided
dominated
dubious
eager
ecstatic
electrified
empty
enchanted
energetic
enervated
enraptured
envious
evil
exasperated
excited

exhausted
fascinated
fawning
fearful
flustered
foolish
frantic
free
frightened
frustrated
full
fury
gay
generous
glad
good
grateful
gratified
greedy
grief
guilty
gullible
happy
hate
heavenly
helpful
helpless
high
homesick
honored
horrible
hurt
hysterical
ignored
immoral
imposed upon
impressed
infatuated

infuriated
inspired
intimidated
isolated
jealous
joyous
jumpy
kind
laconic
lazy
lecherous
left out
licentious
lonely
longing
loving
low
lustful
mad
maudlin
mean
melancholy
miserable
mystical
naughty
nervous
nice
niggardly
nutty
obnoxious
obsessed
odd
opposed
outraged
overwhelmed
pain
panicked
parsimonious

peaceful
persecuted
petrified
pity
pleasant
pleased
precarious
pressured
pretty
prim
prissy
proud
quarrelsome
queer
rage
refreshed
rejected
relaxed
relieved
remorse
restless
reverent
rewarded
righteous
sad
satisfied
scared
screwed up
servile
settled
sexy
shocked
silly
skeptical
sneaky
soft
solemn
sorrowful

spiteful
startled
stingy
stuffed
stunned
stupefied
stupid
suffering
sure
sympathetic
talkative
tempted
tenacious
tense
tentative
tenuous
terrible
terrified
threatened
thwarted
tired
trapped
troubled
ugly
uneasy
unsettled
vehement
violent
vital
vivacious
vulnerable
weepy
wicked
wonderful
worried
zany
zestful

6.1 Experiencing and Expressing Feelings

From our earliest years, most of us have been trained that some emotions are "good" while others are "bad." It was OK to feel happy. That meant that our needs were being met, and made Mommy and Daddy feel good too. But anger, fear, and sadness made people uncomfortable, so they told us, "It's not nice to be angry," "Don't be sad," or "It won't hurt; there is no reason to be afraid." At school we often saw smiling, passive behavior rewarded, and other emotional expressions—from anger to high levels of enthusiasm—punished. Anger was usually more acceptable from boys than from girls, and fear or sadness more acceptable from girls than from boys. It didn't take us long to learn that some feelings were approved of and should be sought after, and others were disapproved of and should be avoided or denied. The "bad" feelings continued, however, and now we had fewer and fewer acceptable ways to express them.

To help in coping with this confusion, many people have dulled their awareness to emotions in general; accepted the idea that feelings are bad; developed indirect ways of handling them; and lost trust in their own experience. Then they wonder why their lives aren't richer and more satisfying!

Emotions are not good or bad, they simply *are.* The constant interruptions of the telephone in the middle of a project that requires quiet and concentration may arouse anger. A loud crash in the middle of the night usually triggers a fear reaction. Watching a tragic movie may result in tears of sadness. How a person chooses to act in the presence of these feelings may be subject to praise or censure, but the important thing to remember is that the emotions themselves are amoral. It is the judgments we learn to connect with feelings—this one is good, this one is bad—that lead to problems. It is running away from them or holding them inside that can make us sick.

Children in all cultures evidence four basic emotions: anger, fear, sadness, and joy. These emotions blend into the whole spectrum of human feelings. Emotions may be considered separately, but it is important to understand that they are each only part of the whole of our experience. The fully alive human being is capable of feeling all the emotions. Increasing our aliveness, our wellness, means becoming aware of our feelings, accepting them as OK, and developing healthy ways of expressing them. Life would be awfully boring without the creative tension of sadness and joy that any moment may hold.

You can increase your emotional awareness if you stop and ask yourself "What am I feeling?" frequently throughout the course of a day. Awareness in general can be enhanced by using any number of creative cues—signs, strings around the finger, colored dots on keys or wristwatch bands, computer screen pop-ups—that remind you of the issue that you may currently be working with.

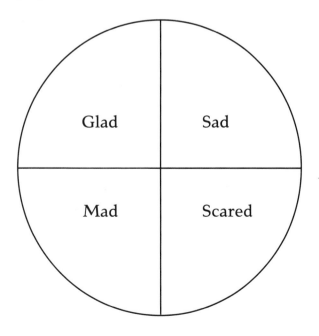

6.2 Different Feeling Styles

Some of us are bigger "feelers" than others—we use a feeling vocabulary with ease, naturally speaking about our emotional inner life, including our immediate intuitions about a person or situation. We are quick to express our sadness through tears, our anger through strong words, our happiness by clapping our hands or jumping up and down. Regina finds that she is strongly affected by nuances of mood or energy of which her husband Jere claims to be completely unaware. She likes to talk about her feelings; about what she is "going through," emotionally. He feels nervous whenever she brings up the subject or asks the question, "How do you feel?" or "What are you feeling?"

Like many couples, and those who work together on a common project, Regina and Jere have discovered that their "feeling styles" are enormously different. It is not that Jere doesn't have feelings or doesn't feel things very deeply—he does! It does mean that he expresses his feelings in a way that is often completely different from his wife's way.

For some, talking about feelings is a type of self-therapy. It is comforting to be able to air what is going on inside. It is satisfying to be able to label the stuff that is swimming around in the emotional gut or the mind. Talking about and sharing feeling states is, for some people, a way of deepening the bonds between them, and two close friends might use this approach as their primary access to intimacy. For others, however, silence and withdrawal are the primary healing modality. John Gray, in his insightful book *Men Are from Mars, Women Are from Venus,* speaks of the need (especially for men) to retreat temporarily into their "cave," where they can sort out the strong and strange emotions that are bearing down on them. His advice to their female partners or friends and coworkers is, "Don't go in there!"—at least, unless requested. It is respectful to leave other persons free to work out their pain, their anger, their fear, their sadness, in their own way, in their own timing.

When the situation is reversed—that is, when someone talks to you about painful feelings—the respectful way to respond is to avoid trying to "fix" the person with an easy piece of advice or some quick platitude. When people express their feelings or talk about their pain, they are helping themselves to gain clarity, not necessarily looking for resolution. In this situation, Gray recommends caring attention, the practice of active listening, and refraining from the cheap closure of easy advice.

Other analysts of human behavior have described our communication styles and our varying degrees of ease with emotional expression in different terms. It is good to keep in mind that our feelings are essentially our gifts and our responsibilities. We can't and shouldn't force—or even expect—others to deal with their feelings in the ways that we deal with ours.

We encourage everyone to deepen their self-awareness, self-responsibility, and self-acceptance of feeling states. We support the choice to express feelings (or to refrain from expressing feelings) in ways that bring people together rather than drive the sexes, races, differing social and economic classes, or nations, further apart. We appreciate that there will always be differences in the ways in which people and nations handle their emotional lives.

On one hand, beware of becoming an emotion junkie.

On the other hand, beware of becoming numb to your feelings!

Getting Reacquainted with Lost Feelings

Here's an exercise that has been invaluable to me. While looking through my baby book I closely examined some of the photos and saw indications of that inner beauty in myself as a child, a presence and light that I had forgotten or didn't know was there. I took some of the pictures out of the book, had them enlarged, and arranged them so I could see those parts of myself I had forgotten or disowned, and reincorporate them into my self-image.

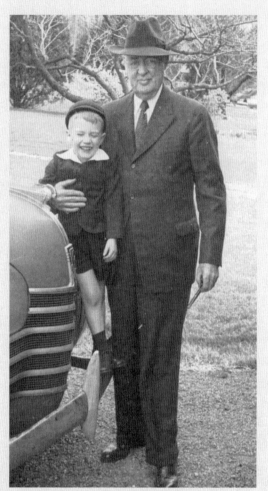

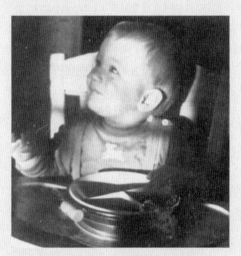

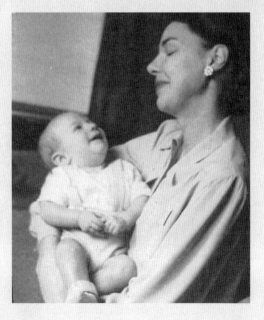

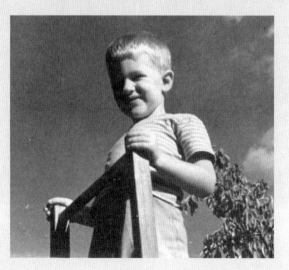

In other photos I saw fear, withdrawal, sadness, pensiveness. Nowhere did I see anger, although I believe that I was really angry when some of them were taken.

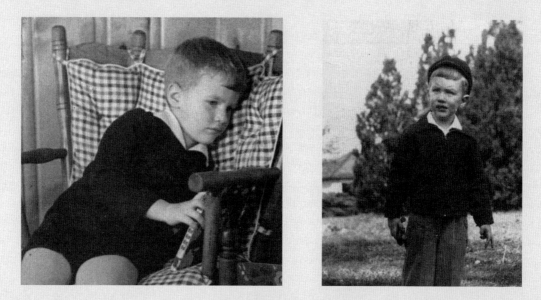

In others I found whimsicalness, silliness, and aliveness that I don't often remember. This exercise has helped me to reconnect with those feelings. Why not do a similar exploration of your early photos? Perhaps you will see something about yourself that you may have forgotten about or lost touch with.

—JWT

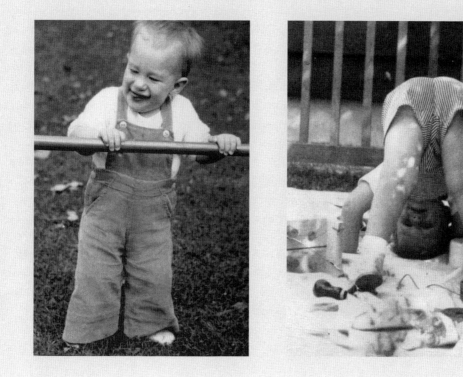

Certain personality tests and type systems have attracted popular attention in the past few decades. Some, like the Enneagram, are based on a centuries-old understanding of human types. Others, like the Myers-Briggs Type Indicator (MBTI), evolved from the work of Carl Jung, are more recent. Essentially, each system demonstrates just how different (but not special!) we are from each other. People see the world and respond to it from many perspectives. Our brain chemistries, our cultural environments, our childhood influences, our metabolisms—among dozens of factors—make us so unique that almost any culture's stereotypical generalizations about norms become highly questionable. Knowing this can also help us to gain compassion, both for ourselves and for others, as it reassures us that we don't have to fit in with one set of prevailing norms. Not our not meeting one set of standards doesn't mean there's something wrong with us.

The Keirsey Temperament Sorter (a simpler alternative to the Myers-Briggs Type Indicator) is widely used in business and education today. Corporations and institutions are finding that productivity and learning may benefit if people accept their own working and learning styles, appreciate the styles of others, and capitalize on differences for the sake of creativity and dynamic learning, rather than engaging at cross-purposes.

This Keirsey Sorter assesses personality according to four dimensions: Extroversion/Introversion (E/I), iNtuitive/Sensing (N/S), Thinking/Feeling (T/F), and Judging/Perceiving (J/P).

Extroversion/Introversion (E/I) is a big factor in human relationships. Imagine a couple, in which one member thrives in group interactions, while the other gets completely drained. (Sound familiar?) Each one can easily assume that the other is crazy, just because they like such different social circumstances. In reality, however, they are each unique and OK. Their challenge is to accept one another's style while finding ways to get their individual needs met. Since the culture of the United States is essentially extroverted (75 percent), introverts are challenged in school, in dating, or in the business world, where so much emphasis is placed on self-promotion—that is, getting out there and mixing with lots of people in order to further your "success."

The iNtuitive/Sensing (N/S) scale, while somewhat similar to the T/F, deals with the differences between an ideal, theoretical but possibly ingenious appreciation of the task (the N) and a hands-on, immediately practical, "show me" view (the S). These approaches have enormous implications in learning, as they tell us how we best receive information and how we best process it.

The Thinking/Feeling (T/F) dimension tells us whether head or heart tends to rule in an individual. Would you feel comfortable having an intimate conversation about someone's recent loss, or would you strive to keep cool and advise them on the best course of action? Big differences here. The Keirsey scale asks, for example, "Are you more concerned with being nice or being fair?" Differing orientations to this issue would make life difficult in relationships or in some working partnerships.

Where Judging/Perceiving (J/P) is concerned, we are talking about the contrast between the person who wants things under control, manageable, orderly, and settled (the J), and the person who is essentially happy in an open-ended, loosely structured situation (the P). Just imagine how that affects the ability of a J and a P to work together on a project with deadlines. Unless they have a huge tolerance for the other's divergent approaches, there is going to be breakdown as the deadline approaches.

You can learn more about the Keirsey system from *Please Understand Me II* and can take the test online at www.keirsey.com (registration is required).

6.3 Confronting and Accepting Fears

Fear is a nonspecific reaction to a real or imagined threat to our security—physical, intellectual, psychological, emotional, or spiritual. It serves as protection by causing us to retreat and pull back into ourselves so that we may reassess the situation and accumulate a needed supply of energy for fighting or fleeing. For example, in one timeless instant you hear an unfamiliar sound, visualize an attacker, freeze, feel weak in the knees, scan the environment for weapons and exit doors, and turn around with an upraised fist.

Fear happens when we can no longer trust something or someone, or when we anticipate the breakdown of one of our security systems. It can be a physically painful emotion because it involves contraction and constriction of the body. For those who deliberately engage in high-risk activities—such as race car drivers and hang glider pilots—fear can be accompanied by high exhilaration that can clear and free the emotional channels to allow the flow of life energy. This is one paradox of fear.

People handle their fears in a variety of ways. Sometimes they run from them by transferring out of a difficult class in school or by leaving the cemetery before the casket is actually lowered into the ground. Many children have learned to keep quiet about fears because of their parents' angry reactions. "There is no monster under the bed. Now turn off that light and go to sleep!" But the fears remained and sometimes showed up in bed-wetting or sickness, which quickly brought Mother to the bedside.

As we mature, we engineer strategies for masking our fears. Some people frantically fill their homes with appliances and furniture, their closets with new clothes or shoes, their calendars with activities, or their mouths with food when what they are really searching for is a way to deal with fear. Others withdraw into fantasy, hide behind computer screens, or build walls of books and papers to protect themselves from the world of real live people who can hurt them. The paradox is that an immense amount of fear is *created* as we spend our lives trying to escape fear.

Once you are willing to admit to having fears, you can begin to face your monsters. Generally you find that the reality is far less scary than the fantasy. One gentle way to begin addressing fears is by taking a class that deals with expanding the scope of your relationships. Assertiveness training is a good way to learn to "stretch your comfort zone"—meaning to take small risks, tiny steps in facing your fears. Every step taken enhances your confidence and builds your strength and ability to challenge your fears. You may start with phoning a business in town to register a minor complaint. The next day you progress to talking with a friend with whom you've had a disagreement.

It takes courage to confront fears, so it helps to share them with others and give yourself lots of positive acknowledgment for each bit of progress realized. Keep in mind, however, that the point is not to eliminate fear, which is a natural human response. The point is to recognize it and befriend it. People who accomplish great things are those who move forward *with* their fears, not because they have no fear.

6.4 Experiencing and Expressing Anger

Anger is the emotional response to what we see as injustice or frustration. While society doesn't approve of injustice, it also doesn't approve of anger. As children we heard, "Don't fight," or "It's not nice to get angry," or "Hold your temper!"

Anger energy is powerful, and ignoring it will not make it go away. Often it will smolder until it bursts into flames, or dam up until it seeps out like poison in ways that encourage illness. If repressing anger is your habitual response, you are likely to get into trouble. For example, a chronically tense jaw can misalign the dental bite, induce headaches, destroy teeth, and detract from a person's physical appearance. Unexpressed anger can feed resentment and lead to unpredictable explosions that upset your relationships and your mental balance. Many "nice guys" and "sweethearts"—those whose behavior in public is exemplary—are often hiding intense anger. Instead of sharing openly, they become covertly hostile, smiling as they stab you in the back. Because there are such strong cultural proscriptions against the expression of anger, this passively aggressive activity has become standard operating procedure in many societal institutions, including the workplace. If we were courageous enough to tell the truth—to respectfully and constructively communicate our anger—our world would very likely be a much more honest and peaceful place.

It's OK to feel angry. It's OK to express it in ways that don't hurt others or yourself. Here are some suggestions for how to use your anger to solve problems, rather than to create new ones.

Feel it! Accept the fact that you're feeling angry. Don't try to deny or explain away that tightness in your gut, those hot tears in your eyes, or that rush of energy in your hands or arms. Do your best to stay focused on your body. "Thinking" about being angry isn't the same as *feeling* your anger. Observing your anger and being with it, like a news reporter on a hot story, is more immediately useful. Accept that something strong is moving through you. Feel it without assuming that you should immediately "do" something to get rid of it in yourself or to make it known to somebody else. Learn about how your body actually feels under the influence of anger. Notice your breathing, your heart rate, your posture. How does your skin respond? How does this feeling state start to affect your thinking or your motor skills?

The longer you can keep yourself attentive to the physical domain without acting out your anger, the more you'll learn about yourself. Although the mind can and will keep you endlessly agitated if you feed it with rationalizations and explanations, or reruns of the event you've just endured, the body itself seeks equilibrium. Observe the body long enough and without a lot of mental intervention (easier said than done) and you'll notice a change in those reactions.

Let off some steam first. Sometimes anger leads to an internal clarity or focus that actually *moves* the body into positive and beneficial action—acts of bravery are the result of such focus. More often, however, anger can cloud the brain, making rationality fuzzy. It may provoke a desire for striking back with violence, more anger, or a plot for revenge.

If you're still "hot" about the situation that has provoked your anger, it is best not to try to negotiate with your perceived "attacker" immediately, if it can be avoided. In many more situations than we might imagine, leaving the scene, at least temporarily, is a viable and valuable option. It is next to impossible, while still in the throes of an anger episode, to speak or listen to someone else without offensive or defensive overtones or blockages. Letting off some steam is an important intermediate step. It's certainly better than swallowing and internalizing the anger, turning it into poison or violence to yourself. A deep, rich, full breath (or two or three) may be all you need to gain a bit of perspective and to soften a tone that would otherwise provoke the other person even more.

If you are indoors, stepping outside for a change of scenery and some fresh air, or merely opening a window and looking at the sky or the trees, for instance, can be enough to alter your mood and maybe the mood in the room. If you don't have to face the other person right away, you can take a fast walk around the block, take a bath, listen to some music, stroke your cat. Perhaps you need to beat on your bed with a tennis racket, park your car on a back road and yell, or conduct a mock argument or "negativity" session with a friend. Discharging some of the energy first may clear your head and makes it easier to identify the problem. Monitor for yourself whether catharsis (yelling or beating on something) is helping you to get clear or not. If it does, use it. If it builds more anger or fear or frustration, don't do it. A hard game of tennis or other aerobic activity, or simply talking to a tree or a willing friend, are helpful ways to deal with the raw edge of anger.

Question what you're angry about. We have found that people are rarely clear about why they are angry, since blame and defense are so closely tied in with anger responses. Many of us put the blame for a situation on someone or something because we're afraid to admit our own culpability in the matter (or conversely, we blame ourselves rather than imagine that a loved one pulled the trigger of our anger). At this stage it is OK to not know *exactly* what lies at the root of the anger. It is OK to admit, "I don't really know who or what I'm angry at, yet. . . ." In other cases, there will be no doubt about the reason for the anger.

EMOTIONAL AWARENESS AND EXPECTATION TRACKDOWN

Often, our emotions are a result of some unfulfilled expectation (in the form of an internal or external desire or demand). Asking yourself the next few questions may help clarify the connection between feeling states and expectations. Using these questions several times in the course of a day, or whenever you're feeling unhappy, may increase your emotional awareness quotient.

1. What am I feeling?

   Am I mad/sad/scared?

   What is happening in my body?

   How, if at all, is this feeling affecting my thinking now?

   How, if at all, is this feeling affecting my overall mood right now?

2. When did this feeling start?

   What was happening at the time or what occasioned it?

3. Was there a desire/demand I had that was unmet, thus giving rise to this feeling?

   What expectation was unfulfilled? (For example: I expected/demanded that Frank would shower me with compliments for my cooking, and I felt angry when he didn't. Or, I secretly hoped for a problem-free workday; when frustrations arose, I became depressed, thinking there was something wrong with me.)

4. How realistic is/was this expectation?

5. Are you able or willing to relax this expectation/demand/desire, even a little?

6. What happens when you ease up a bit on the expectation, allowing things to be as they are?

Congratulations! Investigating these questions may lead you into some challenging or even uncomfortable places—but taking the risk is generally worth it.

Question what you're sad or scared about. Anger is sometimes the surface reaction that reflects a deeper feeling state that we are unable or unwilling to express. Carla's husband Frank readily admits that he becomes angry when she gets hurt or sick. The anger hides his *fear* that something serious is going on for her, and his *sadness* at his inability to fix it.

Recognition of the root of anger as sadness or fear is a much more honest platform from which to speak or negotiate with another person. Sadness and fear inspire vulnerability and openness to support and compassion from the other. When one is standing in these domains, there is less likelihood of counterattack and more pain.

Share the fact that you are feeling angry—or sad, or afraid—with the person or persons involved, and let them know how you see the situation. Remember to take the other person's feelings into account. Ask them how they see things, and if they want to share what they are feeling. This is an important step, as it keeps you from assuming that you know how other people feel and it helps to clarify the situation so you know you're both talking about the same thing.

Be effective, rather than right! As we will discuss at length in chapter 9, it helps to realize that whether you are right or wrong is not the real issue in working through a "feeling" situation. The real issue is, will the problem be effectively addressed? As to who is at fault *really,* that's a waste of time. To be effective may require that you "get off it," and fast. In other words, you drop self-righteousness and aim at understanding the other.

Decide what you're going to do. After the other person has shared her feelings, and you've each had a chance to see the situation from another perspective, you're in an ideal place to apply your best problem-solving skills to the situation. Strive for a win-win solution—one that allows both or all involved to maintain dignity and self-respect while getting their needs met as much as possible.

Not all problems or people are easily dealt with, nor will every sharing session have a happy ending. Be patient with yourself and others. This feeling domain is often a scary place for those unfamiliar with the terrain. Try to stay focused on one issue at a time. If you try to deal with *everything* about your relationship in one session, you're bound to be frustrated. If you demand that others feel as strongly or deeply about something as you do, you're setting yourself up for disappointment.

WHY ARE YOU ANGRY?

The metaphysical system known as *A Course in Miracles* wisely suggests, "I am never upset for the reasons I think." Such a confrontational statement, while not immediately obvious, hides a deep truth. While people (the authors of this book included) may casually talk about "being in touch with their feelings," we are often grossly unaware of what our true motivations are and even less aware of the reasons for our hair-trigger reactions, which we then tend to sanctify by calling them our "true feelings." Given the time and attention that self-observation entails, we may recognize that our present anger is more a result of wounded self-importance, or some flashback to a time when we were misjudged or mistreated by Mother twenty, thirty, or forty years ago. Immediately acting out our anger or even "sharing our feelings" with someone else may be a perfect way to distract ourselves from—and delay—the sort of self-understanding that can only come with time and intention.

Angry Answers

Messages I heard about expressing anger:

_____

_____

These things/events/people stimulate anger in me:

_____

_____

The last time I felt anger was:

_____

_____

Is it OK for me to feel angry?

_____

_____

I express anger by:

_____

_____

Unhealthy ways I express anger:

_____

_____

Healthy ways I express anger:

_____

_____

What I've learned about myself from these questions:

_____

_____

_____

_____

Share with a friend.

6.5 Saying No without Feeling Guilty

Although guilt is not one of the primary feelings (anger, fear, sadness, and joy), it is so pervasive in our culture that it needs some primary treatment. Guilt is a mixture of both fear and anger and acts like an internal smoke screen. It allows us to feel bad about something but prevents us from seeing alternatives and doing anything effective to change the situation.

Regina reports that when she was a regular cigarette smoker she always felt guilty about her habit. She remembers how smokers would often admit to one another, "I hate myself for doing this. I should stop." This little "confession of sins" became almost a ritual that punished and absolved her all in one step. She was then guilt free—until the next nicotine urge struck.

Guilt is rampant among those who have been trained (often since birth) to feel "not OK" about themselves. Guilt usually covers up anger about all the "shoulds" they have swallowed that can never be adequately digested; all the demanding and disapproving parental voices, both within and without, that can never be silenced. Those who are preoccupied with guilt miss the opportunity to constructively channel the energy of their rage into actually alleviating or solving the problem. It is much more comfortable to keep one's familiar misery and perpetuate the cycle of self-depreciation than it is to risk the unknowns that come with being effective and powerful.

Learning to say no and stand one's ground, rather than overadapting to others, is a good starting point in breaking guilt patterns. The next steps include telling the truth about our anger, admitting our fears, and refusing to perpetuate negative self-talk that keeps "not-OKness" alive.

While we may view guilt as a useless waste of energy, there are some important related emotional states that can be confused with guilt. Guilt results from doing something that we knew was wrong *at the time*. Regret comes from learning *later* that we made an unwise choice. Understanding this difference allows us move beyond blaming ourselves for what we didn't know or weren't able to do. Still another feeling close to guilt is remorse—a genuine variation of sadness. Remorse is a healthy human response to the recognition of our responsibility for something that has been harmful or hurtful to ourselves or others. A drunk driver who kills a pedestrian may rightly feel remorse for such behavior, as difficult as this is to face. We feel true remorse when we acknowledge that our self-serving actions have caused pain to someone else—for example, when we have lied, or when we denied our loyalty to a friend. Feeling our remorse—*without* drowning in self-recrimination—is necessary if we are to grow as honest human beings. It hurts to face up to ourselves at times, and that's OK.

6.6 Experiencing and Expressing Joy

You experience joy when you realize some gain: anything from finding a dime on the sidewalk, to receiving a compliment, to understanding that people love you. Joy is a state of in-tune-ment, a feeling of expansiveness, a deep appreciation of the beauty all around. While some see it as a treasure to be searched for and then carefully guarded, it is simply the natural state of living with your eyes fully open—the gift and grace of being human. If this is true, you may wonder why you don't feel it more often.

Joy can be sabotaged when we mistrust having too much of a good thing. You have probably observed this scenario happening among young children: laughter and excitement build to a critical level, the energy gets intense, somebody hits or pushes somebody else, and the next thing you know, one of the crowd is crying, or the whole group is fighting. Adults are familiar with this pattern and often caution children: "Calm down now," "Don't get too excited," "Somebody is going to get hurt." And sure enough, someone does.

It is easy to continue this way of thinking in our adult lives. We often find ourselves expecting the worst so we won't be disappointed. Someplace deep inside, many of us are afraid to open up to joy because we are afraid of losing it. Sooner or later, we think, it's got to end. The result of this closing down can be emotional dullness, a gray world, a guarded heart, and a lonely existence even in the midst of abundance.

Much poetry has been written about the joy to be found everywhere—in looking at a flower, breathing sea air, touching a leaf. Yet many of us miss these moments, and the possibility of joy, because we are too busy, too tired, too "mature," or too bored. One of the magical benefits of setting our sights on wellness is an opening to this richness—a heightened sense of joy in all aspects of our lives.

Whatever road we take to You, Joy.
However one is received, Honor.
With whatever eye one beholds You, Beauty.
In whatever language Your Name spoken, Joy.

—Shaikh Abu-Saeed Abil-Kheir

Although joy often seems to arise naturally and spontaneously as a result of some attunement to the wonder of existence, joy may also evolve as a consequence of our choices, activities, or behaviors, such as these:

- *Recognizing a problem (fatigue, overweight, and the like)*

- *Deciding to confront a problem*

- *Following an early morning jogging program*

- *Feeling a sense of wellbeing or joy*

The infusion of joy into the body-mind is one of the best disease-preventative and curative strategies we know.

A Circle of Joy

Fill the circle with names of people/events that are currently sources of joy for you. Also list people or events that have created joy for you in the past. Show your circle to a friend, or simply share one story of your joy with someone you trust.

STAMP OUT "OUGHTISM"

Oughtism is a disease of the oughta-nomic nervous system. The unfortunate victims oughtomatically do what others tell them they *ought* to do. If left untreated, Oughtism can eventually result in a total loss of the ability to think.

Are *you* Oughtistic?
Take this simple test.

Yes/No

____ Do you feel obligated to give blood even when you're down to your last pint?

____ Do you put on clean underwear each day just in case you get hit by a car and have to go to the hospital?

____ Are you reading this only because somebody said you ought to?

If you answered "yes" to any of these questions you could be Oughtistic. But don't feel bad. You aren't alone. Forty million Americans suffer from this silent crippler. And most of them don't even *notice*.

Yes, Oughtism *can* be cured. But first, you must know its warning signals:

- Any involuntary nodding of the head up and down—especially when someone asks for volunteers.

- Sharp pangs of guilt after digesting a single chocolate-chip cookie

- An enlargement of the onus

- An empty feeling between the ears

- Constriction of the intestines; that duty-bound feeling

So join us, won't you? Let's stop this epidemic before we all become ough-tamatons.

6.7 Sadness and the Grieving Process

The other side of joy is sadness or grief. It is the emotion that arises from a loss, either real or imagined. When someone special, or something important, or some cherished belief is lost, you feel a gap or a hole in your internal reality. This may lead to a variety of physical symptoms, from loss of appetite to tightness in the chest to insomnia, fatigue, or even hyperactivity. Loss also affects your thinking and ways of behaving.

Since the 1970s, supported by the pioneering work of Elisabeth Kübler-Ross, M.D., and the growing popularity of the hospice movement, a greater understanding of the nature of grief and loss has pervaded the culture at large. The psychology of grief and loss informs us that grieving is part and parcel of life as much as it is of death. Kübler-Ross, in her classic book *On Death and Dying,* indicated that there are identifiable stages in the grief process—whether we are grieving the loss of a job, a loved one, or our dreams. Knowing the progression of these stages can be a great help in moving through them and building some sense of security, since there is frequently a tendency to fear that you are going crazy; that you are all alone; that no one else has ever gone through this before; and that there will be no end to it. Realizing that these are very natural responses to loss can provide much-needed encouragement, a tiny ray of sunlight in the midst of so much darkness.

Denial is commonly the first stage in the grief process. You hear yourself or others saying, "I can't believe it," or "This can't be happening to me." When facing loss or death, the organism's natural balance is challenged. It's normal, in the early stages of grief, to go into shock, withdraw, become numb, or act feverishly to block out the harsh reality—these reactions give the body-mind some necessary distance from trauma. They can offer a chance to awaken more gently to a difficult truth. When the world has been temporarily turned upside down, it naturally takes some time to adjust.

Anger follows denial. People get angry at the employer who fired them, the husband or wife who left them, the God who permitted this tragedy to happen. Since anger may not be an "approved" emotion, it is often swallowed and stored away. This can be harmful for both physical and psychological health.

After denial, and along with anger, many people go through a stage called "bargaining" in which they try every strategy they can think of to change their situation. They try to make bargains with God, the fates, or the supernatural, either directly or implicitly, in which they promise to be good or perform some heroic deeds if only their sentence of loss can be removed. Grieving people may undertake a pilgrimage, become extremely religious, make donations to charities, start new health regimens, write letters of apology in which they beg a separating partner to return, and so on. Such bargaining is a last-ditch effort to avoid immersion in the well of deep pain that accompanies facing the loss head-on.

When these strategies fail, the real grieving usually takes place. Sadness touches you at the very core of your being and from that place you mourn the loss. The deep sighing or primitive moaning sounds that come with crying are healthy indications that you are confronting the pain right down to its roots. It doesn't mean that the pain goes away, but that you are doing the grief work necessary to healing.

There are two ways of dealing with grief—"hard and fast" or "hard and slow." The healthiest way you can heal the wound created by your loss is to face it squarely—to cry through the pain you feel and to tell the story of your loss to caring listeners. Allowing yourself to swear or scream is OK too, if that would feel good to you. Such energetic expressions can help some people to loosen the floodgates that hold back tears. However, approach extreme catharsis (like screaming and swearing) with caution, as for some it can intensify into a state that is undesirable, possibly causing even more harm.

All of these stages lead to the final phases—at the least, resignation, and at best, acceptance. Sadness and grief, like other deep emotions, stir up internal waters that may have grown stagnant; this can be cause for profound celebration, since they call for a reassessment of life values, and they raise questions that might otherwise have gone unasked for years.

ONE WOMAN'S GRIEF REACTIONS: REGINA'S JOURNAL

September 11, 2001, Arizona

The news of the attacks on the World Trade Center and the Pentagon reached me early this morning. My friend, Sally, met me at her door with tears in her eyes and told me that something terrible had happened. The shock took many forms. At first, denial, as I couldn't quite understand the words. She spoke clearly, of course, but it seemed like a foreign language. I didn't want to hear such stories. She must be mistaken.

A hot rush of fear hit my belly, my face grew warm, my arms and legs tingled. There was a feeling of breathlessness. All morning long I kept sighing deeply, gasping for air. The sensation in my body is hard to describe—something like cotton candy in the veins. I was simultaneously excited and numbed. The reality did not penetrate for several hours. Since I had no television, I didn't see what most of the world saw immediately, but my sadness and fear grew as the reports came in. I never really felt angry, but I tend to repress anger, so maybe I had it but didn't show it.

As the day progressed, I observed the responses of my friends. Some wept openly. Others, with sharp words, angry tones, described the horrors. Others, with trembling hands, tried to get through by cell phones to loved ones in New York. I tried to keep myself fiercely under control, my typical strategy for handling the unknown.

When I finally saw my husband, we were both shaken. As we spoke, I allowed the first few tears to flow, and then we both became silent. We held each other for a long time. What could we say?

—RSR

The Crying Quiz

Self-awareness about emotional expression may be useful in expanding your emotional vocabulary; it may even lead to great freedom in this domain. Use these questions to spark your emotional memory.

What messages do I remember hearing about crying?

_____

_____

When was the last time I cried?

_____

_____

How do I really feel about crying?

_____

_____

These things make me cry (include songs, movies, events, etc.):

_____

I could cry with these people around:

_____

Because:

_____

I could never cry with these people around:

_____

Because:

_____

What I have learned about me as a result of doing this exercise:

_____

_____

Earn bonus points: share with someone else!

6.8 Positive Attention/Negative Attention

When someone gives us attention, it generally provides a form of stimulation or recognition that arouses feelings in us. The attention may appear in brightly colored packages as smiles, hugs, and loving words (the positive attention), or in dingy paper bags as brush-offs, cold stares, and reprimands (the negative attention). Whenever people acknowledge you in any way—perhaps with applause, maybe with censure—you are moved—"touched," so to speak.

To be attended in these ways is to be confirmed in the realization that we exist. And this realization is absolutely essential for survival. If we aren't successful in getting our needs met in life-affirming, positive ways, we will seek satisfaction in death-promoting, negative ways, rather than suffer the intolerable condition of being a nonentity. As the saying goes, "Negative attention is better than no attention at all." We should try to keep the ratio of positive-to-negative attention we offer ourselves, loved ones, and coworkers close to ten to one.

Let's consider a few examples. Marilyn invests energy in a project to help the poor of the country. She receives the support of her coworkers, the gratitude of her clients, and the powerful self-reward of knowing that she is making some impact on the world. Jeffrey defaces property with spray paint. He brags about it and finally gets arrested. In this way he affects his world by frustrating or horrifying others, and he receives a short-lived, sensational focus of public attention from his parents, the press, and the police. In Jeff's view, to go through life unnoticed would be far worse than suffering the consequences of his destructive acts. But he would be the last one to describe it this way.

Matt, at age six, starts acting out in school. His work reflects it. He immediately reaps benefits from conferences with the principal and counselor, and lots of attention from his parents.

Children and adults need emotional and psychological attention for happiness and health, as much as newborns need physical touch for survival. Our need for both receiving positive attention and learning to cope with negative attention is inextricably linked with our general state of health.

In his work with cancer patients, Carl Simonton, M.D., observed: "The biggest single factor that I can find as a predisposing factor to the actual development of cancer is the loss of a serious love object, occurring six to eighteen months prior to the onset of the disease." The love object—frequently a child or spouse—is a primary source of attention. When that is lost, it can lead to destructive means of compensation. Nobody wants cancer or another serious disease, but everybody wants attention!

Sometimes a problem develops because we have collected a poisonous supply of negative attention. Many of us tend to store it up until it eats away at us from within. Hurts, anger, fear, deep sadness—these create an energy that will look for an outlet somewhere in the body if it doesn't get conscious recognition or expression. Such outlets include:

- *Smoking or overeating*

- *Driving recklessly*

- *Gritting teeth*

- *"Getting" a sore throat, an asthmatic attack, or a headache*

- *An extra rush of adrenaline into the bloodstream that makes us feel wired*

- *A stress-related condition such as constipation, a skin disorder, eye fatigue, or an ulcer*

• Building defenses, by withdrawal and depression, to keep us from being hurt again

When we don't understand our real needs or how to fulfill them, we are left with a void that is all too easily filled by illness or dangerous habits. As children, many of us got some of our most nurturing attention when we were sick. Some of us still use the same tactic as adults. We think we have to break down totally before we can get the help and attention we need. Claudia, at age forty-seven, reported that she had never realized how caring her husband and children could be until she developed cancer. While it would be simplistic to assume that serious illness is the result of one factor alone, many health conditions are significantly improved when friendship, attention, and a support system are added to treatment or healing methods. Attention heals!

6.9 Close Friends

It is important to have several close friends with whom you can talk about anything—friends who will support you in being the best possible person you can be. To create a supportive network may require that you keep extending yourself, meeting new and stimulating people, potential members of your "family." And, it is important to keep in mind that support does not exclude negative feedback or even criticism from others. It is a mark of greatness to be attuned to the truth and willing to hear it, no matter how clumsily it is expressed, how painful it may feel. It is possible, especially among caring friends, to move beyond the realm of winning and losing, being wrong or being right.

This is probably the single most important piece of information for you to remember about wellness and feelings. Life is tough anyway. Alone, it may appear to be intolerable. Remember that it is absolutely necessary to ask for and be open to help, just as it is essential to ask for and be open to love.

A twenty-year survey of adults in the United States reported that, regardless of health problems, people who participated in formal social networks of some type outlived those who did not. An affiliation with a social network was found to be the strongest predictor of longevity, even above age, sex, or health. When people are counting on you, you have a reason to get up in the morning.

Love is giving people the space to be who they are, and who they are not.

—Werner Erhard

NEGATIVITY SESSIONS

Back in the seventies, when John and I managed the Wellness Resource Center, our staff had an agreement that we could call each other day or night and request a negativity session. If the other agreed, the one who had requested it then had full permission to be *totally* negative, without fear of being judged, without worrying. Nothing said in this session was taken "for real." It all went down the drain with a big flush! Now, over twenty-five years later, even though we are scattered all over the globe, several of us still use this process with each other (by phone, of course).

Here's how it worked:

One person is a talker (sometimes more like a "ranter") and the other person is a listener. The talker proceeds to lay it *all* out in no uncertain terms—complaints, fears, problems—everything. Genteelness is not the order of the day in a negativity session. It takes some practice to be able to say what you're thinking and feeling without editing, but the more you do it, the clearer you become, and the faster the negativity dissipates.

The listener's job is just to *be there,* without judging or evaluating what is being said. If the listener doesn't hear or understand something, she will let the talker know, but extraneous conversation is discouraged. The talker has the freedom to say anything! And it doesn't even have to make sense! The listener's responses are ones indicating that the talker has been heard and understood. The only other communications made by the listener, other than acknowledgments, are things like, "OK, what else?" or, if the talker gets into apologizing or rationalizing or philosophizing, the listener can good-naturedly say something like, "Cut the crap and get on with the negativity." The agreement is that positivity is *not allowed* until all the negativity is "dumped." The listener keeps things moving, gently and unobtrusively.

The session concludes when the talker either starts laughing, or says, "Enough!" The listener then says, "Good! Now tell me something beautiful about yourself, or something beautiful that has happened lately." The session is always ended on a positive note.

By using the negativity session for clearing away the unnecessary garbage of our minds, we've established a warmth and a deep trust in our relationships as a staff. The more we can realize that we are all in this together—being human—and the more compassion we cultivate for ourselves and others, the more we can get on with the miracle of living . . . well!

—Bobbie D. Burdett

6.10 Expressing Concern, Love, and Warmth

Studies have clearly shown that people who can experience and express their love and concern live longer, healthier lives. Being able to express our feelings of love doesn't just cause us to feel better—the other person gains a sense of wellbeing as well.

What more powerful attention could you get than to have someone you care about say "I love you"? And what greater impact could you have on your world than to give your love freely, without reservation, without fear? Unfortunately, few of us dare to open up enough to give or receive love. Typically, we tie up much life energy in restricting the flow of love because we are afraid—we fear rejection, fear strong emotions being aroused, fear intimacy, or fear vulnerability.

Like the ground we walk on, love supports us in all we do. Blocking love, whether it be self-love or love for or from others, will inexorably have a negative effect on our happiness and health. Love is not something you can analyze and define. In fact, attempting to do so is likely to keep you from being able to experience it. Love is letting go—letting go of fears, grievances, and judgments. The secret is simply to allow it to happen.

SUGGESTED READING

Amini, F., R. Lannon, and T. Lewis, *A General Theory of Love.* (Vintage, 2001).

Colgrove, M, H. Bloomfield, and P. McWilliams, *How to Survive the Loss of a Love* (Mary Book/Prelude, 1993).

Buscaglia, L., *Love* (Fawcett, 1996).

——, *Living, Loving, and Learning* (Fawcett, 1990).

Epstein, M., *Going to Pieces without Falling Apart* (Broadway, 1999).

Goleman, D., *Emotional Intelligence* (Bantam, 1996).

Gray, J., *Men Are from Mars, Women Are from Venus* (HarperCollins, 1993).

James, M., and D. Jongeward, *Born to Win* (Perseus, 1996).

Jampolsky, G., *Love Is Letting Go of Fear* (Celestial Arts, 1989).

Keirsey, D., *Please Understand Me II* (Prometheus-Nemesis, 1998).

Keyes, K., *The Handbook to Higher Consciousness* (Love Line, 1989).

Kübler-Ross, E., *On Death and Dying* (Scribner, 1997).

Riso, D., *Discovering Your Personality Type: Essential Introduction to the Enneagram* (Houghton-Mifflin, 2003).

Rubin, T., *The Angry Book* (Touchstone, 1998).

Tavris, C., *Anger: The Misunderstood Emotion* (Touchstone, 1989).

For an updated listing of resources and active links to the websites mentioned in this chapter, please see www.WellnessWorkbook.com.

CHAPTER 7

Wellness and Thinking

Thinking depends on the production of electrochemical energy in the brain, and thus, is a type of energy output in the Wellness Energy System. While thinking draws energy from all three of the Wellness Energy System input sources, it is particularly dependent upon sensory data. Thinking energy is intimately connected with the energy of feeling/emotions in mapping our internal version or interpretation of external reality.

**Each thought is a nail that is driven
In structures that cannot decay;
And the mansion at last will be given
To us as we build it each day.**

—George Eliot

Thinking is the art and the craft of the human brain. Like the lungs, heart, and stomach, the brain's work is one of transforming energy. We feed the brain both with the nutrients carried by the blood and with the energy from millions of daily impressions gleaned from what we read in books, watch on television, learn from other people, and experience in sights, sounds, and movement. Some of this energy is used to file away data for later use, and the rest is available for the internal signaling that goes on from brain to nerves and everything else throughout the body, for creating dreams, and for making new connections—for thinking.

Various instruments can demonstrate the energy patterns of the thinking brain. For decades this was done with the head hooked up to an EEG (a machine that measures brain electrical activity), which revealed the various patterns of thinking or nonthinking through electrical impulses detected through the scalp. Think "hard"—and the EEG registers an increase in the frequency of energy. Think "soft"—and see that the brain waves slow down. Now there are many more sophisticated instruments that can reveal the inner workings of the brain, all of which verify why, after a day of mostly headwork, you will often feel physically tired. Thinking takes energy!

Most would agree that what goes into the mouth will affect overall health and wellbeing. Yet few seem to understand that what goes into the mind affects what comes out of the mind. Mental nutrition is every bit as important as oral nutrition. We are repulsed by rotten, moldy food, stagnant air, and polluted water, yet tolerate a good deal of rotten, stagnant, and polluted impressions that leave us with distorted or stagnant thinking. The images and energies that fill our minds affect our physical bodies, influence the people around us, and move the world at large.

YIN-YANG

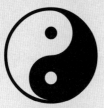

This is an ancient Chinese symbol called the T'ai-chi T'u, which means the "Diagram of the Supreme Ultimate." It is often simply called the *yin-yang*. It is a representation of the way the world works.

Notice first that it is a circle. There is no point at which it starts, no point at which it stops. Half of it is black or darkened; the other half is white or light. These areas represent the opposites: night and day, darkness and light, wet and dry, male and female, attraction and repulsion, expansion and contraction, right and left, sun and moon, heaven and earth . . . the list goes on and on. The dichotomies are separated from each other but also blend together, one flowing into the other.

What it means is that the whole is made up of the opposites. The force of life, of creation, is one of dynamic tension created by the union. It is in the coming together of the male and the female that new life is created. The mysterious play between sound and silence creates the rhythm that we recognize as music, as intelligible speech. One side represents all that is scientific— the logical, the rational, the mathematical, the verbal. The other is the artistic—the musical, the intuitive, the sensual, the nonverbal. Put the two together in one person and you create a genius, an "erotic scientist": the Einstein who was both physicist and poet; the balanced, integrated female who is both strong and gentle; the male who is both nurturing and powerful.

7.1 Thinking about Thinking

Have you ever paused to examine the many thoughts that pass through your mind during a given period of time? Typically, this kind of observation gets quickly short-circuited because instead of simply witnessing our thinking, we start *reacting* to our thinking and soon have to deal with feelings of insecurity or an upset stomach. Instead of simply *observing* the events of some mental scenario as it passes through our mind, we identify with it as if it were real. We actually get up on the stage in our own minds and start interacting with the other mental characters in our internal play, mistaking our fantasy for reality.

Socrates said that to "Know thyself" is the greatest of human endeavors, yet most people are regrettably ignorant about the operation—as well as the moment-to-moment content—of their minds. Since consciousness is related to self-awareness (or knowing that we are alive and knowing what we are doing as we are doing it) the bottom line is that most of our actions and thoughts are not entirely conscious. We live most of our lives automatically. We even *think* automatically, as you probably realize when you notice a familiar thought pattern cropping up for the ninety-ninth time in two weeks. For instance, every time your friend does that one gesture—or doesn't do the gesture—your mind is off and running: "There he goes again, trying to embarrass me. He doesn't like me, or he would not do that! If he doesn't like me, then I don't like him ..." and on and on. The Sanskrit word is *samskaras*—somewhat like grooves in the brain created by habitual ways of acting and thinking. Once we fall into one of the grooves, it can be surprisingly difficult to extricate ourselves.

When we pause to think about thinking, we realize how many different activities are going on in our head. Stepping into the stream of consciousness, we discover that we have memories—some sharp, some hazy; some happy, some sad. We become aware that we daydream about anything or nothing. We rehearse our lives and create expectations for the future, and then plan out these expectations step by step: "After I finish writing this paragraph I'm going to get a cup of tea, then go for a walk, then come back to my desk and work again until six o'clock. And after that ..." We talk to ourselves (self-talk) and to others (internal dialogue) via some projection of them in our own minds, and we then make up potential outcomes of these conversations. We form concepts—of everything from galaxies to subatomic particles—by sorting through masses of concurrent sensory data: some coming from outside sources, including the reactions of other people, and some arising within our own bodies, like what we call our "gut feelings." We then compare and contrast what we have most recently received with what we've already filed away. We create mental images, we analyze, we evaluate, we make unlikely associations and call it art or poetry, we render judgments of good and bad on everything we see, feel, hear, or think about. We create a composite internal picture or description of who we are—the self-concept—and, for better or worse, we call it *me*. Depending upon our focus—a spreadsheet to analyze or a beautiful image in an art gallery to enjoy—we will experience ourselves differently. We tend to solidify our most recent descriptions of ourselves and others, and often much to our own detriment, despite the fact that we are all changing from moment to moment. Then we venture out into the world, attempting to live from these descriptions as if they were "the whole truth and nothing but the truth."

Many philosophers and consciousness researchers today support the idea that consciousness is not singular.[1] Even though it makes things simpler to speak as if "I" means the same thing all the time, even our casual speech reflects our appreciation that we are a multitude: "Well, one part of me likes the idea, but another part is really against it; but then again, another part wants . . ."

Early in the last century, Georg Gurdjieff, an astute teacher and explorer of the human psyche, pointed out that we are run by a vast number of "I's" all vying with each other for attention and dominance. He identified three centers of consciousness, each with its own "I's": the intellectual (thinking or mental), the emotional (feeling), and the moving (action-based) center. Gurdjieff explained that one or more of our thinking "I's" can often be at odds (if not at war) with our feeling-based "I's," and either or both can be in conflict with our action-based "I's"; for example, the "I" that set the alarm clock last night, firmly intending to get up for that early-morning jog in the park, is not the same "I" that heard the ringing in the morning, turned the clock off, and rolled over for an extra hour of sleep. In other words, not only is there potential confusion in the intellect about who's running the show, but that confusion can spill over into our emotional responses and actions as well.

Ordinarily, we limit the idea of "thinking" to something that happens in the cortex of our brain. Yet, the more we learn about the nature of the body, the more we find that our cells have a type of consciousness, a type of memory, a type of intellect that makes connections and directs activity. Author Carolyn Myss (*The Creation of Health* and *Anatomy of the Spirit*) sees evidence in people's lives for how our memories are literally stored in the cells of our tissues throughout the body.

As we explore the interrelatedness of thinking and wellness, it is vital that we get to know our own minds. Learning to pause, to observe, to "listen" without judgment; learning to identify and recognize recurring mental patterns that lead us into depression or anger; learning to drop identification with the mind's constant stream of illusions, while still nurturing the creative flights of fancy—these and many other skills related to self-observation are available to all of us through awareness and practice. Unless we can appreciate how powerfully our thoughts direct our experience of reality, we are doomed to an unconscious existence filled with automatic responses.

7.2 **Thinking Molds Experience**

Living in the sea of our old memories and beliefs, buffeted by the waves of conflicting thoughts, intentions, and impressions from the past, we are forming our present thoughts, words, and deeds, and thereby shaping our future. Little wonder that often things don't seem to change as we might like, either for us as individuals or for the world in which we live, since the past is generally determining the present for better or worse. To become more conscious participants in our life and health, and the life and health of the planet, will mean attending to our thoughts and the ways in which they ultimately either de-energize or benefit us.

The universe begins to look more like a great thought than a machine.

—Sir James Jeans

We see the world through glasses colored by our assumptions and beliefs—our thoughts about the way things are or should be. When we look at the world through glasses tinted with love, trust of others, and optimism, we tend to find examples of goodness and generosity everywhere. When we look through lenses clouded with suspicion and fear, we find hundreds of reasons to be paranoid. Thinking, therefore, will color and even determine our relationships—with ourselves, others, and our environment. For example, many of us are involved in a relationship with another person that has begun to deteriorate in some way: the parent losing faith in the child; the wife suspecting the husband of "playing around"; the friend jealous of another friend. The injured party, wearing "glasses" of victimization, can always find scores of clues to reinforce the belief that he or she is being wronged.

7.3 Shaping Our Own Realities

What we find in the world around us is definitely a function of what we go looking for. In the domain of science, a research study will start with a hypothesis, then attempt to prove it. Often, however, this type of focused looking will cause the researcher to miss another bit of data that might be extraordinarily significant, though not immediately related to the hypothesis. Regina tells a story that dramatically demonstrates that we can't see something for which we don't have a point of reference. A young Tibetan farmer left his ancestral village in the company of an American peace activist; they took a plane to California. The Tibetan man had never seen the ocean—nor any massive body of water, for that matter. As the two men strolled along a boardwalk in Long Beach, the young Tibetan was overwhelmed with impressions. The thousand-foot-long ocean liner the *Queen Mary*, docked at the pier, elicited no response. Even when the American pointed it out, along with many other wonders, the younger man seemed dazed and noncomprehending. When a small dinghy with a loud and sputtering outboard motor moved into view, however, the Tibetan youth began waving with excitement. Pointing at the small boat, he shouted, "A jeep riding on the water!"

Researchers in the field of human consciousness tell us that our senses are actually data-reduction devices, filtering out vast amounts of information that would otherwise create undue confusion. What we end up perceiving in the world around us is largely the stuff we need for survival, for comfort, and for stimulation, as well as the stuff that reinforces our beliefs. All these things create a sense of safety and continuity for us. Therefore, we will often hear what we need, expect, or want to hear, rather than what the other person is actually saying. We will see what we need, want, or expect to see. We will even experience physical sensations, including discomfort, illness symptoms, or the relief of symptoms, because of what we think or need to believe.

Imagination is more important than data collecting, since there is shortage of the former, and a surfeit of the latter. Indeed, information by itself will rarely give a good idea. It is the imaginative skill applied to looking at data that makes the big difference.

—Nicholas Berry

7.4 Thinking Changes the Body

The placebo effect is one of the clearest demonstrations of how thinking affects the body. Believing that someone has given you an effective cure for a problem (although they have only given you a sugar pill or waved something over your head) can not only cause emotional calming, but actually change the physical experience within the body. For example, a study of prostate disorder symptoms reported a two-year improvement among the men who were given a placebo and informed that it would help.

In a more common example of how thinking influences the body, have you had this experience? You went to bed late one night during the work week, looked at the clock, calculated the hours until you had to get up, and thought to yourself, "I'm going to be exhausted tomorrow." In the morning, you felt miserable as you climbed out of bed and dragged yourself to work. All day long you reinforced this feeling by repeating "Am I tired!" Sound familiar? Now replay the same scene, but this time it happens when you are on vacation. You stay out late into the night, dancing, partying. Going to bed, you anticipate the exciting prospects of the next day—new adventures, new sights, new people. You remember that some people thrive on only a few hours of sleep a night and, armed with this thought, you retire happily. The next day you leap out of bed ready for the magic, barely giving a moment's reflection to the amount of sleep you've had. Your thoughts have energized your body.

There are other examples. Years ago, when we were sharing dinner at John's house in Mill Valley, California, we heard a rumbling noise. John, who had been through three earthquakes in eleven months, immediately labeled the rumbling "earthquake." The thought of an earthquake was enough to get our hearts beating faster, blood flowing with greater intensity, hormones activated, stomachs churning. There was no earthquake, but it took a lot longer to convince our shaky hands and queasy stomachs than it did to reassure our minds. Our bodies responded as actively to the imagined danger as they would have to a real one.

7.5 Body Awareness

In the mid-twentieth century a Russian scientist, A. R. Luria, demonstrated that imagining running uphill actually increased his subject's pulse rate.[2] In the 1960s, the newly emerging field of biofeedback research took observations such as Luria's and raised them to a new level, affirming our understanding of the body-mind connection. After fostering the creation of the science of the body-mind connection—known as psychoneuroimmunology (PNI)—biofeedback is today more accurately called *neurofeedback*. We now know that we can not only slow or quicken heartbeat, but affect a whole host of other physiological functions by merely thinking about stressful—or relaxing—conditions.

Under hypnosis, individuals can create blistered skin when given a suggestion that they have been burned. Simply believing you are in danger, or maybe harboring a deadly tumor or virus, can create extreme changes in your body. Bob, who was a medic during the Korean War, tells the story of a young soldier who had a badly lacerated leg. His vital signs were excellent as the corpsmen worked on him. When the doctor arrived on the scene, he took one look at the leg and exclaimed, "Oh my God, this is bad." The young patient immediately died.

Accounts of this nature are common. Doctors and nurses are continually confronted with the reality of the will to live or the wish to die in seriously ill people. Two individuals with the same symptoms. Prognosis for both is the same. One lives. One dies. Why? The Greek philosopher Socrates answered the question in 500 B.C.E.: "There is no illness of the body apart from the mind." In modern times, Arnold Hutschnecker, M.D., in his book *The Will to Live*, reinforced this: "Anxiety is a whisper of danger from the unconscious; whether the danger is real or imagined, the threat to health is real . . ."[3]

WHAT IS BIOFEEDBACK?

Biofeedback is a treatment technique in which people are trained to improve their health by using signals from their own bodies. Physical therapists use biofeedback to help stroke victims regain movement in paralyzed muscles. Psychologists use it to help tense, anxious clients learn to relax. Specialists in many different fields use biofeedback to help their patients cope with pain.

Chances are you have used biofeedback yourself. You've used it if you have ever taken your temperature or stepped on a scale. The thermometer tells you whether you're running a fever; the scale, whether you've gained weight. Both devices "feed back" information about your body's condition. Armed with this information, you can take steps you've learned to improve the condition. When you're running a fever, you go to bed and drink plenty of fluids. When you've gained weight, you resolve to eat less (and sometimes you do).

Clinicians rely on complicated biofeedback machines in somewhat the same way that you rely on your scale or thermometer. Their machines can detect a person's internal bodily functions with far greater sensitivity and precision than a person alone can. This information may be valuable. Both clients and therapists use it to gauge and direct the progress of treatment.

(continued)

For clients, the biofeedback machine acts as a kind of sixth sense that allows them to "see" or "hear" activity inside their bodies. One commonly used type of machine, for example, picks up electrical signals in the muscles. It translates these signals into a form that clients can detect: it triggers a flashing light bulb, perhaps, or activates a beeper every time muscles grow more tense. If clients want to relax tense muscles, they try to slow down the flashing or beeping.

Like a pitcher learning to throw a ball across a home plate, the biofeedback trainee, in an attempt to improve a skill, monitors the performance. When a pitch is off the mark, the ballplayer adjusts the delivery so that he performs better the next time he tries. When the light flashes or the beeper beeps too often, the biofeedback trainee makes internal adjustments that alter the signals. The biofeedback therapist acts as a coach, standing at the sidelines, setting goals and limits on what to expect and giving hints on how to improve performance.

The Beginnings of Biofeedback

The word *biofeedback* was coined in the late 1960s to describe laboratory procedures then being used to train experimental research subjects to alter brain activity, blood pressure, heart rate, and other bodily functions that normally are not controlled voluntarily.

At the time, many scientists looked forward to the day when biofeedback would give us a major degree of control over our bodies. They thought, for instance, that we might be able to will ourselves to be more creative by changing the patterns of our brainwaves. Some believed that biofeedback would one day make it possible to do away with drug treatments that often cause uncomfortable side effects in clients with high blood pressure and other serious conditions.

Today, most scientists agree that such high hopes were not realistic. Research has demonstrated that biofeedback *can* help in the treatment of many diseases and painful conditions. It has shown that we have more control over so-called involuntary bodily function than we once thought possible. But it has also shown that nature limits the extent of such control. Scientists are now trying to determine just how much voluntary control we can exert.

How Is Biofeedback Used Today?

Clinical biofeedback techniques that grew out of the early laboratory procedures are now widely used to treat an ever-lengthening list of conditions. These include:

- Migraine headaches, tension headaches, and many other types of pain
- Disorders of the digestive system
- High blood pressure and its opposite, low blood pressure
- Cardiac arrhythmias (abnormalities, sometimes dangerous, in the rhythm of the heartbeat)
- Raynaud's disease (a circulatory disorder that causes uncomfortably cold hands)
- Epilepsy
- Paralysis and other movement disorders
- Stress reactions

Specialists who provide biofeedback training range from psychiatrists and psychologists to dentists, internists, nurses, and physical therapists. Most rely on many other techniques in addition to biofeedback. Clients usually are taught some form of relaxation exercise. Some learn to identify the circumstances that trigger their symptoms. They may also be taught how to avoid or cope with these stressful events. Most are encouraged to change their habits, and some are trained in special techniques for gaining such self-control.

Biofeedback is not magic. It cannot cure disease or, by itself, make a person healthy. It is a tool, one of many available to health care professionals. It reminds physicians that behavior, thoughts, and feelings profoundly influence physical health. And it helps both clients and doctors understand that they must work together as a team.

Excerpted from Bette Runck, *Plain Talk Series*, DHHS Publication No. (ADM) 83-1273, U.S. Department of Health and Human Services (Division of Communications and Education, National Institute of Mental Health Public Health Service—Alcohol, Drug Abuse, and Mental Health Administration, 1983).

7.6 Psychoneuroimmunology

Research in the modern science of psychoneuro-immunology (PNI)—literally meaning the interrelationship among the psyche, the nervous system, and the immune (glandular) system—verifies what folk healers and metaphysicians have known for centuries: that thoughts and their resulting emotional states directly affect the body's chances of healing. Since the immune system is the body's first line of defense against disease, if we can strengthen the immune system we have a much better chance of maintaining the health of the whole body.

For ages, teachers of Ayurveda have known that passionate desires and emotional states could sometimes overwhelm the body's ability to maintain homeostasis. Patients who were unwilling or unable, physiologically, to make the changes necessary to heal their disease were rejected as candidates for treatment.

The pioneering research of neuropharmacologist Candace Pert, Ph.D., revealed that naturally occurring chemical messengers called *neuropeptides,* found in both the brain cell walls and the immune system, constantly circulate throughout the body in the blood, lymph, and cerebrospinal fluid.

This knowledge opened the door between body and mind much wider. Basically, neuropeptides (nerve proteins) regulate almost all life processes on a cellular level and thereby link all body systems—glandular, immune, muscular, and so on. There are dozens of different neuropeptides that send numerous chemical messages from the brain to receptor sites on cell membranes throughout the entire body. These messages affect not only physiology but also emotional states. The neuropeptides known as *endorphins* and *enkephalins,* for instance, are known to be triggered by thought patterns, as well as by physical exercise. Their release by the brain promotes a sense of wellbeing throughout the body.

Many popular programs for cancer patients make use of the cutting-edge research in this revolutionary science. Such programs inspire people to visualize an outcome they desire, keep a strong affirmative attitude, and uphold an exercise and fitness regimen as a means of stimulating the immune system through neuropeptide activity.

If you can relate to what we have been discussing, then you have a good appreciation for the vital connection between thinking and wellness.

7.7 Beware of Your Programmers

Broadly applying the definition of the transitive verb *program*—"to predetermine the thinking, behavior, or operations of as if by computer"—everything programs you. You are influenced in some way by every single event on life's path—every word you give or receive; every chance meeting or intense interaction with another; the room and the chair you sit in, the view from your window, the route you take to work or play, every TV show, even the weather pattern. You are also highly programmed by the tribe or culture into which you are born—and certainly by the people who raised you. Your brain operates like a highly sophisticated computer, your memory banks filing away each experience.

Wilder Penfield, M.D., found that when a certain portion of a subject's brain was electrically stimulated, the subject could describe minute details of an event that had happened when he was four years old. Not only did the subject recall cognitive data, but the emotional responses to the scene were also recalled. Aldous Huxley was able to induce a trancelike state in himself, then recite, verbatim, the contents of a page in a book he had not read in twenty years. Under clinical hypnosis you could likely remember an event that your conscious mind had seemingly forgotten. Most people can remember certain injunctions given to them by parents or teachers (even ten, forty, or sixty years ago) that still cause some internal stress or reactivity today, especially when the injunctions are being violated. It may be something as simple as advice not to swim after eating, or as serious as the admonition never to date somebody outside your religious faith.

Advocates of conscious parenting tell us that the first two years of a baby's life (beginning at conception) are the most crucial in terms of development and growth. These are the stages in which children are literally absorbing their environment, receiving both initial impressions and reinforcements that will determine their view of the world.[4] Children are programmed by the adults in their world, at all levels—physically, emotionally, intellectually, spiritually. They learn, based on the way they are treated, that the world around them is safe or threatening. They learn to speak and assign meanings to things as their parents do. They learn what will gain approval and what will elicit distress. In the domain of health, parents constantly orient their children for illness or accident by telling them: "Don't do that—you'll fall, you'll cut yourself, you'll get sick, you'll get hurt . . ."

As adults, we are being influenced daily by the stuff we incorporated into the body-mind in these first two years and beyond. Therapies abound for helping people face and cope with aspects of their early childhood programming that are presently causing dysfunctional behaviors, irrational thought patterns, and impaired relationships. When you realize that everything, everywhere, all around you is interacting with you, and you realize how influential these interactions can be, you may feel overwhelmed. But you may also be moved to examine the sources of your present-day programming and start taking more responsibility for what you take in.

THE BRAIN-HEART CONNECTION

The Institute of HeartMath (Boulder Creek, California) has conducted research on how the brain functions. Their findings show that our perceptions, mental and emotional attitudes, immune system, and decision-making abilities are all related to the electromagnetic frequencies broadcasted by our heart. These frequencies are many, many times stronger than brainwave frequencies and can be measured from several feet outside the body. They influence our own brain rhythms as well as the brain rhythms of others nearby (bad vibes?), especially those of in-arms infants. It is through this mechanism that the heart appears to influence the brain and live up to its popular reputation of being more than just a pump. Studies show that the heart is a powerful agent for transforming perceptions, resolving challenges, and manifesting values that benefit everyone.

Recurring feelings of frustration, worry, stress, and anger cause heart rhythms to become unbalanced and disordered (incoherent). These feelings are detrimental not only to the physical heart but also to the brain, hormonal production, and the immune system. Even remembering an upsetting experience can reduce the heart's pumping efficiency by 5 to 7 percent and decrease the immune system's potency for many hours. On the other hand, forgiveness, appreciation, and love engender coherent, harmonious heart rhythms and affect the physical heart's electrical output, as seen in an ECG. These feelings generate heart frequencies that are radiated to every cell in the body and boost the immune system. One five-minute episode of feeling genuine care or compassion enhances the immune system, causing a gradual climb in IgA (an antibody and one of the body's first defenses against colds, flu, and infections) for the next six hours. Feelings of happiness and joy benefit the white blood cells that are needed for healing and defense against invading pathogens, including cancer and virus-infected cells.

Take a few minutes to consider the implications of this data. For example, the next time a flu bug is making the rounds, John will ensure he and his daughter take several strong doses of nurturing and fun-filled time together, even for five minutes every couple of hours, rather than just reaching for the vitamin C or echinacea!

Doc Lew Childre, *A Parenting Manual: Heart Hope for the Family* (Planetary Publications, 1995).

7.8 Choosing Your Impressions

Impressions are the brain's food. Some impressions you don't have much control over—like it or not, you are going to be affected by the sights in your neighborhood unless you lock yourself in a windowless room and never come out. Many other forms of impressions are entirely under your control. Looking around at all the possible input sources in the environment, you can decide which ones to attend to, which ones to ignore. Say you decide to watch television. Turn it on. Ah, your favorite soap opera! The scene is a hospital waiting room. The distraught woman standing beside the window is being informed by the doctor that her husband has cancer. Symbolically, the woman reaches for the cord of the venetian blinds, closing them. Fade to black. Commercial. Once again you get a message loud and clear: "Cancer equals death"—the dimming of the light. A very strong impression has been made. Now, if this happened rarely, you would have little cause for concern. But because similar depictions are made constantly in the media, you can easily begin to believe them. The fear of cancer has become a national epidemic.

Television, the Internet, magazines, and newspapers are powerful forces in programming our thinking. From these sources we learn that people look happy when they take drug X for headaches or drug Y for impotency. We actually get to see acid indigestion eating away at the stomach lining, then watch as drug Z coats it all rosy again. We are shown hundreds of images of ultraskinny women who look sultry but unhappy, yet still have fabulous jewelry, beautiful clothes, and lots of adoring men. The inference is that skinny is good, and that "things" will ultimately satisfy us. Even though we may laugh at the simplistic nature of the inferences, we are still affected by them. In a relaxed or highly susceptible state—the near-hypnotic trance that TV or computer-screen watching creates—we can be easily persuaded that we need these remedies or these goods. When we enter a supermarket, the repetitive lines of color and shapes produce a similar trancelike state. One study indicated that grocery shoppers blink only six or eight times per minute, whereas in an alert state they blink about twenty times a minute. So, when you find yourself reaching for the product that you saw advertised, you may be carrying out a hypnotic suggestion.

Surrounding ourselves with a negative climate of worry, constant complaints, and continual expectations of the worst possible outcome drains us of energy and fills our biocomputer/brain with garbage that will come out in some way as illness, accident, depression, whatever. Think about your own energy levels and how they vary with your moods. After a day filled with emotional tension or negative impressions, do you sometimes feel exhausted or like you are "coming down with something"?

What is called for is conscious selectivity in choosing the data—the forms of impressions—that we feed into the mind. If we feed it with impressions that inspire compassion in the face of suffering, with encouragement in the face of difficulty, with beauty and humor, we will help to balance the many forms of energy and pain that cannot be controlled, and we will orient ourselves to realize high-level wellness.

Perhaps the fundamental freedom that anyone possesses is the choice of where to put their attention.

—Albert Einstein

7.9 Programming Illness— Programming Wellness

Worry is one of the biggest energy drains around. Worries, often closely related to a sense of guilt or shame, typically run as strong background programs in our minds. While they usually run with little intentional direction from us, they drain us of a tremendous amount of energy that could be put to much better use. When you create negative mental pictures or repeat worry messages to yourself about illness, accident, failure, or weakness of any kind, it impacts your body and influences the reality you create.

Mind and body are connected, and worrying about illness wears down the body's natural defense mechanism. Remember the experience of a severe headache? Say, for instance, you wake up with it: "Damn, headache!" Repeat over and over "I've got a headache!" These messages from the conscious mind create a whole range of responses that become established in the body. You are likely making your headache even worse, increasing your chances of having it all day. We've all done this. The job interview presents another clear example. You know that next Tuesday you will be meeting a prospective employer. You create a mental picture of him or her, design the office in your mind, and visualize yourself seated opposite your inquisitor. If your self-concept has suffered some harsh blows lately, you probably start worrying about your inability to answer the questions asked. You actually hear or see yourself stumbling over words, moving your hands nervously, drawing a blank. The face that looks across the desk at you is frowning, or aggressive, or smiling condescendingly. The whole experience is one of anxiety, and you will have from now until Tuesday to anticipate making a total fool of yourself. If your thinking continues in this way, that is in all likelihood what will happen. There is no magic involved. The power of your thinking has produced just what you have programmed it to produce. Your whole presence will communicate the invisible message "I'm a loser."

Well-Thinking

Well-thinking is our term for a response-able and creative means of dealing with counterproductive thinking or worry. Well-thinking includes deciding on a course of action that will move us toward our desired outcome. It means using the mind to relax and/or substitute more intentional thinking about a problem or a condition in your body. Applied to worry, well-thinking might work like this:

Recognize the worry. As long as the worry or the counterproductive image remains as background noise or sensation, it will insidiously and unconsciously color everything in your life. The first step is acknowledging that this buzz or drone in your head, or that knot in your gut, is worry or negativity at work.

Ask whose problem it is. A lot of our worry is unnecessary. Many people take on the problems of others (or make problems of the actions of others) and simply ruminate about them, neither helping the situation nor the other person. Instead, they drain their own energies going around in circles in their minds. One way to short-circuit this pattern is to ask yourself the question, "Is this mine, or does this worry, this problem, or this situation rightly belong to someone else?" For example, a college math instructor may certainly hope that her students will all pass their exams, and may do whatever she can to facilitate this. But it does neither her students nor herself any good to spend her nights worrying about the potential consequences of their failures.

Take one small step. If the "problem" is yours, pause a moment and determine if there's any action you could take *right now* that would improve the situation you are worrying about. Hours of procrastination mingled with worry can create a backlog of tension, which may be dissipated with simply making one "baby step" in a long-overdue task.

Maybe a phone call to make an appointment with your doctor is all it will take to get the ball rolling.

Maybe a moment of relaxation, or a deep breath, would break the ultraserious nature of your approach.

Maybe a moment's prayer would serve to shift the context from complete self-absorption to an appreciation of the big picture. In some worldviews, people are encouraged to give up the problem to a higher power.

Maybe the heartful creation of an image or affirmation statement that incorporates the desired result is the best thing you can do.

Take one small step again and again and again. Each time you realize that you are thinking about the problem, or creating an unproductive picture, use this as a cue to substitute the one small step you've determined—perhaps a healthy or nurturing image, prayer, or affirmation. These steps need reinforcing, so be creative in coming up with new ways to work with them. Write out your verbal statements or draw the desired pictures. Make several copies and place them around where you will see them often. Especially when dealing with illness, spend several short relaxation periods each day re-creating the healing images or repeating your words of healing. Put other cues in your environment to remind you to plug in the positive: colored stickers, small pictures, or perhaps spiritual or religious images.

Postpone worry. If the situation is one that can't be helped today because all the facts aren't in, or all the planets aren't in alignment, or whatever, postpone your worrying! Determine to think about it tomorrow, and get on with the business of today. Is there an action you can take at a particular time in the future that will improve the situation? If there is, make a commitment to follow through on that action. Many people find it helpful to ask themselves what would be the worst possible outcome should the situation they are worrying about eventuate. Often, it's not that big a disaster, not worth the attention they are giving it. Or, maybe otherwise. Maybe the outcome would be death or worse, for themselves or a loved one. In this case, it is necessary to make some degree of peace with the "worst," however that is possible. The next two steps may aid you.

Grieve when nothing will change. Maybe there's nothing anyone can do about the situation that is disturbing you, ever! If that's the case, each time the painful thought arises you may want to take a few moments to acknowledge the loss that you may be feeling at the irreparable nature of the problem, then do your best to open yourself up to the next moment. This may mean releasing yourself into the hands of a "higher power," or remembering all those throughout the world who are suffering a loss similar to yours, and taking some comfort and strength in knowing that you are not alone; or it may mean taking whatever action you can to redirect your mind to move in a more hopeful direction.

Practice gratitude for what is. Instead of becoming preoccupied with the future or worrying about the past, wrestle (if you have to) your attention into the present moment in all its richness. Instead of focusing on what you don't have, focus on what you do have. Attend to the gifts and graces around yourself all the time. Look at the sky. Look at the trees. Look at children.

Forgive yourself for any failures, difficulties, or compulsions experienced or encountered in your efforts to change your mind's direction.

Accept yourself as you are, as gently as you would accept a friend in the same situation.

Kay's story testifies to the value of this well-thinking approach. Kay had a lump in her breast and was scheduled for surgery. She reported that the picture in her mind was of a black mass with tentacle-like arms. She thought of it as cold and hard and evil. She played that picture over and over, day in and day out, becoming more and more fearful as she actually imagined the lump growing in size, eating up everything in its path. When instructed in the process of well-thinking, she drew a picture of what a healthy, clear breast would look like. She used yellows and golds and wide, free, circular, spiraling movements. She placed copies of the picture everywhere. This was the picture she used in breaking her negative programming. Each time she noticed it, she paused momentarily and allowed the positive image to sink into her. She did this for two weeks. When she next saw her doctor, he examined the lump and, in amazement, reported that it simply seemed to dissolve under his fingertips. He had no rational explanation for it. But Kay knew why.

Of course, there are many factors involved in any disease situation. It would be foolish to say that imagery alone "cured" Kay. But it would be equally foolish to deny the body-mind connection. Current research shows that an optimistic attitude helps surgical patients to heal faster and diminishes their need for pain medication.

Imaging Flip—For Self-Healing

Your thoughts help to keep you stuck in pain, in tension, in depression, but they can be flipped over and used to alleviate the very same conditions.

Focus in on one problem area to which you devote energy. Perhaps it is the chronic tension in your right shoulder, or the nausea you experience riding in a car or plane. Note as many aspects of it as you can:

- *Is there a picture associated with the problem or pain? (For instance, tight, knotted nautical ropes, or a murky, stagnant pool.)*

- *Is there a sound connected with the problem or pain? (For instance, a grinding or gurgling sound.)*

- *Is there a texture associated with it? (A sore throat, for instance, might feel like rough sandpaper; an upset stomach might feel slimy.)*

- *Is there a temperature associated with it? (A headache might feel hot; a broken arm might feel cold.)*

- *Is there a smell or taste associated with it? (For instance, curdled milk or some nasty-tasting medicine.)*

- *Is there a movement associated with it? (Churning, pounding, stabbing?)*

Now comes the flipping part. The essential question here is what the problem or pain will look, feel, smell, sound, taste like when it is alleviated or cured. For the image, substitute its opposite.

- *Knotted ropes are slowly untied and loosely laid out on the deck.*

- *A stagnant pool is drained and filled with clear, sweet water.*

- *A dark cloud of pain in the head is penetrated with sunlight.*

- *A pounding sound is replaced by the sound of a waterfall.*

As you relax, substitute a positive, healing image for each negative, painful one. Use words if necessary to reinforce the stimulus, like, "My head is filled with billowy white clouds."

Put up reminders for yourself around the house, in the car, at your place of work. Whenever you see them, flip into your new set of images.

Don't be discouraged if you can't conjure up all the types of images we have suggested. Use the ones that are strongest for you. Be patient with yourself in anticipating results, but know that other people have used this exercise to great advantage. Give it a try.

7.10 Right Brain, Left Brain

The diverse functions of our two brain hemispheres have been the subject of some of the most exciting research findings about human anatomy and behavior in the last sixty years. First identified in the late 1950s by Roger Sperry and Ronald Meyers, in experiments first with cats and then with monkeys, the data became important to consciousness study when it was applied to human subjects. In the 1960s, at the California College of Medicine (now the University of California at Irvine) and the California Institute of Technology, a group of severely epileptic patients underwent operations in which their brain hemispheres were surgically separated. The nerve fibers known as the corpus callosum, which joins the two halves of the brain and serves as the primary information pathway between the two, was severed in an attempt to keep seizures isolated to one hemisphere. (The hemispheres are still connected at the brainstem, however.) As a surgical and therapeutic technique it was effective. What was learned as a result of this intervention continues to have a profound impact on our knowledge of the human brain, particularly in the areas of perception, speech and language, and human learning and creativity.

The "split-brain people," as they came to be known, acted quite normally, but exhibited some curious behaviors when subjected to certain tests. For instance, they were seated behind a screen that blocked their view of the objects on the table in front of them, then asked to identify an item placed in one hand. If a comb, for instance, was put in the right hand, it was recognized as such and verbally labeled. If, however, the comb was first placed in the left hand, the subject could indicate, through gesturing, how it might be used, and recognize it from among other items, but drew a blank when asked to name what it was.

The researchers concluded—and later studies verified—that the right hemisphere of the brain controls the left side of the body, and the left hemisphere controls the right side of the body. When the left hand was sending information about an object, the right hemisphere didn't have a word for it. With the object in the right hand, however, the left brain recognized it as *comb* and named it as such.

The left hemisphere of the brain seems to be the verbal genius, the logician, the part that focuses on the individual phenomenon. The left brain is the researcher, the mathematician, the scientist who looks to cause and effect. The right brain gets the credit for the opposite traits: not irrational or illogical, but nonrational or nonlogical. The right brain is the domain of intuition and holistic thinking. This is the side of the brain in which the dreamer and the artist dwell, where creativity rules. This is where "I don't know why I thought of putting those two things together, but isn't it wonderful that I did?" comes from. Or "Don't know how I knew it, just had this weird feeling in my gut!" Music, art, dance, psychic impressions, symbols, metaphors, seeing the whole picture in an instant, grasping the fullness of the present moment, experiencing the sunset without the need to analyze its component colors or talk about it—this is the stuff of the right brain.

Split-brain research indicates that we may have been correct in thinking of the two different sides of our bodies as being distinct in some ways. The right side of the body, controlled by the left hemisphere, is generally stronger—and it is dominant in most of us. In French, "right" is *droit,* from which we get the word *adroit,* meaning, "skillful." In Latin, it is *dexter*—the source for *dexterity* and *dexterous.* The left side of the body, ruled by the right hemisphere, has perennially been associated with the darker, more mysterious aspects of the personality. The French word for "left" is *gauche.* In Latin it is *sinister.*

Split-brain research today is highlighting the role of the brain stem as a "lower-pathway" site for the sharing of hemispheric information. In other words, the corpus callosum is not the only information highway between the hemispheres. This understanding of the brain stem is also offering researchers additional insight into the evolution of human consciousness, as they try to explain the stages of the brain's development. In a more immediately practical application, educators are constantly looking at the ways in which individuals process information:

some seem more inclined to right-brain skills, seeing the whole, working concretely; others have great difficulty without more linear, verbal approaches that rely almost exclusively on the written word. The implications for learning and education are tremendous—one style does not fit all!

Since wellness means wholeness, which means integration, it's helpful to pay more attention to both brains, utilizing a variety of approaches to education, to relationship building, and to working together. Tapping the latent powers of the neglected half of ourselves will provide us with exciting new approaches in all fields of endeavor, as well as in self-healing.

MANY KINDS OF SMART

Our society generally focuses on the highly linguistic person who reads and writes well and on the logical thinker. Yet the other forms of intelligence are equally important to the wellbeing of the individual and our culture.

Research conducted over many years by psychologist Howard Gardner at Harvard University has shown that there are many different ways of being smart. Gardner has identified eight different kinds of intelligence:

- Linguistic (word-smart)
- Logical-mathematical (number/reasoning-smart)

- Spatial (picture-smart)
- Bodily-kinesthetic (body-smart)
- Musical (music-smart)
- Interpersonal (people-smart)
- Intrapersonal (self-smart)
- Naturalist (nature-smart)

Every person has all eight intelligences, but in different proportions. Some people excel in several, others have special difficulties in many of the intelligences, and most of us are somewhere in between, with one of more intelligences that we find very easy to use, others that are so-so,

and one or more that we may have great difficulty in using.

Gardner's identification of multiple intelligences encourages us to look at an individual's potential in a more holistic way than by simply focusing on IQ. It also gives us a way of looking at the complete picture of a learner's potential so that any neglected abilities will also be honored and developed.

Howard Gardner, *Intelligence Reframed: Multiple Intelligences for the 21st Century* (Basic Books, 1999).

7.11 **Training in Attention**

While our education may have trained us in certain cognitive skills, others have been sorely neglected. The ability to pay attention is one of those undeveloped abilities. Perhaps because of the media's approach to keeping us always stimulated by changing images every few seconds or because of the enhanced pace of life in today's techno-culture, the mind's ability to focus and keep attention is rarely addressed. Most of us know that we've got a "wild monkey" running around in our brains, jumping from tree to tree, from thought to thought. If we have ever tried to simply watch one phenomenon for more than just a minute, we know how incredibly taxing and even impossible that can seem. The typical example used is that of trying to watch the second hand on a clock with full attention. In a short time we are feeling edgy, tapping our fingers or shaking a foot. Most people can't keep such focus for even a minute. Try it and see, noting when your attention wanders or your thoughts take you to another time and place altogether.

Yet the ability to pay attention is a treasure worth cultivating. Not only can paying attention be relaxing—as happens when attention can be focused solely on the movement of breath—it can be transcendental, as when the painter or sculptor becomes utterly immersed in the work.

The martial artist first sharpens and then diffuses attention to the point where he or she appears to be responding even without thinking. In healing, the ability to focus attention is also essential, for picking up on subtle cues from our inner experience or for directing energy from one area of the body to another. Many of the mind techniques for enhanced health require an exceptional placement of attention and continuity of practice. But the effort is well rewarded. You can practice paying attention in any activity of your day: preparing a pot of tea and drinking a cup with mindfulness; working in your garden, experiencing all the sensory input that is flooding you even amidst a barren patch of earth. The possibilities are endless.

Paying attention is a prelude to living life in the present moment. And the present moment is the *only* place wherein the fullness of life can be experienced—the only place where power, love, and creativity coexist.

Mindfulness is the capacity of being present in the here and now. When I eat an orange, I can eat the orange as an act of meditation. Holding the orange in the palm of my hand, I look at it mindfully. I take a long time to look at the orange with mindfulness. "Breathing in, there is an orange in my hand. Breathing out, I smile at the orange." For me, an orange is nothing less than a miracle.

—Thich Nhat Hanh

He always wanted to say things. But no one understood.

He always wanted to explain things. But no one cared.

So he drew.

Sometimes he would just draw and it wasn't anything. He wanted to carve it in stone or write it in the sky.

He would lie out on the grass and look up in the sky and it would be only him and the sky and the things inside that needed saying.

And it was after that, that he drew the picture. It was a beautiful picture. He kept it under the pillow and would let no one see it.

And he would look at it every night and think about it. And when it was dark, and his eyes were closed, he could still see it. And it was all of him. And he loved it.

When he started school he brought it with him. Not to show anyone, but just to have with him like a friend.

It was funny about school.

He sat in a square, brown desk like all the other square, brown desks and he thought it should be red.

And his room was a square, brown room. Like all the other rooms. And it was tight and close. And stiff.

He hated to hold the pencil and the chalk, with his arm stiff and his feet flat on the floor, stiff, with the teacher watching and watching.

And then he had to write numbers. And they weren't anything. They were worse than the letters that could be something if you put them together.

And the numbers were tight and square and he hated the whole thing.

The teacher came and spoke to him. She told him to wear a tie like all the other boys. He said he didn't like them and she said it didn't matter.

After that they drew. And he drew all yellow and it was the way he felt about morning. And it was beautiful.

The teacher came and smiled at him. "What's this?" she said. "Why don't you draw something like Ken's drawing? Isn't that beautiful?"

It was all questions.

After that his mother bought him a tie and he always drew airplanes and rocket ships like everyone else.

And he threw the old picture away.

And when he lay out alone looking at the sky, it was big and blue and all of everything, and he wasn't anymore.

He was square inside and brown, and his hands were stiff, and he was like anyone else. And the thing inside him that needed saying didn't need saying anymore.

It had stopped pushing. It was crushed. Stiff.

Like everything else.

—Anonymous

7.12 Right/Wrong Thinking— The Old Paradigm

Being right is, for most of us, a cherished value— albeit one we generally hold and pursue unconsciously. At its root, being "right" is the basis of all prejudice, and leads to acts of discrimination ranging from bullying and ridiculing to segregation and murder, torture, and war. Thinking that we are right while others are wrong and acting accordingly is no small thing. Although these manifestations may seem minor, they may occur dozens of times a day. You know how it feels when someone self-righteously declares, "I told you so!"—or more subtly exhibits their right/wrong attitude by "looking down their nose" at you or anyone else who does things differently than they do. In whatever form it appears, right/wrong thinking is an energy drain, yet one that usually goes unnoticed. After all, as far the perpetrator is concerned, those others really *are* wrong!

Right/wrong thinking is deeply embedded and actively encouraged in cultures such as ours, in which everyone—from students in school to employees in the workplace—is "graded" according to external standards that have little or nothing to do with our innate and unique personal worth.

Right/wrong thinking is a reflection of the zero-sum fallacy: the belief that if one person (or group of persons) succeeds, or wins, someone else (the other team, the other guy, the other nation) must necessarily lose. Once you learn to look for these patterns of right/wrong or better/worse thinking, you can see and hear them everywhere: in media headlines, in daily conversations, and definitely in your own mind. The programming is so strong, and one that people align with so closely, that some of us would rather be dead than wrong.

If you look closely at the workings of your mind, you will probably notice that for everything you see or know in your world, along with having a name to label it, you have a judgment about it—formed from a connection from the past or to the anticipated future, an association with something similar, and the like. Each of those judgments is associated with a feeling, positive or negative. All of this mental processing usually goes on in a split second, completely out of our awareness.

We are not suggesting that you become soft in your head, taking everything as the same. Judgment or distinction making is a precious function of your mind. There really *are* differences among things. Some things, like carrots, are generally good to eat. Other things, like arsenic, are not good to eat. But if you are allergic to carrots, they are not good to eat either. What we are pointing to is the tendency to separate the world into categories of good and bad based on our own views of things, and to label others as less worthy or less good than we are, because they don't abide by the same opinions. When presented with two options, most people unthinkingly take the option that will further their own immediate survival or satisfaction.

Rather than striving to eliminate your judging mind—an accomplishment to which followers of many spiritual disciplines aspire, but few attain—see if you can separate yourself from your judgment. This means that you first have to catch yourself "judging" and then watch that judgment without acting on it in any way. You don't move toward it or away from it. You don't talk about it or deny it. You don't berate yourself for it or congratulate yourself about it. You simply note it: "Ah, judging is happening." You are, in that moment, taking a step back from totally identifying with your thoughts, simply noting that judgmental thoughts are passing through your mind. When it comes time to act, you make your decision clearly, without being pressured by your identifications. You simply choose what seems like the most beneficial "right" thing to do in the moment.

Black-and-white thinking is a variation on the right/wrong theme. No shades of gray are allowed in this world. A person is either a demon or an angel. Period. Can you see what an irrational belief system this supports? Look around you and see it in operation.

Once our automatic judgments are seen for what they are—usually habits or associations from long ago, not based on the genuine needs of the moment—they cease to have full power over us. We free up energy to be used for other things—things that lead us in a direction we *consciously* or intuitively choose.

7.13 Other Thought Patterns That Hurt Us

In addition to the right/wrong paradigm of thinking, there are many other patterns or irrational belief systems that we fall into—and being "educated" is no safeguard against such unhealthy thinking. In fact, our schools and work environments actually encourage many of these damaging and futile patterns. For instance, those of us who learn to strive for perfection know the drill on this one: no matter how hard we try, we are never good enough.

Consider the following common, dysfunctional thought patterns to find your familiar ones:

Unrealistic expectations. This is the mode of thinking at which perfectionists excel. They take on too much, then berate themselves when they can't accomplish it all perfectly. Their external speech is filled with "Absolutely," and "I must" and "You have to." Their internal speech (self-talk) is filled with fear and worry and self-hating. Perfectionists will not accept second prize. They will not abide the compassionate maxim "just doing the best I can"—because "best" for the perfectionist is translated into a completely unrealistic standard, set higher than any god could achieve! They are hard on themselves and hard on others. If life doesn't conform to their expectations, they just push harder.

Jumping to conclusions. Many folks follow this pattern to think themselves into deeper and deeper levels of suffering. They assume that they know the end of the story when they are only on chapter 2— and in their own cases, the story will usually have an unhappy ending. They tell themselves, even before they ask, that people will say no to their requests. They make up scenarios in which they will get left with the short stick, no matter what the issue is. When the phone rings, they assume it is someone calling to berate them. When the phone doesn't ring, they assume it is because people don't like them.

Catastrophizing, a variation on jumping to conclusions, happens when we make a mountain from a molehill. When my spouse is late from work, I automatically visualize an accident on the highway. When I notice a sore throat, I think immediately of cancer. Can you see how much unnecessary pain we carry around?

Taking it personally. While all of these hurtful patterns are forms of self-obsessive thinking—

reflecting a core belief that "Everything is about *me!*"—this one takes it to the extreme. It assumes that the weather, the traffic, the crowds, the price of tea in China . . . is *all* either aimed at me, or my fault, in one way or another. If there is a traffic jam, my irrational belief system offers one question: "Why is this happening to *me?*" "Everything conspires to make *my* life miserable!" "If my daughter isn't invited to the school dance, it must be because of something *I've* done wrong!"

Equating feelings with facts. Here we take our emotional state and give it a life of its own. If I feel dull, it means I am dull. If I feel sad, it means I'm hopeless. If I feel confused, it means I'm not a good person.

These are just a few of the ways in which negative thought patterns show up, and we each have our own unique ones. Regina knows her "tapes" about needing to be good at all costs, as John knows his about justifying his existence by constantly having to prove his worth. The important thing is to learn to recognize our own patterns, or "tapes," ideally before they sink their teeth into our guts; then, to take a step back from them, to reject identification with these unhealthy judgments. Finally, we need to keep choosing to live mindfully and heartfully in the reality of what is, rather than in the self-created pain of our illusions.

Sounds simple enough. It is simple, but not easy. The practice of self-observation, whereby we recognize our thought patterns, requires intention, attention, diligence, and a hearty dose of courage. It isn't fun to keep seeing how uncontrolled and unhealthy our minds can be. Yet, slow, persistent efforts bring rewarding results. We can get support from others by asking for occasional reality checks, especially when the thought patterns seem stronger than we are. "I've been thinking that all my efforts are going nowhere. What do you think?" Those of us who possess a religious or spiritual faith can trust that we are ultimately the reflection of God or Spirit as a way to counter the irrationality of our beliefs. Whether we are spiritually inclined or not, we can all contemplate a sense of basic goodness.

7.14 Whole-Brain Wellness

Reflect upon what you have been doing in the course of this day. Chances are that most of your activities have focused around planning, communicating verbally, following directions, staying on the proper side of the road. Our educational institutions have done a reasonably good job in training us in these skills. But at what expense? In the feeding of the mind, we have often neglected the body. How much time have you spent today in intuitive and creative endeavors? In nourishing logical reasoning, we have often starved these nonlinear, right-brain faculties. As a result, we are only half alive.

Giving attention to the neglected half of our being/brain means greater wellness for the whole. People from a diverse range of backgrounds are becoming aware of this fact. When American businesses realized that worker productivity could be increased through stress-management techniques, programs teaching these techniques began springing up everywhere. Some of these methods of stress-management require people to do seemingly nonrational things, such as repeating a meaningless sound, which has the effect of quieting the "thinking" brain. This relaxation spills over into the whole body and can open up previously untapped creative potential. Thus, top-level executives are signing up for workshops in which they meditate and exercise their way to new and livelier ideas.

Through neurofeedback training, people are learning that lowering blood pressure may be as simple as imagining vapors rising from a sun-warmed lake. Migraine headaches can be relieved when the subject creates a mental picture of heat flowing into the fingertips.

The practice of eurythmy, as taught in Waldorf education, involves children in learning to read by moving their bodies in a dance that corresponds with phonetic sounds, thus bringing the right and left hemispheric abilities into harmony.

In their book *Superlearning 2000,* Ostrander and Schroeder report the amazing possibilities for gaining proficiency in a foreign language, often in less than half the time previously necessary. The method, originally called *suggestology,* was developed by a Bulgarian educator named Lozanov. Subjects, reclining in chairs, listen to vocabulary being read to classical music in a unique rhythmical cadence.

Artistic creativity explodes when students are taught to draw, paint, or write from the right side of the brain. This work is discussed and illustrated by Betty Edwards in her remarkable book *Drawing on the Right Side of the Brain* and by Gabriele Rico in *Writing the Natural Way.* A book by Tony Buzan, *Use Both Sides of Your Brain,* suggests similar possibilities in many other areas. So, what are the implications for health?

A mountain of research has singled out stress as the great killer, the unbalanced condition that makes us ripe for accident and disease. Learning to calm tensions creates a state of mind that is receptive to healing visualizations and suggestible to new and more-positive mental programs. Let's note some examples here:

- *A review of forty-six studies conducted from 1966 to 1998 by the American Cancer Society found that guided imagery was effective in managing stress, anxiety, depression, pain, and the side effects of chemotherapy. Many of these guided-imagery approaches are offshoots of the work of oncologist O. Carl Simonton, M.D., and Stephanie Matthew-Simonton. This approach makes use of periodic relaxation coupled with visualizations of healthy, energetic cells fighting and destroying the weaker and disorganized cancer cells.*[5]

- Psychology Today, *March-April 1998, discussed a study of sixty-five patients who listened to guided imagery tapes for three days before and six days after surgery. The patients reported less stress and physical pain than a control group and needed only half as much pain medication as those who had not listened to the tapes.*[6]

- The American Journal of Health Promotion, *July 2001, noted the effects of a "mindfulness training" program on thirty-two highly stressed individuals. Following the two-month program, during which participants learned stress-coping and meditation methods, an average 54 percent reduction in psychological distress was reported, together with a 46 percent drop in medical symptoms, compared to the control group.*[7]

- *Meditation has an excellent record for reducing pain; it is the core of a successful pain program developed by Jon Kabat-Zinn, founder of the Stress Reduction Clinic at the University of*

Massachusetts Medical Center. His many books tell wonderful stories about integrating mindfulness practice into the ordinary stresses of daily life.

Close your eyes for a moment and imagine a beautiful natural setting in which you experienced a sense of restfulness or awe. Take a slow inhalation as you say to yourself—"Ease and peace," and with the exhalation, "Ease and peace." Try doing this for a few minutes and see if it relaxes you.

LATERAL THINKING

Edward DeBono, Ph.D., has devoted his life's work to the study of the thinking process. His term *lateral thinking* describes a process that attempts to counteract the limitations and errors of logical thinking, but not to replace it. Lateral thinking is a way of rearranging available information to form a new and better pattern. Others have called it *creative thinking* or, more recently, *right-brain thinking*. Here are some examples:

Random input. DeBono says, "A random input from outside can serve to disrupt the old pattern and allow it to reform in a new way." For instance, you could take your question to an antique store, a mall, or an art museum, or try opening a dictionary, Bible, or almanac at random, and look for connections. Intrigued? Try it.

Quotas. We often limit ourselves by wrongly imagining that there is only one right answer. To use quotas means to challenge yourself to come up with a minimal number of alternatives, giving yourself the pressure of a limited deadline; for example, ten minutes of concentrated time.

Rotation of attention. The man who tries every new diet fad in his attempt to lose weight is placing all of his attention on the one connection of food and flab. In any given situation, one element will naturally monopolize our energy unless we consciously attend to the less dramatic, or subsidiary ones (our dieter, for example, might pay attention to his boredom, hours of netsurfing, unhappy relationship, and so on). Make *each factor* in the problem or question the focus of attention and learn as much as you can by examining it as if it were the only one.

Reversals. Sometimes it helps to turn a situation completely upside down in order to see it from a different point of view. Often we are not sure of what we want, but we are very clear about what we don't want. ("I don't want to have to do homework every night of the week," "I don't want the full responsibility for the cars," "I don't want to swallow pills to keep up on my vitamins and minerals," and so on.) To determine what we want our job to be, we might do better by listing the things we *don't* want it to be. To determine what wellness is, we may learn a lot by asking ourselves what we are sure it is *not*.

Cross-fertilization. This step involves getting input from a variety of other sources, books, and people. Sometimes it is most helpful to talk to someone who holds an opinion opposite to the one you support. Ideas generate ideas. The more input you have, the more discriminating you can become in your choices.

7.15 Creative Thinking and Wellness

So many of the challenges of life involve getting *unstuck*. You may find yourself stuck in a job that is unstimulating, in a relationship that has ceased to nourish you, on a vacation that promised excitement and developed into boredom, with a headache that no longer responds to two aspirins.

"Stuck" is the state of finding a brick wall in the maze, then retracing your steps only to take the same path again. It happens because you believe your options are limited to what has worked in the past, or because you are afraid to consider or chance the alternatives. You may choose to stay where you are because it seems safer. It is the known, the home court, the backyard. Afraid of uncertainty, ambiguity, dynamic tension, you try again and again to apply the old solutions, and end up frustrated, or at least dissatisfied with the results.

William James defines genius, or creativity, as "the faculty of perceiving in an unhabitual way." Habits can keep us stuck. Breaking habitual ways of thinking gets us unstuck. The process is essentially one of making new connections. When we create the opening for two previously unrelated elements to come together in an uncharacteristic way, a new form emerges. Or, we open our eyes for the first time and really see something entirely different from what we have seen before, and we're off and running on a new track. Sandburg feels the fog and watches a cat move and writes a poem that connects the two. Picasso likes blonde women and baskets of fruit and so paints the two together. Newton gets hit on the head with an apple. You eat raspberry and tangerine ice cream and go home to repaint your bedroom in pink and orange. It can happen anywhere, anytime. Do you allow for the possibility?

When we examine some of the characteristics of the creative process we find some very strong similarities to characteristics of the wellness process. The creative process is often ambiguous and almost always incomplete. Many artists and writers say that they know they could always do more to a work, that it could always be perfected in some way. Yet they also know that the imagined perfection might stifle the creative energy of the piece. The challenge, then, is finding the moment at which they can release their hold on their piece, declare it complete, and "put it on the mat," as our friend George Leonard, the author and aikido master, loves to say.

The process of wellness points to this same kind of satisfaction with "imperfection," urging us to accept and honor ourselves with compassion, as we are, regardless of our current state of health. Wellness also means a balanced view, knowing when "enough is enough"—which can serve us well when we are trying to change our diet or attempting to work with our mental programming.

Wellness, like creativity, is a sensuous process, one that incorporates mind and body and spirit. Yeats has stated: "Art bids us touch and taste and hear and see the world, and shrinks from . . . all that is not a fountain jetting from the entire hopes, memories, and sensations of the body." Wonder, awe, and curiosity—those traditionally childlike qualities of mind—these are characteristics of creative thinking and of wellness.

Both processes call for play and energy and passion. The exact opposite of a closed, indifferent approach to life, creativity means openness and receptivity—and the same is true of wellness. We take risks, we try new options, we keep the lines of communication open, within ourselves and with other people.

Finally, the creative process is, like wellness, a courageous one. The ability to be creative and well is an ability to be analytical and critical of yourself in the most positive sense of the terms. It takes knowledge of the self, an ego strength, to be able to reveal your dreams and visions and thoughts to the world at large, to stand by them in the face of opposition. And it requires persistence to stick to something for long periods of time, to pursue a goal with no guaranteed results.

We all possess the potential to be creative, but some of us have simply never been encouraged, even allowed, to develop this potential. Typically, creativity means coloring outside the lines, and is actively discouraged by many of our schools and institutions. So it is with wellness! It takes courage to tell your doctor about the guidance concerning your condition that you received in a dream, through your own intuition, or through prayer. More so, to refuse conventional medical treatments may leave others thinking that you are crazy.

When we learn skills of creative thinking, we learn to improve ourselves and our world as well. We invite you to accept this challenge.

7.16 Brainstorming

Brainstorming is a thinking process that helps in getting unstuck. It allows you to tap into your own internal resources, to recall previous experiences and past successes, to fantasize new connections; in short, to play with possibilities without judgment. You can always discard the impractical and unworkable, but without the excitement and possibility generated by creative new ideas and more data, you will easily fall back into old patterns, hoping that maybe *this* time they might work out. Here's how brainstorming works.

1. *Formulate a question, or state your problem as simply as possible: "What can I do on my summer vacation this year?" or "How can I cut down on my smoking?" or "I hate my job."*

2. *Let go of the need to come up with the "right answer"—or the most logical, least expensive, or easiest alternative.*

3. *Relax yourself—with deep breathing exercises, a walk in the woods, the visualization of a crystal clear lake, perhaps vigorous exercise.*

4. *Repeat the question or statement to yourself, and tape record or write down every suggestion or answer that comes into your head. Doing this with a friend who simply writes down what you say without comment will allow you to speak freely. Do not judge any suggestion. Do not reject any idea for being dead wrong, silly, impractical, too expensive . . . whatever.*

5. *Continue throwing out ideas as fast as you can for a limited period of time—say five minutes. This will force you to think fast, and it will minimize evaluation.*

6. *Set the material aside. Let it rest, simmer, gestate for a while.*

7. Go back and review your data with new eyes and an open mind. What surprises you? What delights you? What hits you hard? What elements can be combined? Which ones are possible—and easy? Which ones generate new ones? Which ones are worth a try?

Here are some responses generated around the question "How can I make more time for myself?":

• *Get up earlier.*

• *Go to bed later.*

• *Unplug the phone.*

• *Hire a babysitter.*

• *Quit my job.*

• *Eliminate one meal a day.*

• *Give away the television.*

• *Turn back the clocks.*

• *Buy a dishwasher.*

• *Hire a maid.*

• *Shop by phone.*

• *Go on strike.*

• *Overlook the mess.*

• *Organize the house better.*

• *Build bigger closets.*

Brainstorming is a good way of revealing the hidden needs that are manifesting themselves as problems. As we have asserted in previous chapters, it is not enough to treat the symptoms. You must also find out why you have the problem in the first place; you need to interpret the body's messages.

Start by asking yourself not "Why?" but "What can I learn from this . . . *whatever it is?*" "Why?" questions often lead us to a dead end, as there are rarely clear answers to anything. So instead of "Why do I have a cold now?" or "Why did I sprain my ankle?" try asking: "What is this cold telling me now?" Or "What is this sprained ankle doing for me?" Proceed from there. Answers may generate new questions—answer them. But keep in mind that there will be a tendency to move into familiar territory by answering in such a way as to reinforce self-hatred or a sense of helplessness. Stay aware of this, and look instead for more information, rather than more judgment.

Questions can be repeated until any lead is exhausted:

Q. What can I learn from my current eating patterns?

A. When I overeat I have less energy.

Q. What have I learned about having diminished energy, specifically?

A. My thinking gets cloudy. My enthusiasm dwindles. I want to take a nap and skip my work.

Q. What would I like my eating patterns to encourage?

A. . . .

Once you've brainstormed and set the answers aside for a while, review the material; this may furnish you with valuable clues to your real needs and wants. Don't neglect to use material from your dreams, too. With a little practice and attention (see chapter 12), these nightly brainstorms are readily available for your conscious use. Brainstorming is a powerful way of practicing self-responsibility and taking charge of your life.

The ideas generated from brainstorming lend themselves well to a form of organizing called *mindmapping*—a clustering of ideas on paper in two dimensions (instead of the usual one-dimensional linear style of outlining). A mindmap often looks like groups of circles, each representing an idea, with lines connecting them to show their various relationships. For more information on mindmapping, see Tony Buzan's *Use Both Sides of Your Brain.*

7.17 Brainstorming a Big Question

If you can accept that your thinking is shaping your reality, can you also accept that it is similarly shaping planetary reality? Fear can be contagious. As fear is shared with more and more people, panic can result. Panic can immobilize people; it can cause them to be short with each other; it can encourage them to sell all their stocks, arm themselves, or commit murder. These actions affect increasingly larger circles of other people. A "group mind" about an issue becomes an overwhelmingly powerful force. If folks believe that Communists are everywhere, they will find them everywhere, as happened in the early 1950s in the United States. If we believe that war is inevitable, poverty is unconquerable, cancer is incurable, we easily lose heart for attempting to do anything about them. Our inaction feeds our feelings of inadequacy and impotency. Can we recognize that we have contributed, by our inaction, to the spread of that which we feared?

Thinking, then, molds the reality we will experience—individually and collectively. What would happen if, tomorrow, millions of people across the globe chose hope or love instead of fear? What if people started thinking that hunger can be eliminated? What if millions chose to believe that peace is possible? What changes would we see in our schools—and in our children—if thousands of teachers across the country accepted the unique beauty and innate wisdom of each child? Skeptics among us may scoff at these possibilities as idealistic dreams—and immediately challenge "how?" And "how?" is a very important question. But it is misplaced when it is the first question. The "how?" questions flow from our belief—or lack of belief—in possibility. A better question is "what?"—that is, "What *are* my beliefs?"—because *what* you believe will play a primary role in determining your way of being and working in the world. If you do not believe peace is possible, it is highly unlikely that you will experience peace.

THE HUNGER PROJECT

An example of using our collective powers of mind is the Hunger Project, a strategic organization and global movement committed to the sustainable end of world hunger. Begun in the 1970s, the Hunger Project has transformed the way many people view hunger in the world today. Their website (www.thp.org) describes who they are and what they do.

In Africa, Asia, and Latin America, we empower local people to create lasting society-wide progress in health, education, nutrition, and family incomes. We apply a two-pronged strategy: mobilizing grassroots self-reliant action, and mobilizing local leadership to clear away obstacles to enable grassroots action to succeed.

Our highest priority is the empowerment of women. Women bear primary responsibility for family health, education, and nutrition—yet, by tradition, culture, and law they are denied the means, information, and freedom of action to fulfill their responsibility. The Hunger Project is committed to transforming this condition.

A NEW WAY OF THINKING ABOUT WAR

The unleashed power of the atom has changed everything save our modes of thinking and we thus drift toward unparalleled catastrophe.
—*Albert Einstein, 1945*

Our precious lives, and the fate of our planet, are at stake in every moment. The ongoing development, stockpiling, and threatened use of nuclear weapons has involved us all in a deadly game in which there can be no winners. Even if we eliminated all the weapons tomorrow, we would only have bought ourselves some time. We will always know how to build nuclear weapons. We will always be able to discover new weapons if we want them. The only permanent solution is to change our thinking to see that war of any kind is no longer an acceptable method for resolving conflict.

Many groups today are focused on the necessity of changing our minds about the efficacy of war as a means of conflict resolution. One such agency, the Beyond War movement, begun in 1982 as a grassroots response to the need for a change of heart and a change of thinking, was revived in 2003 as a special project of the Foundation for Global Community. The movement is based on three foundational ideas:

- War is obsolete.
- We all live on one planet together.
- The means are the ends in the making.

The commitment to building a world beyond war involves a hard look at our individual lives and the national and international policies we support. We cannot create a world beyond war while we still harbor the mindset of fear; think that conflict and violence can solve our problems; create "enemies" of others; and overshadow the core issue of our oneness with all life. Everyone can make peaceful efforts to counteract these ways of thinking and take constructive action to support a greater sense of global community. One person does make a difference. That person is you.

For information about Beyond War 2003, see www.beyondwar2003.org or contact the Foundation for Global Community, 222 High St., Palo Alto, CA 94301, (800) 707-7932.

SUGGESTED READING

Achterberg, J., *Imagery in Healing* (Shambhala, 1985).

Borysenko, J., *Minding the Body, Mending the Mind* (Bantam Doubleday Dell, 1993).

Brown, B., *New Mind, New Body: Bio-Feedback, New Directions for the Mind* (Irvington Press, 2000).

Burn, D., and A. Beck, *Feeling Good: The New Mood Therapy* (Avon, 1999).

Buzan, T., *Use Both Sides of Your Brain*, 3rd edition (E. P. Dutton, 1991).

Childre, D. L., *A Parenting Manual: Heart Hope for the Family* (Planetary Publications, 1995).

Criswell, E., *Biofeedback & Somatics: Toward Personal Evolution* (Freeperson Press, 1995).

DeBono, E., *Lateral Thinking* (HarperCollins, 1990).

Dossey, L., *Healing Words: The Power of Prayer and the Practice of Medicine* (HarperSanFrancisco, 1997).

Edwards, B., *The New Drawing on the Right Side of the Brain* (J. P. Tarcher, 1999).

Gardner, H., *Intelligence Reframed: Multiple Intelligences for the 21st Century* (Basic Books, 1999).

Gawain, S., *Creative Visualization* (Bantam, 1995).

Houston, J., *The Possible Human: A Course in Enhancing Your Physical, Mental, and Creative Abilities* (J. P. Tarcher, 1997).

Liedloff, J., *The Continuum Concept* (Perseus, 1986).

Lozowick, L., *Conscious Parenting* (Hohm Press, 1997).

Maltz, M., *The New Psycho-Cybernetics* (Prentice-Hall, 2002).

Ornstein, R., *The Right Mind: Making Sense of the Hemispheres* (Harvest Books, 1998).

Ostrander, S., and L. Schroeder, *Superlearning 2000* (Island Books, 1997).

Peale, N., *The Power of Positive Thinking* (Ballantine, 1996).

Pearce, J., *Magical Child* (Plume, 1992).

Pert, C., *Molecules of Emotion: The Science behind Mind-Body Medicine* (Simon & Schuster, 1999).

Robbins, J., *A Symphony in the Brain: The Evolution of the New Brain Wave Biofeedback* (Grove Press, 2001).

Rossman, M., *Guided Imagery for Self-Healing: An Essential Resource for Anyone Seeking Wellness* (Kramer, 2000).

Samuels, M., *Healing with the Mind's Eye* (Random House, 1992).

Simonton, C., S. Matthews-Simonton, and J. Creighton, *Getting Well Again* (Bantam, 1992).

Van Oeck, R., *A Whack on the Side of the Head: How You Can Be More Creative* (Warner, 1998).

Zinn, J. C., *Full Catastrophe Living: Using the Wisdom of Your Body and Mind to Face Stress, Pain, and Illness* (Delta, 1990).

For an updated listing of resources and active links to the websites mentioned in this chapter, please see www.WellnessWorkbook.com.

NOTES

1. Tart, C., *Waking Up: Overcoming the Obstacles to Human Potential* (iUniverse.com, 2001).

2. For more information, see Luria, A. R., *Working Brain: An Introduction to Neuropsychology* (Basic Books, 1973).

3. Hutschnecker, A., *The Will to Live*, rev. ed. (Cornerstone Library, 1972), 24.

4. This is the subject of many diverse books and websites (see the Alliance for Transforming the Lives of Children, www.aTLC.org). Two basic sources are Pearce, J. C., *Magical Child* (Plume, 1992); and Liedloff, J., *Continuum Concept: In Search of Happiness Lost* (Perseus Publishing, 1986).

5. Simonton, C., S. Matthews-Simonton, and J. Creighton, *Getting Well Again* (Bantam, 1992).

6. Murphy, P. and A Murphy, "Reality Goes under the Knife," *Psychology Today* (March/April 1998), www.psychologytoday.com/htdocs/prod/ptoarticle/pto-19980301-000012.asp

7. Williams, K. A., et al., "Evaluation of a Wellness-Based Mindfulness Stress Reduction Intervention: A Controlled Trial," *The American Journal of Health Promotion*, Vol. 15, (July/August 2001), 422–32.

CHAPTER 8

Wellness, Playing, and Working

Playing and working are directed, focused energy expressions. The energies of thinking and communicating, enhanced by the energy of movement, combine to create a form of energy in which human beings interact with others and their environment, produce goods and services, and structure their time and, thus, their lives.

It takes one a long time to become young.

—Pablo Picasso

Work and play are the stuff of our lives. Almost all your waking hours are spent doing one or the other. Because these activities are so dynamically connected with self-concept, a sense of meaning and purpose, and, in some cases, your very survival, they are strong determinants of wellness. If there are significant, ongoing problems in either your work life or play, your state of health will usually reflect it. The list of stress-related diseases grows daily. And many of us are employed in highly stressful jobs. Moreover, we can hardly be living life to the fullest if we have no energy with which to play, no inclination for simply "fooling around."

As we begin our exploration of playing and working, let us make it clear that the two are not necessarily separate categories of activity. What is play to one may be work to another (compare a sandlot baseball game to a major-league game, for instance). Some people don't consider their jobs as work at all, because they enjoy them so much. And others make a chore out of their recreation.

In any case, rather than changing *what* you do for work or play, what's important is increased awareness and a change in attitude. Stop long enough to examine the roles that working and playing take in your life. If they do not enhance it, you may want to make some changes.

8.1 Redefining Play

The dictionary refers to play as recreation. This is a very significant word. Hyphenate it and it becomes *re-creation*. This is play in the fullest sense of the term: to make new, to vitalize again, to inspire with life and energy. This is "creativity" at its best. Everything creative contains some element of play.

Playing is a form of self-nourishment. Playing is not something you do. It is rather an *attitude* you create, at any time, in any place, that transforms the mundane into the divine, the boring into the joyful, the required into the desired, and the present moment into a sacrament. With this type of nurturance we are more likely to experience equilibrium and to conserve the energy that is often wasted in frenetic activity. In this way, playing strengthens us.

Take a moment to identify the words that are associated with play: laughter, frolic, fun, exciting . . . and lots of other similarly active words. But play can also be described as absorbing, fascinating, peaceful, beautiful, flowing, and restful. Perhaps one of the reasons we don't play more is that we have defined play inadequately. We have looked around at what the society tells us is "fun" to do, and we've accepted this as the meaning of play. We have remembered our childhood and have sought out swings and slides to give us pleasure. We have forgotten natural abilities we had for enjoying a rock, an abandoned tire, or a cardboard box. We frequently consider play as the opposite of work, thus solidifying the dichotomy between the two. Play must take a backseat to purposeful, "meaningful" activity. It is something to be done after hours, or on weekends, or with children. And it frequently costs a lot.

Mary recently posted a list of goals on her bathroom mirror. One of them was to save more money so that she could "do fun things." This attitude is far from uncommon. Many people are frustrated during their vacation periods and only too glad to get back home. They have accepted the notion that play is something you do, some place to go, an expensive camper or piece of sporting equipment. When it doesn't prove "fun" for them, they feel disappointed and out of sorts. (*What's wrong with me, anyway?*)

What has happened to us in our maturation process that makes adult play so different from child's play?

Life's door, love's door, God's door—they all open when you are playful. They all become closed when you become serious.

—Osho

8.2 Learning by Playing

One of the most important reasons for being alive is to *experience* life, for without the sense of wonder, the excitement, the emotions—joy, sadness, anger, fear—life is hardly worth living. And children teach us about the full-throttle experiencing of life. If we are willing to watch children play in their natural interactions with the world around them, we can learn a great deal about what has been temporarily obscured by our adult seriousness. We will see what it means to be in touch with our essential goodness, our innate sense of wonder, our free range of emotions. For the more serious "head cases" amongst us (John counts himself as one of these), learning to play again can be a means of getting in touch with yourself.

When a child plays, or works (since many children love to imitate and create what they call "work"), she does so spontaneously, she puts her whole self into the task at hand. When they feel safe, children, especially younger children, embrace all these behaviors:

- *Joyful experimentation with life*

- *Fascination with anything in their environment— a bumblebee, a ray of sunlight*

- *Unlimited reign of the imagination*

- *Trying out various behaviors; imitating others*

- *"Being" everything—an airplane, a famous ballerina*

- *Learning consequences naturally*

- *Freedom to be silly, fantastic, wrong*

Playing (or working) in this way nurtures children immensely. Through play, they learn about the world, and along with the growth of their confidence, self-esteem, strength, and experience, they experience the mastery that is both impetus and foundation for further learning. Children learn consequences naturally. Depending on the feedback they receive from people or things in their environment, they sometimes adapt, sometimes seek help or nurturance, sometimes cry—expressing their needs, their displeasure, or their frustrations. Generally, within a short time, however, they are ready to start something new, or tackle the old problem again as if for the first time. Either way, what we often see is a "no problem" attitude, even with the most challenging tasks. Isn't that what we all want?

8.3 Nourishment for the Spirit

Most of us suffer some guilt when taking time for ourselves. We are often embarrassed by our enjoyment of pleasure; we need to justify it to others and ourselves. We persist in repeating life-negating or energy-draining messages to ourselves, such as, "You're wasting time!" or "Watch out when things are going well," or "This is selfish," or "You *should* be doing something more productive." They have come to us from our parents, our church leaders, our employers, or our teachers, and they are often hard to turn off.

If you still need justification to allow yourself to play, then try this one:

Nourishment of yourself is the best preventive medicine currently available!

From all sides we are constantly being challenged: Change! Grow! Move! Volunteer! Contribute! Boycott! Picket! Diet! Exercise! In order to respond to challenge, we must have the energy to follow through. Decidedly, some challenging activities will generate their own sources of energy. Many people who work in highly stressful jobs report that the feedback from clients and coworkers, or the knowledge that their work is making a contribution to the life of all, seems to build their energy reserves, rather than depleting it. However, even in the most ideal circumstances, we will generally need to give attention to receiving nourishment in order to have adequate energy to meet a challenge. That energy comes from breathing, from moving, from eating well, and all the other energy channels mentioned throughout this book. In the context of work and play, it also comes from doing things that feed the soul, the sense of joy, the wonder, the awareness of belonging.

What nourishes you may not nourish me. One person retreats into the quiet and comfort of home; another gets energy from moving out into a crowd. Your needs may vary from day to day. We all need to be good to ourselves. Wellness includes this balancing of challenge and nurturance. When we are loved and cared for, almost anything is easy. When we are deprived, tired, needy, even the smallest detail becomes a monumental task.

The alternatives and possibilities for nourishment are limited only by our old habits, by our fear of trying the untried. Nourishing yourself is well worth the risk involved.

What Nourishes Me

When I consider nourishing myself, I think of strengthening, stretching, and celebrating through activities and nonactivities that get easily pushed aside when I'm in my habitual, no-nonsense "work" mode. I see these things as play, in the truest sense of the word. These activities feed my soul, and my body too.

What do you consider as play or nurturance? Here is my list today. Tomorrow it may be totally different. I share it as a way of encouraging you to write your own. I am nurtured by:

Long periods of silence
Short periods of silence
Exploring somewhere, with no agenda, with a child
Creating a surprise treat for the children in my life
Being alone in nature
Taking an energetic hike on a cold day
Dancing, nonstop, for half an hour or more
Writing in my journal
Writing a letter to Michelle or Brenda
Having a picnic lunch, anywhere, with Lynn
Sitting in the silent presence of my Teacher
Traveling, especially to foreign countries
Enjoying a planned evening at home with my husband, Jere
Doing something specific and tangible to support a friend in need

As I look over this list, I am reminded of these many fine activities that give me strength, joy, and courage. I also see that I haven't done some of them in a long time. So, when you make your list, you might note when you last did the thing you listed. When you've completed and read over your list, resolve to do one of those things today. And how about doing another one tomorrow?

—RSR

Now, write your own list:

_____

_____

_____

_____

_____

_____

_____

8.4 Competition and Play

If you operate from the philosophy that all of life is a game in which some people come out winners, then it follows that some people must come out losers. From our earliest years we are taught the connection between playing and games. Children soon learn that winning means bettering someone or something. Winning is praised or rewarded; losing means being a failure.

The link between playing and competition is a strong one. Competition means rivalry, challenge, and excitement. It can be wonderful, exhilarating, inspiring our best efforts. But it may also mean cheating, pressure, putting down the opponent, agreeing to the decisions of referees, and the privilege of the skillful few. It is sad that much of the physical education provided in schools involves training children to take part in competitive sports—in which few will ever engage in later life.

The other side of competition is cooperation. We recognize it as an essential part of the curriculum of our education programs and all of life. We ask our children to work together, and we reprimand them when they fail to share with others. It is little wonder that they are often confused. The messages they get are so often contradictory to them. "Win this." "Help others with that." "Win that, but when you do, share it with the rest of us." As adults we can appreciate that competition and cooperation need not be mutually exclusive. Young children don't see it quite so clearly.

Defining play as competition, as so many of us do, is not only limiting, but actually harmful. The attitude "If I'm not good enough to make the team, I'm not good enough, period" pervades our lives—in our business and economic affairs, our education, our politics, our recreation. When our self-concept comes from measuring ourselves against the skills and abilities of others, judging ourselves by the rules that society has set up, and comparing ourselves with our parents, brothers, sisters, and friends, it is very easy to come up wanting. Most of us hear these internal messages: "Be the first, the strongest, the best, and the brightest." "Too bad, you didn't make it." "You lose."

The pressures that result from playing in this dog-eat-dog world, the realm of cutthroat competition, encourage a wide range of stress-related ailments that are often climaxed with suicide or heart attack. We need to take a good, hard look at these old games if we are to survive and flourish individually as well as collectively. But, at the same time, we must be careful of compounding these "serious" issues by getting more serious, or more righteous, about what constitutes play and what does not. The opposite of play is not work. The opposite of play is excessive seriousness.

8.5 Seriousness

The weight of the burden is the seriousness with which we take our separate and individual selves.

—Thomas Merton

This job of becoming healthier is serious stuff—or so we have been led to believe. Just take a look at some of the books that deal with the subject. What you frequently find are predictions of dire consequences for failure to follow certain methods. "Authorities" supply you with horror stories of what specific foods, or lack of vitamins, or traditional techniques can do to you, along with lists of do's and don'ts, and diets, and warnings about the cancer-causing qualities of almost everything. It's enough to make you crazy!

And the subject of health is not the only one to be taken "seriously." The same attitudes and beliefs permeate our approaches to religion, education, family affairs, politics—our whole approach to life in general. Everybody is giving us the same message: "You've really got to start taking this more seriously!" And we do . . . and that is probably the main cause of our problems.

Seriousness breeds anxiety and creates the tension that is one of the chief causes of the problems we experience in body, mind, and spirit. Seriousness is the parent of fear, and fear is a deadly child. Seriousness is the generator of judgment. It demands that we assign meaning to mystery, that we leave no question unanswered, that we catalogue, evaluate, and institutionalize every aspect of our lives. Even if we are playing, we've got to get serious and play hard, always try to win, and above all—do it right.

Seriousness is actually an aspect of overblown self-importance, as Thomas Merton mentions above.

When we can't laugh at ourselves, it is because we are guarding our defenses, trying to be right, or good, or healthy. Trying to keep to some schedule that can't ever be broken. This is not sanity; this is self-obsession at its best. When every little thing about ourselves and our world is assigned some super-critical importance, we have lost perspective. We've placed "me" at the center of the universe, and determined that nothing must move us off our spot.

Whatever breaks undue seriousness opens us to play and to the revitalization that play brings. Bearing that in mind, you may want to try out some of the following strategies for breaking seriousness.

Strategies for Breaking Seriousness

"Lighten up." Choose a good-natured phrase that you can say to yourself often as a remembrance to drop the seriousness. (Be careful in your selection of this phrase, however, as repeating something can be a way to attract it. In the first edition of the *Wellness Workbook* Regina recommended the phrase "Give me a break" for this exercise. She herself used it a lot. Two years after publication, she fell on the ski slope and broke her leg in three places. It definitely gave her a much-needed rest, but she says now that there are many more positive ways of getting her needs met than by inviting physical traumas. Today, Regina uses the phrase "Just doin' the best I can." It helps her to be realistic about her limitations, and gives her permission to be less than perfect.

The president-on-the-toilet technique. Our fears and anxieties about other people frequently result because we hold the other in higher esteem than we hold ourselves. Remembering that we are all "just folks" may be as easy as conjuring up a picture of the other performing the most mundane of operations, those that everybody has to do. (Or as Mamie Eisenhower used to say to Dwight: "Ike, for God's sake, will you take out the garbage?")

Mirror, mirror. For some people, the simple act of looking in the mirror is enough to break a serious mood. Look at the wrinkles you are forming. Mothers sometimes tell children: "Watch out or your face will freeze that way." Now make ridiculous faces at yourself and just try to keep from smiling.

Monkey meditation. There is a Zen Buddhist technique that suggests that you jump out of bed first thing in the morning and spend ten minutes assuming the most absurd postures you can achieve. This is enhanced by laughing at yourself the whole time. Try it.

Get off my back. This exercise is good for you not only emotionally, but physically as well. Form your hands into fists; bring them together at the center of your chest. Raise your elbows on a line with your fists. Thrust your elbows back, expanding your chest and drawing your shoulder blades together. As you do so briskly for several minutes, say to yourself, or scream out loud, "Get off my back!" Imagine that you are releasing all the heavy burdens that have been weighing you down—people, jobs, fears, and so on.

Screaming in the car. With your car safely parked, roll up the windows and scream, rant, and rave at the top of your lungs.

Dance off. Put on the wildest music you can find. Dance until you exhaust your seriousness. (This is also good for weight control and breathing.)

Poor pitiful Pat. For a brief period, exaggerate your mood, or your fears, to the point of absurdity. Dress up. Act out the most pitiful, burdened, suffering creature you can become. Give yourself a name. Be ridiculous. Start laughing as soon as possible.

Red-flag technique. This is a method for talking yourself out of getting even more serious. The dialogue:

Helen: Hey, Helen, haven't you been down this road before?

Herself: Yes, many times.

Helen: Then you remember where it leads?

Herself: Only too well.

Helen: You realize what a dead end it is?

Herself: I sure do!

Helen: Do you really want to take it again, knowing what you know?

Herself: No! Let's go make some cookies (or take a shower, or . . .).

Take off all your clothes. Look at yourself in a full-length mirror. Now take a shower and wash off your seriousness.

8.6 Healing Laughter

It was in 1964 that Norman Cousins, editor of *The Saturday Review,* checked out of the hospital a few weeks after having been diagnosed with a very serious illness, a rare condition that affects the body's connective tissues. His chance of recovery, he was told, was one in five hundred. Barely able to move, and in intense pain, Cousins had two very important realizations. One was that the pain medication he was receiving was worsening his condition. The other was that the hospital was a bad place in which to be sick. So he stopped taking the medication, and he checked into a hotel and began a regimen of high doses of vitamin C and "laughter therapy."

His reading of several classic books on the subject of stress convinced him that disease was fostered by the chemical changes in the body produced by emotions such as anger and fear. Would an antidote of hope, love, laughter, and the will to live do the opposite? He was determined to try it and to be *the one* of the five hundred who successfully recovered.

In a remarkably short time, he found that short periods of hearty laughter, encouraged by watching Marx Brothers movies and *Candid Camera* TV sequences, were enough to induce several hours of painless sleep. He read books of humorous stories and jokes and continued his "laughter therapy." It was working. Slowly but steadily he began to regain control of his body. He could move without excruciating pain. He could turn his head. He could live again!

The whole experience created in him an overwhelming respect for the ability of the body-mind to heal itself, when nourished by the conditions, the environment, that allow it to reestablish its natural balance.

Worldwide interest in establishing the benefits of laughter and humor in health continues to grow, supported by wide-ranging scientific research. The Humor Project Inc., based in Saratoga Springs, New York, one of many associations dedicated to tickling the funny bone, publishes *Laughing Matters* magazine in twenty countries, and offers Daily Laffirmations through its website, www.humorproject.com.

Therapeutic humor is any intervention that promotes health and wellness by stimulating a playful discovery, expression, or appreciation of the absurdity or incongruity of life's situations. This intervention may enhance health or be used as a complementary treatment of illness to facilitate healing or coping, whether physical, emotional, cognitive, social, or spiritual.

—The American Association of Therapeutic Humor

Raymond Moody Jr., M.D., the author of *Laugh after Laugh: The Healing Power of Humor,* has used this approach with his patients for many years. Humor works, he claims, because laughter helps take your mind off pain and problems and catalyzes the basic will to live.

Critics of this "mind over matter" approach credit the placebo effect for its positive outcome. If you believe something strongly enough, they say, you will produce it. Hooray for that! If that is the mechanism that is working here, then we all need to learn the skills for fostering such belief. As we begin to understand the secrets of the brain, we learn that our thoughts do trigger the pituitary gland, which directs the rest of the endocrine system. The role that these glands play in establishing the body's equilibrium has been known for centuries. Perhaps now we will gain some insight into how it all happens. In the meantime, let's keep laughing.

8.7 Defining Work

The first definition Merriam-Webster offers for the noun *work* includes the words *effort, exerted, to do purposeful activity, labor,* and *toil.* The next definitions include: *employment, business, task,* and *duty.* It's enough to tire you out by simply reading about it! It sounds so very serious and difficult—and that's often the crux of the problem with it.

We use work to give structure to our time and meaning to our lives, to earn our livelihood, to express our talents, our dreams, our creativity, to change ourselves and the world at large. As such, work is both necessary and desirable. But when it becomes hard and serious to the point of causing excessive stress, or depression, or a sense of personal frustration or worthlessness, it undermines both our health and our happiness. That's why we consider work in the context of wellness.

If you listen to yourself or other people talk about work, you get a sense of what it means for vast segments of the population. People describe work as:

- *The rat race—the grind*
- *Dog-eat-dog competition*
- *Publish or perish*
- *Meeting deadlines*
- *Killing themselves to complete a project*

When Barry leaves his home each morning to teach at the local school, he talks of entering the "madhouse." When Tina goes to the office, she leaves word that she can be reached "in the dungeon." Kids refer to school as "prison"—and in fact, many of our educational institutions look that way.

When work is this serious and this hard, it robs energy from mind, body, and spirit and contributes to the creation of an internal environment in which illness can easily develop. Work creates illness when:

- *It becomes so serious that we assume we can't not do it. ("If I don't teach these poor kids, who will?")*

- *We allow it to slowly suffocate us because we think we have no choice, no alternatives. ("If I quit this job, what else would I do?")*

- *It is based on unrealistic expectations and demands that ignore the physical, emotional, and spiritual needs of human beings. ("My boss expects me to do the work of three people.")*

There are countless real-life examples that illustrate these attitudes and conditions and what they lead to. Take Dennis, for instance. He says he wants a meaningful relationship with a woman. He would like to settle down and have a family. But for the past twelve years he simply hasn't had the time or energy to pursue this goal. As a caseworker for a social service department in a large rural community, he has allowed his work to eat up his life. Even on his day off he is never without his cell phone, checking with his clients. If you ask him whether he is really happy in his life and work, he will candidly, and sadly, admit that he isn't. He simply doesn't know how to break the pattern.

Tom complained that he had had three colds over the course of one long winter. One cold had just barely cleared up when the next one happened. When a friend asked Tom if things were going well at work, he was startled by the question. Was his friend really implying a connection? As they talked, Tom disclosed that he hated his job as a reading teacher in a large city school. Work had become increasingly tedious over the past winter, and he was really looking for any excuse that would allow him to quit without feeling guilty.

Gene was employed by the U.S. government and his own health and welfare were at stake on the job. He suffered a continual battle with stomach ulcers, had hypertension, and had trouble sleeping. The pressures on him were enormous, and he disliked his work. But he liked his large salary very much! He wanted his second car, he wanted his boat, and he wanted his financial security. He would have preferred to be healthier—but assumed that since that wasn't possible in his present job, he would simply tolerate the symptoms.

Changing our ways includes changing the way we define work, the way we compensate work, the ways we create work, and the way we let go of work and learn to infuse it with play and ritual. A paradigm shift requires a shift in the way we think about, talk about, and undergo work. We should not allow ourselves to be deceived that today's crisis in jobs is just about more jobs; it is not. The job crisis is a symptom of something much deeper: a crisis in our relationship to work and the challenge put to our species today to reinvent it.

—Matthew Fox

Mary described herself as "bored to death." She was a bank teller, but she wanted to be a pilot. She wanted to work in an environment in which her abilities would be challenged, in which she would be stimulated to grow, in which she could develop more in-depth relationships with other people. Most Monday mornings found her with a headache. But what to do?

Burnout is an all-too-familiar phenomenon in all jobs, at all levels. It happens when people are stuck in jobs they do not like, in jobs that fail to satisfy their needs. Burnout is quite common among those in the helping professions. The "helpers" often turn out to be "rescuers" who take on unnecessary and unrealistic burdens and actually undermine their own health.

Here are six ways to prevent burnout:

- *Self-care—nutrition, exercise, creation of a supportive environment*

- *Regular deep relaxation and frequent mini-relaxations*

- *Awareness of rescuing tendencies (doing for people what they should be doing themselves) and victimized feelings*

- *Directly asking for what you want and need (especially appreciation and attention)*

- *Regular exercising of your creativity*

- *Acceptance of your limitations—with compassion*

Take one method that appeals to you, because you probably need it most, and focus on that one alone, drawing your awareness to it as you go through your day. Your awareness will build the foundation from which change will happen more easily.

8.8 Stress, Work Choices, and Alternatives

Stress-reducing activities can transform your attitudes toward work and enliven your state of health. Here are some of the many techniques that can help you cope with stress and transform your attitudes toward work:

- *Moving and breathing exercises designed to reduce stress (chapters 2 and 5)*

- *Using well-thinking and creative brainstorming to relieve stressful problems (chapter 7)*

- *Asserting yourself to make your needs known (chapter 9)*

- *Breaking typical game-playing patterns in communications (chapter 9)*

You can also use meditation techniques to get in touch with yourself and as an aid in dealing with the pressures of life that confront us all (chapter 12).

Creativity in bringing a playful attitude to bear on your work may help you to get a new perspective on your job. This can mean something as simple as rearranging your office, giving a flower to your coworkers, inviting your boss to play tennis, or changing the music station on the radio. One small company in Colorado found that weekly staff meetings could become brainstorming sessions in how to personalize and relax the working environment. Productivity increased at the same time.

Applying the principles of wellness to working means that you assume responsibility for yourself and your choices and continue to love yourself. Wellness means that there are alternatives. There are other jobs. There are ways of dealing with stress in your present job. There are ways of transforming your work by incorporating the attitudes that enhance play. There are ways to give up being so serious—to stop being the rescuer for the whole world. There are ways of discovering your real needs and fulfilling them; of discovering your real talents and using them; of discovering your many options and trying them out.

The field of life-work planning is devoted to helping people clarify what it is they really want to do, what they do best, and how to design a plan for doing it. In his brilliant book, *What Color Is Your Parachute?* Richard Bolles presents practical guidance in how to find out about yourself, in how to assess the job market, and how to put the two together.

Continuing education programs through large universities, community colleges, and technical schools list courses in everything from computer programming and small business management to jewelry making. Thousands of folks just like you are taking advantage of these low-cost (sometimes even free) opportunities to develop themselves in new ways. Darla, for instance, was a dissatisfied typist who, at one point in her life, took evening classes in shoemaking for less than one year. She went on to open a thriving shoe store that specialized in custom-made sandals. Darla loved this work. Even so, she went on to study auto mechanics, just so she'd be prepared if she again wanted a change of pace. She was determined not to be stuck again!

8.9 My Work and My Self—The Same Thing?

There is little doubt that your self-concept and the work you do are intimately connected. Typically, when people meet, the first question they ask each other is, "What do you do?" To which each responds with a job description: "I'm a butcher." "I'm a baker." "I'm a candlestick maker."

The trouble is, when we are temporarily out of work, or when we lose enthusiasm for our work, or even when we are merely on vacation, many of us feel that we've lost our identity. While it is true that meaningful work enhances your sense of self, it is dangerous to tie up all your self-worth in your work alone. As you are more than your physical body, so you are more than the work you do. Regardless of what you do, you are a complex, unique, powerful, and beautiful human being. The more you open to your truest self—the more you accept yourself for who you are, not just for what you do—the more open you become to reading the signs that point you in the direction of meaningful and satisfying work.

A DIFFERENT VIEW OF NURTURING PLAY

I had some additional thoughts about play today, as I took a dynamic walk in the mountains, with a strong biting wind blowing at my back. I call my walks my play. They really are for me. However, in writing this chapter with John for the first edition of the *Wellness Workbook* many years ago, we talked about the inner child and how that child needed nurturance. At the time, I think I equated nurturing the inner child—or the nurturing aspects of play—with comfort, and the two are not the same thing for me anymore. Nurturance might not be comfortable, but it would provide food and sustenance in a very vital way. For instance, when I hike or climb I am nurturing my body, my emotional life, my soul, my prayer. I often have a smile in the midst of huffing and puffing. I am playing in God. I am worshipping creation. Sometimes the harder the hike, the more my soul is stretched and then filled. I think many people will report that assisting at the bedside of a dying friend can be one of the hardest things they've ever done, but at the same time that it had provided more nurturance, in the sense of sustenance and food for the being, than almost anything else they've ever done, too.

While I wouldn't call all these things play—and I do think that it might also be important to point to play as lighthearted, spontaneous, silly—I wouldn't rule out things that might be seriously taxing at times, yet provide overall a kind of lightness and joy that touches us at a deeper level. A joy that is reminiscent of the breath of God.

—RSR

8.10 The Planet at Play

In discussing competition, we saw how it can become a destructive force in our personal lives. As a national policy it can lead to devastation. Where was the satisfaction in winning the "arms race" if we continue to live in constant fear as a result? Where is the joy in having the world's highest standard of living if we do so at the expense of the poorer countries that we exploit? Does happiness mean becoming an island of plenty surrounded by a sea of poverty and misery? These are hard questions. But they are real issues nonetheless. If we need to learn to play and work cooperatively on the corner lot, we need to learn to play and work, cooperatively, on the planet-field if we are to survive.

In Hindu cosmology, the term *lila* refers to the Divine play. All of creation, as we perceive it, is said to be the result of the Creator at play. The work of creation is not separate from the play. In fact, the Divine actually transforms Itself into the earth, the waters, the animals . . . and dances with all of it— Itself. Everything then is sacred.

In Christianity, the doctrine of the mystical body of Christ says that we are all cells in one larger body—the body of God. We are all working together in order to bring about the perfection of the whole.

Our work and our play can serve the realization of our interdependence as a species and our reliance on other species, or it can undermine it. Most people desire a form of work that serves some meaningful purpose, even though in the short run they may operate as if they are only in it for personal gain. The Buddhist concept of "right livelihood" speaks to this, urging us to engage in forms of work (and play) that move us forward toward the realization of unity and happiness and freedom from suffering, instead of increasing our separation, unhappiness, and pain with one another.

Work that harms the earth and its resources, work that creates weapons of mass destruction, work that generates greed, jealousy, and fear, and alienates people one from another . . . this is work that also harms the worker, if not in body, then in soul and spirit.

If we are to genuinely enjoy the fruits of our labors, we must examine their impact on the planet as a whole, and reaffirm our commitment to letting everybody win.

SUGGESTED READING

Bolles, R., *What Color Is Your Parachute? A Practical Manual for Job-Hunters and Career-Changers* (Ten Speed Press, revised annually).

Covey, S., *The Seven Habits of Highly Effective People* (Simon and Schuster, 1990).

Felible, R., and C. W. Metcalf, *Lighten Up: Survival Skills for People under Pressure* (Perseus, 1993).

Fox, M., *The Reinvention of Work: A New Vision of Livelihood for Our Time* (HarperCollins, 1994).

Houston, J., *The Possible Human: A Course in Enhancing Your Physical, Mental, and Creative Abilities* (J. P. Tarcher, 1997).

Huber, C., *There Is Nothing Wrong with You* (Keep It Simple, 2001).

Kapit, W., and L. Elson, *The Anatomy Coloring Book* (Addison-Wesley, 2001).

Koch, R., *The 80/20 Principle: The Secret to Success by Achieving More with Less* (Doubleday, 1999).

Lakein, A., *How to Get Control of Your Time and Your Life* (New American Library, 1996).

McGee-Cooper, A., *You Don't Have to Go Home from Work Exhausted!* (Bantam, 1992).

Matt, M., *Human Anatomy Coloring Book* (Dover Publishing, 1982).

Moody, R., *Laugh after Laugh: The Healing Power of Humor* (Headwaters, 1978).

Ornstein, R., and D. Sobel, *Healthy Pleasures* (Perseus, 1990).

Pirsig, R., *Zen and the Art of Motorcycle Maintenance: An Inquiry into Values* (Bantam Books, 1984).

Simon, S., L. Howe, and H. Kirschenbaum, *Values Clarification* (Warner Books, 1995).

Terkel, S., *Working* (New Press, 1997).

For an updated listing of resources and active links to the websites mentioned in this chapter, please see www.WellnessWorkbook.com.

CHAPTER 9

Wellness and Communicating

Feeling and thinking together lead to communication. Communicating involves the organization of feeling and thinking energies and their transmission in the form of a message, verbal or nonverbal. Communicating is an energy output that allows us to share our internal maps of reality with others, and thus forms the foundation of culture.

You think it's a secret, but everybody knows.

—Fortune cookie

Human communication is simply an exchange of information, verbal or nonverbal, between a sender and a receiver. (A rather cold description for what can be poetry or lovemaking.) However, because we humans are so fantastically complex, it is virtually impossible for us to communicate isolated bits of data, despite what you may have experienced from your high school history teacher. Every time you speak to (or write to, or look at) someone, you are revealing yourself. You can't avoid it. Your tone of voice, selection of words, facial expression, even the clothes you wear and the way you comb your hair, all these are messages in themselves, messages about you. Furthermore, the person you are addressing interprets what you share in the light of his or her own beliefs and values. Sometimes there are so many variables, so many hidden messages, that the original information is deeply buried, and a map is required to recover it.

When you are not busy communicating with someone or something else, you are carrying on a running conversation with yourself, even though you may not be aware of it. These internal conversations are as vulnerable to distortions and misrepresentations as any other conversation. Because internal conversations direct the way you view the world and the way you view yourself, they have a momentous impact on your health and happiness. If you tell yourself enough times that the world is a terrible place, if you tell yourself enough times that you are weak and susceptible, then very likely the outcome will be just so.

In this chapter we will focus almost exclusively on verbal communication, exploring the dynamics of how people talk to themselves (intrapersonal communication) and one another (interpersonal communication). We will also study the breakdowns that can occur. As you come to understand and appreciate this process, you may simultaneously understand and appreciate yourself. The clearer the channel (you), the better the possibilities for a meaningful encounter—a dynamic energy exchange.

COLLECTING GOLD

What might happen if you were to devote the next three days to listening and looking for the acknowledgments and serendipitous gifts that seem to be aimed in your direction? What if you were to accept them with nothing more than a simple "thank you"? Here are some of the experiences you might notice:

- The thank-you's of bus drivers
- The admiring looks of your children
- The comment of a coworker, a client, a student, a customer

- A stray dog following you home
- An obliging motorist who stops to let you through the traffic
- A wink, a whistle, a second look
- An acquaintance remembering your name
- A letter from home
- A phone call from a friend
- A hug and a kiss
- A discount, a bargain, a quarter in the soft-drink machine
- A grateful waitperson
- Your newspaper left in a plastic bag on a rainy day

- A luncheon date
- A sunset more dramatic than any you can remember
- A cool evening; a warm fire; a feeling of wellbeing . . .

Why not try and make up your own list? You may even find that you have written a poem.

9.1 Intrapersonal Communication

You communicate with yourself more than you do with anyone else. Talking to yourself is more formally referred to as *intrapersonal communication,* and it's sometimes called the *internal dialogue,* although it is often more of a monologue. These conversations actually structure your reality. Since they will influence what you find "out there," they will have an impact on your health and happiness. So, as we discussed at length in chapter 7, be aware of what you tell yourself.

When you were a child, the world was described for you and you got attention for repeating these descriptions. "Nice doggy!" "Bad cold." "Pretty girl." "Ugly mess!" You soon came to understand that words were symbols for things and that some things were good and necessary; others were bad and should be avoided. As you asked "Why?" and "What is it?" you received not only a verbal message, but also a whole range of more subtle, nonverbal cues about what was approved and what was not. Since you didn't comprehend all the words used in these descriptions, you relied more upon the emotional tone that accompanied them. You were very perceptive in picking up these nonverbal cues. Your parents and others around you used tone of voice, facial expression, and physical touch (such as a restraining touch on the shoulder as you approached the stove) to teach you, to protect you, or to control you.

As you grew older, you moved from a simple awareness of a few things into the process of talking to yourself about everything. You began to draw on your rapidly developing linguistic skills to describe your world. Any white stuff that fell from the sky was called snow. You *understood* snow. Or so you thought. The fact that some of it was heavy and very wet, while some of it was light and powdery may have escaped you. Snow was snow, falling, piling up on the fence or trees, frozen into ice, turning gray as it was trampled underfoot. All of its textures, its infinite patterns, its many stages may not have been appreciated. Snow was snow! This is what we mean when we say that the way in which we describe the world limits us.

As you look around the room right now, you are talking to yourself about everything you see. Your language is structuring your reality. Furniture and pictures are not good or bad in and of themselves; they become beautiful or ugly, valuable or tacky, based upon your descriptions of them. The "real" world simply *is,* but *your* world is created by *your* judgments.

Let's use a common example to illustrate this concept. Remember a time in your life when you were in love? Perhaps you had just met the person of your dreams, or held your first child or grandchild. Do you remember what the world was like for you then? Typically, you found beauty everywhere. The sun was brighter and warmer, or the clouds more dramatic. Colors were deeper. You laughed at situations that formerly annoyed you. People in supermarkets let you ahead of them in line. Others smiled at you as you walked down the street. Without effort, you found the perfect greeting card, or the ideal restaurant, or the best spot at the concert.

We say "love is blind" not because it diminishes our sight. On the contrary, it usually intensifies it. The blindness refers to the inability to see what formerly you considered bad, ugly, or meaningless. Love causes you to change your perception—and, subsequently, the language you use to describe it. As a result, the world appears to be more beautiful—and what's more, you usually feel better too.

If we really understood this connection between language and our reality, then the focus of our attention on health would undergo a radical change. Instead of talking to ourselves about germs, flu, headaches, arthritis, and senility, we would talk about enthusiasm, strength, balance, energy, and joy. If we appreciated that what we find is really a function of what we look for, our sense of responsibility for our own life and health would increase dramatically.

9.2 Self-Talk and Self-Concept

When you talk to yourself, you are altering or reinforcing your self-concept. *Self-esteem* has become a common term, but the origins of our self-concept often remain lost in the murky memories (or lack thereof) of our first months of life—beginning in the womb.

Michel Odent, M.D., has amassed data showing that our present state of health is more strongly affected by our experiences in our mother's womb than by any of the health-promoting behaviors we have discussed in this book.[1] While there's nothing we can do to alter what has already happened, there is much we can do to recognize and compensate for the damage that may have been done to our developing nervous system in the first months of life (and much we can do about the experience any of our future offspring will have). The sum total of the thoughts you think about yourself, who you are, and what you are worth, are built upon your experiences of yourself and your world, as an infant. The environment you grew up in (nurturing and supportive versus harsh and unsupportive) profoundly shaped the architecture and development of your brain (see module 3.16). It determines your self-concept, and that in turn designs your internal environment. A strong, worthy self-concept goes with a strong, worthy body-mind. Your wellness depends upon your self-concept.

> **You may not remember your early years, but you'll never forget them.**
>
> —Anonymous

Many people have been "trained," from before they could even speak, to turn gold into garbage—using the Midas touch in reverse. Someone says, "I like what you're wearing tonight" and your internal wiring hears "So you didn't like what I wore last night? I suppose that means I'm not OK." A supervisor remarks, "This is good work." The employee with a damaged self-concept remarks to herself, "So everything else I've done has been bad? I'm just an incompetent person."

These inner conversations, internal dialogues, are *you* talking to yourself all day long. What once appeared to be someone else's judgment of you now is your own judgment, not only of yourself, but most likely of everyone around you, from morning till night, and even in your dreams. This is how you furnish the stage on which you act out your personal drama: by constantly judging, endlessly choosing the right category or box in which to safely place each person and situation you encounter. This is a very tiring way of life!

Once you realize how frustrating and exhausting this self-talk is, you can resolve to change it. Try setting aside a few short periods each day in which you simply listen to your inner dialogue. Write out the dialogue or make a list of the negative messages you frequently hear yourself repeating. It is amazing how predictable and uncreative such messages are. Don't try to change them, at first. Just notice them, again and again and again. After a short time, when you get really tired of them, you may be more motivated to try a different strategy to turn them off. Some people say that bursting into song is a good way to turn your attention to something else. Others support strong physical exercise as a way to break the patterns.

In earlier editions of this book we suggested using affirmations, making up positive statements that provide counterarguments to your negative self-assessment. They seem to work well for people who already have a fairly positive self-image, or for whom times seem good, but for others they are not effective because these affirmations are not based in present reality.

Recently a powerful technology has emerged that helps you uncover previously unnoticed evidence about your behaviors. This science is part of the emerging field of positive psychology, as espoused by Martin Seligman, Ph.D., in *Authentic Happiness*. His approach teaches specific skills for collecting this evidence from your life; you can then use it to refute any negative messages that you tend to dwell on. You expand your awareness of yourself by looking "laterally"—in directions different from those in which you are accustomed to looking—to find other truths about yourself that you have been overlooking or discounting.

It's as if you've taken off blinders—you can see "the other side"; that is, the truth of counterbalancing arguments *based in reality*. Over time, use of this approach will reveal a bigger truth that you have likely been ignoring by habitually focusing on one tiny aspect of your reality that has become deeply ingrained.

Seligman describes other techniques for expanding your self-awareness. One is the process of savoring positive experiences that counter your familiar negative ones. You can consciously set up time to have pleasant experiences. Focusing on the pleasure available to you expands your repertoire. You can share these experiences with someone close to you, savoring them together in real time; you can reminisce about experiences from the past (recycling them); you can take mental snapshots while a savored experience is happening, to make it more indelible in your memory; or simply immerse yourself more deeply by describing it to yourself as you experience it.

Building a stronger self-concept might well begin with learning to accept compliments. These gifts, like gems, are being handed to all of us all the time. Even if the people in your immediate environment don't seem to be giving them, nature itself is showering them continually—a fresh breeze, a purple and orange sunset, a spring rain. Simply opening your eyes and cultivating gratitude as a way of being can show you many good things to talk to yourself about. You can make Thanksgiving Day happen every day of the year.

9.3 Interpersonal Communication

We move now to a consideration of the information exchange that happens when you talk to other people—*interpersonal* communication.

People talk to one another because they have needs that must be met. They require direction, or food, or relief from pain, or quiet, or touch, or acknowledgment. Getting our needs met helps give us a sense of mastery in our life. Without shared information you are, like the autistic person, alone in the world. You don't know what to expect. Without the ability to communicate, learning becomes an almost impossible task. Without mutual understanding, relationships break down and jobs don't get done. Lacking the needed energy, life becomes imbalanced. What often results, then, is a state of dis-ease.

While many of us would rather blame others when our communications break down or our directions are interpreted incorrectly, it is important for us to assume responsibility for how we communicate, including some assurance that we are being understood. Although other people have a role in any communication exchange, we can't force them to do things our way, nor can we expect them to change. Ultimately we can only work on ourselves. In line with that, we can maximize the possibility that our communication is free of disruptive roadblocks, essentially nonjudgmental, and even understood.

Aiming for total agreement in communication sets you up for failure. You can't win at that game. Aiming for understanding and mutual respect offers the best chance of ensuring that everybody can win. Actually, the effectiveness of communication is directly related to the degree of trust between two individuals.

In order to trust others, we need to allow trust for ourselves. We nourish trust for ourselves by taking responsibility for our own lives and living with integrity, authenticity, love, and compassion. You'll recognize these attitudes as the chief supports of wellness, too.

Our investigation here will highlight some common causes for breakdowns in communication:

- *Conversations that are really monologues—and thus don't share energy (see module 9.4)*

- *Failure to express real feelings, resulting in dishonesty and nonassertiveness (see module 9.5)*

- *Inflexibility, which shows up in absolutes and generalizations (see module 9.6)*

- *Failure to listen (see module 9.9)*

- *Manipulative communication (sometimes called "game playing")—another form of dishonest communication (see module 9.10)*

We will look at the connection between breakdowns in communication and the potential for illness, and we'll explore ways of using communication in the service of wellness.

Communication Theory: I know you believe you understand what you think I said. But I am not sure you realize that what you heard is not what I meant.

—Anonymous

9.4 **Monologues and Dialogues**

When a character in a play delivers a monologue, it generally serves an important purpose. When two people carry on a simultaneous monologue with each other, or when one person speaks only about himself without ever inviting interaction with the other, very little communication happens. With the simultaneous monologue, I talk about what interests or involves me, while you talk about what interests and involves you. Neither of us really hears the other, so we may each start talking louder, interrupting more, or trying to bring the focus of attention back to ourselves. When this has gone on for a short time, and nobody is truly satisfied, we often give up on conversation altogether and turn on the TV, or suggest going out for a drink. Anything to change the energy or the environment.

Here's a typical simultaneous monologue:

A: "I just got back from the doctor's."

B: "Oh, is everything OK? I have to see my doctor soon too, but I'm not looking forward to it."

A: "Yeah, well, I need to get my prescription changed and he says I have to cut out caffeine."

B: "I could never do that. If I don't have my morning coffee I'm hell to live with."

A: "I've tried herb tea, but I don't like it."

B: "Did you see where that new company just started making green tea ice cream?"

An image this might evoke is that of a couple running toward each other with outstretched arms and longing looks, and then tripping as they run right past each other.

Despite all that we have in common, time and time again we fail to really meet each other. We may spend an evening, a bus ride, or our whole lives together, and never achieve common ground. These unsatisfying relationships lack the energy needed for life and health. They create boredom and joylessness. We leave them with our needs for intimacy, for caring, unmet. As a last resort in our attempts to make these relationships work, some of us even use sickness—because illness demands a response.

It would be far better to use communication for revitalizing, for wellness. To do this, we need to make communication an energy exchange, a dialogue.

Every person alive has a story. When you are open to hearing my story, and I am open to hearing yours, when we are truly aware of one another and sensitive to what each of us needs, then we are experiencing dialogue.

Dialogue is characterized by honesty, true presence, and nonjudgmental listening (honesty will be discussed in the next module, and nonjudgmental and active listening will be described later).

With *true presence,* you attend to the other as fully as possible. You turn your face or your body in her direction. Your eyes are open to more than the movement of her lips. You become sensitive to what is going on inside the words, between the lines. Speakers give much valuable information about the world as they view it through tone of voice, fluency, facial expression, hand gestures, posture, and the distance they put between you when they talk. As much as possible, begin to notice the extent to which you are able to postpone your own agenda and give your attention to the other. Perhaps you think you should give your attention solely to the other, and take no time or space for your own "less important" agenda. Perhaps you tend to dominate, allowing no space for the other person to share. Ideally, dialogue will be a balance, a sharing: your agenda, my agenda, and areas of overlap.

In *nonjudgmental listening,* you try to understand as fully as possible what is being said. If you spend your time calculating your responses, you will miss the full impact of the message being sent. Often one word or expression triggers your disapproval or disagreement so strongly that a conversation becomes a subtle debate. At times, even without saying a word, you may get hooked on that point of disagreement and block out everything that follows. When you become aware that this is happening, it takes courage to stop and admit it.

Misunderstanding is at the root of most of the problems in relationships, personal as well as professional. Yet most misunderstandings can be prevented by dynamic, nonjudgmental listening.

9.5 Truthful and Caring Communications

When communication is too carefully guarded—when we "walk the fence," trying to say what the other person will accept rather than what we really mean; when we say yes when we mean no—we can easily cross the line into dishonesty, so that our interactions with other people become dry and meaningless. Cocktail-party chatter is not bad, but it is generally not all that nourishing. The failure to express our real feelings can rob us of energy. Sharing ourselves honestly with another can provide both parties with a real gift—a gift of energy.

Communicating with others is more intimate when you are able to share your true feelings, rather than merely talking about the weather or hobbies. Feelings are not always pleasant subjects and most of us have trouble expressing negative feelings. Often, when we are upset, we send "you messages" to the person with whom we are upset, rather than state how we feel. Other people are more likely to become defensive if they feel they are being judged. They are more likely to be receptive if, instead, you tell them what you are feeling—an "I message"—rather than make a judgment about them.

Example of "you message" with a judgment:
"You're confusing me. You are not making sense."

Example of "I message" with an emotion stated:
"I'm upset because I don't understand."

Notice how the first can be construed as an invitation to fight, and the second, an invitation to share feelings and solve a problem. These methods are effective with those who are invested in having a healthy relationship with you. Despite your best efforts at wording the communication from an "I message" point of view, some people will probably take offense anyway, especially at first. Defensiveness is a natural response when we feel threatened, or feel like we may have done something wrong. Be patient. In these cases you may need to broach the subject at a more ideal time, giving your partner some chance to adapt to this straightforward means of communication. Do your best. If the relationship is an intimate one or one that requires the building and maintenance of trust, it is all the more vital that clear, truthful, and caring communications be the foundation. By sharing our words with others, we share our thoughts, and thus we share ourselves. As we learn about each other, we learn more about the world at large and more about ourselves. The ability to view our exchange in this way allows us to be open, to learn, and to grow.

The advantage of telling the truth is that you don't have to remember what you said.

—Mark Twain

---

1. **Experiencing what is.** Distinguish between what you actually experience (see, hear, sense, feel, notice, remember) versus what you imagine (interpret, believe, assume) to be true. The statement "I see you looking at the floor" is your own experience. The statement "I see you are uncomfortable" is an interpretation. If you get caught up in believing your interpretations about another person's behavior, you'll be responding to your interpretation of what she did instead of what she actually did.

2. **Being transparent.** To be transparent is to be willing to be seen, warts and all. Contrary to what we may think, most people become more appealing when they reveal their needs and insecurities. This doesn't mean presenting the story of your wounds in misfortunes in vivid detail. It's more a matter of practicing being open about your feelings, impressions, wants, and self-talk about your interaction with the person in front of you.

3. **Noticing your intent.** Do you communicate to relate or to control? When your intent is to relate, you are most interested in revealing your true feelings, learning how the other feels, and connecting heart-to-heart. When your intent is to control, you are most interested in getting things to turn out a certain way—avoiding conflict, getting the person to like you, being seen as knowledgeable or helpful, etc.

4. **Giving and asking for feedback.** Giving feedback is the act of verbally letting the other know how his actions affected you. Being open to receiving feedback means you are curious about and willing to hear how your actions affect other people. Most people don't get very much valid feedback in their daily lives, and they long for it.

5. **Asserting what you want and don't want.** Many of us are afraid to ask for what we want in a dating relationship for fear of either not getting it or of having the other person give it to us out of obligation. Asking for what you want is an act of trust. You are taking a step into the unknown—not knowing how the other person will respond.

6. **Taking back projections.** If some aspect of my own personality is unconscious or suppressed, I may find that I have a pattern of being attracted to men who exhibit this quality in spades. Have you ever been attracted to someone for some wonderfully appealing quality only to discover a few months down the road that this very same quality turned you off? That's a great opportunity to take back or rediscover your own hidden qualities.

7. **Revising an earlier statement.** This means giving yourself permission to revisit a particular interaction or moment in time if your feelings change or if you later connect to some deeper feelings or afterthoughts. For instance: "After I said such and such, I later realized there was more to it than that. What I now feel is _____."

8. **Holding differences or embracing multiple perspectives.** Many people fear intimacy because they fear losing themselves in a relationship. If you know how to practice holding differences, you won't need to fear losing yourself. This is the capacity to listen to and empathize with opinions that differ from yours without losing touch with your own perspective.

9. **Sharing mixed emotions.** Sometimes we want to tell someone the truth but at the same time we are concerned about their feelings. A desire to clear the air might be accompanied by a fear of being misunderstood. If you do have mixed feelings, expressing both feelings can add depth to your communication.

10. **Embracing silence.** Authentic communication depends as much on silence as it does on words—the silences between your words and the silence you experience as you await the other's response. Embracing silence encourages understanding that there are many things that cannot be known all at once or once and for all. These things emerge gradually as we get to know the other person.

Susan Campbell, *Truth in Dating: Finding Love by Getting Real* (New World Library, 2004), www.truthindating.com.

9.6 Avoiding Absolutes, Generalizations, Labels, and Judgments

It is natural to form judgments about the world. As we have already pointed out, we do this continually, whether or not we are aware of it. We all have generalizations about the sexes, other age groups, and other cultures, but if we use those generalizations to stereotype, "write off," or oversimplify our ideas about another person, we miss the opportunity to know them better or to learn from them, and expand our understanding of the world we share. Appreciate that there is some truth in generalizations, but don't make them the sum total of your communications. It can become a problem if we are unable to change our opinions, or if we make the mistake of assuming that everyone else shares our opinions—or would, if they were intelligent enough or better informed.

This tendency to put people or things into convenient boxes commonly shows up in conversations as absolute statements, generalizations, and "is" labels:

"You *never* ask me what *I* want to do."

"Teenagers *all* like that horrible, loud music."

"Coffee *is bad* for you."

"There *is nothing* we can do about it."

"You'll *never* get a decent job."

"Iraqis *can't* be trusted."

Statements like these are communication barriers; they detour our energies in a number of ways:

- *They limit our worldview, and also our alternatives. As alternatives decrease, stress increases.*

- *They set us up for opposition, debate, and confrontation with those who don't agree. As defensiveness increases, so does stress.*

- *They distance other people or cause them to decide, "It's no use talking to her." And it's difficult to cultivate intimacy or friendship when the other moves away.*

Try listening to yourself to see if you have fallen into the habit of speaking in absolute terms. As you catch yourself, let that cue you to substitute a statement that will keep the lines of communication open. For instance:

J: How was the movie?

R: That is the worst movie ever made! [the absolute statement] I mean, I didn't care for it at all. I found the plot confusing, and the characters undeveloped . . .

Or . . .

J: Have you been following the campaign?

R: Yes, Joe is an idiot! [the absolute statement] Excuse me—I mean, I find it hard to justify his policy on energy, especially when . . .

Note how these amended responses actually communicate more data; they also leave the other person free to disagree—and therefore keep the lines of communication open.

9.7 Assertive Communication

Assertiveness basically means the ability to express your thoughts and feelings in a way that clearly states your needs and keeps open the lines of communication with the other. By blocking our feelings, we may create tensions that collect in different parts of our bodies. Eventually they may surface as illness of some sort.

The great majority of us are required to live a life of constant systematic duplicity. Your health is bound to be affected if, day after day, you say the opposite of what you feel, if you grovel before what you dislike and rejoice at what brings you nothing but misfortune. Our nervous system isn't just a fiction; it's a part of our physical body, and our soul exists in space and is inside us, like the teeth in our mouth. It can't be forever violated with impunity.

—Boris Pasternak

As you listen to people talk, you can become aware of how often they assume it is natural and preferable to suppress rather than express their real feelings or the truth:

- *"I was furious, but I wouldn't give him the satisfaction of seeing me blow up."*

- *"Just swallow your pride!" (Which usually means your anger.)*

- *"What a strong woman—she never cried, even at the funeral."*

- *"No matter how tough things get—keep smiling!"*

We tell ourselves that we don't want to hurt other people's feelings. Our friend might be insulted if we were to admit, "I really don't want to go out tonight." So, instead, we smile and say "Sure," or "I'd love to," while inside we churn with anger or sadness or frustration.

It takes a great deal of effort to continually walk the fence, trying to please all the people, all the time. But that's what we must do to remain "nice guys" or "sweethearts." We have to swallow hard, breathe lightly, walk on tiptoe, and maybe end up with stomach ulcers, or arthritis, or cancer. The body will allow just so much repressed emotion to collect. Then it will have its way.

Our reluctance to be assertive often stems from confusing this type of communication with aggression, but they are simply not the same. If someone is talking near your seat in a movie theater, the aggressive response is, "Shut up!" The assertive response is, "I can't hear the film. Would you please be quiet?" The first one is hostile. The second is firm but respectful—and probably does the job much more effectively. Hostility breeds hostility. Firmness with respect leaves the other intact.

Taking care of your own needs, taking charge of yourself (or letting others take charge, as appropriate), expressing an unpopular opinion, saying no when that is what you mean, are among your privileges as a human being. To refrain from doing so in situations of importance to you may undermine your peace of mind, your self-esteem, and your body's natural inclinations towards equilibrium.

9.8 Owning Our Mistakes

It takes energy to try to cover up our tracks if we've made a wrong turn. It wastes energy to procrastinate in our communications when we realize we've made a mistake. It's painful to worry and wonder what might happen if or when somebody finds out about something we've done . . . or neglected to do. Owning up to our mistakes, quickly, is a healthy way to conserve energy better spent in life-enhancing ways.

When it comes to offering apologies or telling the truth about errors in judgment or any other mistakes, it's crucial to make the distinction between the essential goodness of yourself, on the one hand, and your behaviors on the other. Everybody breaks things; everybody breaks down, at times. Nobody fulfills the perfect ideal! We are not defined by our mistakes, however, unless we want to be. (Some folks keep pointing to their failures as if they are proud of them.) But because we have difficulty separating a label from the person/thing itself, we often take on unnecessary guilt or blame because we have identified with our shortcomings or accidents. Certainly this is true in our culture: because of our perceived need to be "right," assigning blame is most likely the first line of response. This form of defensiveness may easily overshadow the more important need to solve the problem that has arisen as a result of the mistake.

Instead of getting reactive when you make a mistake, take a deep breath and a metaphorical "step back" from your behavior, if only by the slightest degree. Sometimes it helps to think of how you might advise another person in a similar situation. You've seen how easily a friend or relative has become twisted up with guilt and self-recrimination for something they've done. You've seen how painful this process becomes. You know that by equating their self-worth with their ability to do things perfectly, they are creating an unrealistic expectation that can never be fully realized.

Ask yourself if your fear of making a mistake is based on the hidden assumption that you are potentially perfect and that if you can just be careful enough, you will not fall from grace. Recognize the impossibility of such a goal. Determine to move forward in solving the problem in the best way you can in the moment, even if you still feel dissatisfied by your imperfect performance. Apologize if appropriate; own up to the truth as necessary; acknowledge your own essential goodness; move on.

But a "mistake" is a declaration of the way I *am*, a jolt to the way I intend, a reminder I am not dealing with the facts. When I have *listened* to my mistakes I have grown.

—Hugh Prather

ASSERTING YOUR RIGHT TO WELLNESS

People often feel timid about questioning "experts," and this is particularly true in the doctor-patient relationship. Here are some suggestions that may help you assert your rights to wellness:

- Ask your doctor to explain fully your condition and what exactly is going on in your body; if necessary, ask for illustrations.

- Ask if there are ways, other than drugs or surgery, to deal with your problem.

- Ask about possible side effects of drugs prescribed.

- Ask for a second, or third opinion, or investigate alternatives for yourself.

- Ask for a generic drug prescription, which is usually less expensive than a brand name.

- Ask for a full description of a procedure suggested before it is used.

- Ask for a lead shield to cover other parts of the body (particularly ovaries or testes) when X-rays are being taken.

- State your displeasure and inconvenience at being made to wait.

- Ask for anything that will provide you with greater privacy or comfort.

- Ask for a fee schedule before you make an appointment.

- If you do not have health insurance, ask for a discount for cash payment.

- Ask about your doctor's previous experience in dealing with a condition similar to your own.

- Refuse treatment if your questions are not answered adequately.

- Tell your doctor what *you* think is wrong or right with you.

THE UGLY FAT GUY

There are probably an infinite number of ways in which to describe the same person, the same event. The description we choose betrays much about our attitudes and our appreciation of the person or scene. I describe the man I don't know or care about as "the ugly fat guy." To his friend, he is the one in the blue jogging outfit or the heavyset one with glasses.

Listen to yourself describe things and people to yourself and others. If you find you are expressing judgments, you might want to plug in a more objective (perhaps kind and compassionate) description. While you're at it, try applying this to descriptions of yourself as well.

—RSR

9.9 Listening Skills

Since more than half the time you spend in communication is probably spent listening, you should be an expert by now. Unfortunately, however, really good listeners are the rare exception. Most people listen passively, because they consider speaking to be the active component of communication. That is because they confuse *listening* with *hearing*.

When you walk through a mall or enter a restaurant, you probably hear music playing in the background. Contrast that with the experience of attending a concert. In the first case you are hearing, in the second you are listening. A similar dynamic exists in communication with others. We hear a lot, but we are less likely to listen with attention.

We all need to develop our dynamic listening (sometimes called *active listening*), because we generally allow much of what we hear to go in one ear and out the other. The semanticist S. I. Hayakawa gave this example of poor listening: "Jones says something, Smith gives a heated response to what he mistakenly believes Jones said, and Jones tries to refute what he mistakenly believes Smith meant."[2]

This enormous energy waste is easily remedied by using a very simple technique called *reflecting back*. After Jones has spoken, Smith recounts what he understood Jones to be saying. If Jones agrees, Smith then continues with his remarks. If Jones disagrees, he can restate his case in another way that leaves less room for misinterpretation. Smith then reports what he has heard. The exchange continues on this level until Jones is satisfied that he has been understood. The conversation might go like this:

Jones: The records in your department are terribly confusing to interpret.

Smith: Are you saying that I keep bad records?

Jones: No, not at all. I'm saying that the complexity of your work makes reporting a difficult task. I'm impressed by what you've done, but I need help understanding it.

Smith: Thanks for the compliment. So you need someone to work with you when you look them over?

Jones: That's exactly it! Any suggestions?

This technique can become ridiculous if used all the time; in talking about the weather, for instance:

Jones: What's the weather like outside?

Smith: Am I correct in assuming that you are asking for my knowledge about the current temperature, humidity, and rate of precipitation?

But it is an invaluable tool to use when taking directions or instructions, when discussing matters that might put the participants on the defensive, or when dealing with problems in a close relationship. For example:

Tom: The children have really been hard to deal with lately. I'm getting fed up.

Terri: You are really frustrated by their behavior.

Tom: Yes—do you think it's just me, or have you noticed it too?

The next time you find yourself embroiled in a heated debate, why not try this "reflecting" strategy? You just might find that there really was no disagreement in the first place. If there is, at least you'll have a clearer understanding of what the problem stems from.

Learning to listen brings tremendous, and often immediate, rewards that contribute to health and happiness on all sides. We relieve stress; we meet the other on common ground; we provide them with caring and attention. To be listened to is to be acknowledged as a worthwhile human being—and that's the best medicine there is.

When you are open to hearing my story, and I am open to hearing yours, when we are truly aware of one another and sensitive to what each of us needs, then we are experiencing dialogue.

Carl Rogers, the eminent psychologist who first coined the phrase *active listening,* said: "Real communication occurs . . . when we listen with understanding. What does this mean? It means to see the expressed idea and attitude from the other person's point of view, to sense how it feels to him, to achieve his frame of reference in regard to the thing he is talking about. . . . If I can really understand how he hates his father or hates the university or hates communists—if I can catch the flavor of his fear . . . it will be the greatest help to him in altering these very hatreds and fears and in establishing realistic and harmonious relationships with the very people and situations toward which he has felt hatred and fear."[3]

When you listen to me without interruption or anything that feels like a judgment, you allow me the time and space to get more in touch with the many facets of me Thank you for never playing with my words, getting a laugh or recognition at my expense. When you allow me to revise or restructure what I have said, I feel that you are truly committed to understanding me and what I'm about. Thank you for not feeling that you necessarily have to do something about what I share. When you listen, I feel that you are listening not only to my words but the feelings behind them. Bless you for being you and thereby assisting me in my journey.

—Bennett Kilpack, M.F.C.C

I Know a Good Listener

Think about people in your life (past or present) whom you consider to be good listeners. What did these people do or not do to earn them this credit? Try to be as specific as possible. For example: Ann D.—She rarely tries to "match" my stories by adding one of her own. Instead, she simply listens and asks insightful questions.

Record your observations or reflections here:

_____

_____

_____

_____

_____

_____

Consider which of these qualities you would like to incorporate into your own listening repertoire.

Listening: The Non–Building Blocks

Communication specialist Jud Morris sums up the ways in which we block or discourage understanding by poor habits of listening:

- *Evaluation, judgment.* We are so busy planning our attack, or criticizing the other's message, that we often do not really hear what is being said.

- *Jumping to conclusions.* We jump to conclusions, filling in our own details before the other has had a chance to explain himself or herself.

- *"We're all the same."* We assume that other people think as we do.

- *Attitude, the closed mind.* We tune out people with whom we don't agree.

- *Lack of attention.* We let our minds wander.

- *Wishful hearing.* We tend to hear just what we want to hear, or expect to hear.

- *Excessive talking.* We interrupt or dominate the conversation so that the other doesn't get a chance to adequately express his or her ideas.

- *Unclear words.* We fail to find out what the other means by the particular words he or she chooses.

- *Lack of humility.* We feel that we must express our superiority by speaking or contradicting the other.

- *Fear.* We avoid listening with understanding because we are afraid that the other may challenge some long-held belief. We are afraid to be threatened by a new idea.

If these are the non–building blocks, what are the building blocks? List some here:

_____

_____

_____

_____

_____

_____

_____

_____

_____

_____

_____

9.10 Manipulative Strategies in Communication

If many of our communication exchanges seem to go around in circles—leaving us feeling power-robbed, angry, dissatisfied—we are probably playing psychological games—manipulative communications. These approaches are manipulative or controlling because the spoken words hide an underlying message, a message of which we may be unaware. You may ask innocently "Where are you going tonight?" when you really mean "I have plans for us tonight." You may ask, "What can I do about it?" when you are already convinced of what must be done.

Sound familiar? We all play games at times—when we are afraid to be honest or to reveal true feelings, or when we want intimacy but fear it, or when we don't trust that another person will attend to us in the way we want to be attended to. Unfortunately, some people make game-playing, or manipulative communication, a way of life, effectively shutting off real communication.

If any of these questions or statements have a familiar ring, you are very likely involved in a game:

- *"Do you expect me to do everything?"*

- *"Are you going to wear those shoes with those pants?"*

- *"I'd really like to teach him a lesson once and for all."*

- *"Whenever I talk to my sister we end up in an argument."*

- *"But I was only trying to help."*

Once you are aware that you're playing a game, and you're aware, too, of just what triggered it, you're in a better position to break the cycle. You can decide not to start a game when you normally would or not to take the bait if someone else initiates a game.

Then you are in a position to seek the support of your fellow game player in getting your real needs met: "Mary, every time we talk about visiting my parents we end up deadlocked or in an argument. I think we may be playing or replaying a game here and I'd like your help in breaking it."

If the other agrees, you've got some excellent alternatives. These include:

- *Dropping the subject when it is emotionally overcharged, while agreeing to consider it when you both feel more balanced*

- *Asking a third party to be present, to help you keep the real issues on the table*

- *Using dialogue—really listening to the other, reflecting back what you think they're saying, until you're both sure that understanding has been achieved*

- *Agreeing that it's OK to disagree*

- *Working together to find out what each person's unspoken needs are*

- *Contracting a workable compromise*

Throughout the process, follow one significant rule: Tell the truth, and tell it with heart, using "I" rather than "you" messages (seeking to learn and grow in the communication, rather than to protect and defend yourself or your position). Honesty is always the antidote to game playing (and to most of the other "wars" on the planet as well). Can you imagine what business would be like if people simply told the truth?

9.11 Checking That Help Is Wanted

Rescuing is a subtle form of manipulative communication, and it's one of the most energy-draining interactions imaginable. A rescuer is a compulsive helper, someone who cannot keep from stepping in to give aid, even when it is not wanted. Many professions are attractive to rescuers—medicine, nursing, teaching, and all the other helping professions. Parents are also notorious for being rescuers, as they do and do and do more things for their kids, trying to save them from the natural consequences of their actions.

It may seem unfair to criticize rescuers or rescuing, but a closer look at the dynamics of the interaction reveals the inequities in the situation. Rescuers will always be left unsatisfied because, in attending to others, they neglect their own needs and eventually become burned out. This is a double blow because a prime reason behind rescuing is to *get* attention—and, more often than not, rescuers are rejected by the same ones they are trying to help. The rescuer is then left feeling like a victim of the other's refusal, and unappreciated. This is a key contributing factor in burnout among helping professionals. The person *being rescued* is also left dissatisfied, because the rescuer's unconscious message is "I'm OK, you're not OK—you're so inadequate I have to do it for you." From this vantage point, the "rescuee" typically turns on the rescuer, thus becoming a persecutor, saying "Leave me alone" or "See what you've done." Such role reversals are the basic strategy at work in all games.

This is not to say that you can never help someone. But you first need to find out if help is wanted, and then you need to find out if what you're doing is actually beneficial.

If you are a chronic rescuer, you would do well to undertake some self-examination. You are probably projecting your inadequacies or needs onto others. Here is a comparison of characteristics of both helpers and rescuers.

The Helper

- *Listens for a request*
- *Presents an offer*
- *Gives only what is needed*
- *Checks periodically with the other person*
- *Checks results:*
  - *—functioning better?*
  - *—meeting goals?*
  - *—solving problems independently?*
  - *—using suggestions successfully?*

The Rescuer

- *Gives when not asked*
- *Neglects to find out whether an offer is welcome*
- *Gives help more and longer than needed*
- *Omits asking for feedback*
- *Doesn't check results and feels good when accepted, bad when turned down*
- *Does the greater share of the talking*

As you can see, rescuing is a weak foundation on which to build a relationship with anyone. It disempowers everyone involved.

Rescuer's Checklist

Completing this checklist can help you become aware of ways you may be rescuing people without realizing it.

    Mark each of the statements below as it applies to you, using to this code:

0 = Seldom or never   1 = Sometimes or occasionally   2 = Frequently

(X designates significant others in your life, such as a spouse, boss, parents, friend, or colleague.)

____ It is hard for me to take time for myself and have fun.

____ I supply words for X when he or she hesitates.

____ I set limits for myself that I then exceed.

____ I believe I am responsible for making (keeping) X happy.

____ I enjoy lending a shoulder for X to "cry" on.

____ I believe that X is not sufficiently grateful for my help.

____ I take care of X more than I take care of myself.

____ I find myself interrupting when X is talking.

____ I watch for clues for ways to be helpful to X.

____ I make excuses, openly or mentally, for X.

____ I do more than my share; that is, I work harder than X.

____ When X is unsure or uncomfortable about doing something, I do it for X.

____ I give up doing things because X wouldn't like it.

____ I find myself thinking that I really know what is best for X.

____ I think X would have grave difficulty getting along without me.

____ I use the word "we" and then find I don't have X's consent.

____ I stop myself by thinking X will feel badly if I say or do something.

____ It is hard for me not to respond to anyone who seems hurting or needing help.

____ I find others resenting me when I was only trying to be helpful.

____ I find myself giving advice that is not welcome or accepted.

____ Total score. More than 10 points: Rescuing is possible. More than 20 points: Rescuing is probable.

Adapted, with permission, from Valerie Lankford (www.valcanhelp.com) and Paschal Baute, Ph.D. (www.paschalbaute.com).

CORNERING QUESTIONS OR "ISN'T IT TRUE THAT . . . ?"

You've probably seen a TV show or a movie in which a crafty lawyer skillfully uses questions to "trap" the defendant into an admission of guilt. You may not realize it, but many times your own questions corner people or subtly trap them. This can set up barriers in the communication process and may even bring a conversation to a swift close. Here are some examples of cornering questions:

- Questions that force a yes or no answer.

Isn't this beautiful?

Wouldn't you like to help me out?

- Questions that are really statements.

You really hate me, don't you?

This is awful, isn't it?

- Questions that require an *all-or-nothing* response or that allow for one of only two alternatives.

Are you joyful or sad?

Are you religious or atheistic?

- Questions that take us off the hook by making the other person responsible.

What do you want to do?

Want to stop asking—or answering—cornering questions like these? Here's a follow-up exercise: Determine to listen attentively to your own conversations over the course of the next few days. Focus on your use of questions. This awareness may prove valuable in improving your communication skills.

NONVIOLENT COMMUNICATION

The purpose of nonviolent communication (NVC) is to strengthen our ability to inspire compassion from others and to respond compassionately to others and to ourselves. NVC guides us to reframe how we express ourselves and to hear others by focusing our consciousness on what we are observing, feeling, needing, and requesting.

We are trained to make careful observations free of evaluation, and to specify behaviors and conditions that are affecting us. We learn to hear our own deeper needs and those of others, and to identify and clearly articulate what we are wanting in a given moment. When we focus on clarifying what is being observed, felt, and needed, rather than on diagnosing and judging, we discover the depth of our own compassion. Through its emphasis on deep listening—to ourselves as well as others—NVC fosters respect, attentiveness, and empathy, and engenders a mutual desire to give from the heart. The form is simple, yet powerfully transformative.

While it is taught through the use of a concrete model, and is referred to as "a process of communication" or a "language of compassion," nonviolent communication is more than a process or a language. As our cultural conditioning often leads our attention in directions unlikely to get us what we want, NVC serves as an ongoing reminder to focus our attention on places that have the potential to yield what we are seeking—a flow between ourselves and others based on a mutual giving from the heart.

Adapted from Marshall B. Rosenberg, Ph.D., *Nonviolent Communication: A Language of Life.* For more information, contact the Center for Nonviolent Communication, 2428 Foothill Boulevard, Suite E, La Crescenta, CA 91214, (800) 255-7696, (818) 957-9393, www.cnvc.org.

9.12 To Control or to Relate/Connect?

We've discussed playing psychological games and described rescuing and other manipulative behaviors, but the underlying issue in communication is the overall *intent* of our communication. Very simply, all communications can be divided into two categories: attempts to control and attempts to relate.

Living in a highly competitive society, most of us have unconsciously been trained to try to *control* either the outcome of a conversation or what the other person does (to get what we want). We make demands, pass judgment, diagnose problems, and blame others. While business, sales, and marketing strongly value this type of communication, it is far more widespread—and so insidious that, like the fish who doesn't understand what water is, most of us have no idea that we've been trained to communicate primarily in this way.

The alternative way of communicating is to *relate* to people and to connect with them. Women often have an advantage in this arena (for more, see module 9.13). The goal of communication with the intent to relate or connect is to arrive at a new conclusion that serves everyone. The outcome is usually something that neither party would have thought of on her own. Good listening skills and openness and flexibility are the hallmarks of this type of communication.

Learning to recognize our patterns of control is the first step. The hard part is changing them. Two popular approaches offer tools to change these deeply ingrained habits.

Nonviolent communication—pioneered by Marshall Rosenberg, Ph.D., in a book by the same name—is probably the most widely available of the two. In addition to the book, videotapes and training courses are offered worldwide (see page 233).

A second approach, pioneered by Brad Blanton, Ph.D., in *Radical Honesty,* and amplified by Susan Campbell in *Getting Real* (see "Ten Truth Skills," page 222) offers fresh perspectives on communicating honestly and caringly, with the intent to connect rather than control.

9.13 Cross-Gender and Cross-Cultural Communication

We commonly interpret other people as being abnormal, weird, or wrong when they do or say things that we do not understand. Such misunderstanding is a cause not only of divorce, but of wars. Consequently, it is vital that we learn to control the human tendency to translate "different from me" into "less than me" or "better than me." We can learn to do this. Investigating the differences in the ways people communicate is one of the primary ways to avoid this type of misunderstanding.

One's own culture provides the "lens" through which we view the world; the "logic" . . . by which we order it; the "grammar" . . . by which it makes sense.
—Kevin Avruch, Peter Black, and Joseph Scimecca

Heredity and environment play a huge role in our communication patterns and our language development; consequently, they affect our ability to relate to others. Communication styles differ greatly. Linguist and author Deborah Tannen, speaking within the American cultural context, claims that men and women speak different languages because they live in different worlds. Like other communication specialists, Tannen observes that men in general (there are always many exceptions) use conversation to give information and to compete. They talk about things—business, sports, and food—rather than people. They are concerned with facts, and less likely to elaborate the details. They are goal-oriented. Solving problems is important to men. Why men are less likely to ask for help or directions has long been an enigma to women. Women in general (again, with many individual differences) use conversation to get information and to connect. They talk about people more than things and are easy with expressing the mood, or feelings, associated with a situation. Their speech patterns are more detail oriented. Relationships are key for many women. They are quicker to ask for and accept help or directions and are more likely to cooperate.[4] These differences are compounded when the communication across cultures is highlighted.[5] Here are a few examples:

- *In some cultures, to point out a mistake or even a slight oversight is practically an insult.*

- *Different cultures have different perceptions of closeness and personal space. To stand too closely or to speak from too far away is viewed as threatening behavior.*

- *A loud voice is viewed in some cultures as a prelude to a fight, whereas in another culture it may be necessary in order to indicate enthusiasm for a subject.*

- *Direct eye contact, which we in the West prize as being the ultimate expression of communication attentiveness and effectiveness, is considered invasive by some cultures. This is especially true between men and women because so much communication goes on through the eyes alone.*

- *While Americans stress the importance of dealing with conflict face-to-face, to approach a personal conflict head-on would be to invite shame, if not embarrassment, in some cultures. Putting something in writing, thus creating some objective distance, is preferable for these people.*

Language use varies greatly among individuals, the sexes, generations, races, socioeconomic groups, and cultures. Even the simple word *yes* can be a source of misunderstanding. Among some groups, saying yes is tantamount to signing your name in blood. For others, a yes means "Probably I'll consider it." When dealing with others in a situation that demands common understanding, it may be necessary to ask for further elaboration.

Decision-making styles are different depending upon your cultural upbringing. Some cultures prize unanimity above all; for others, a simple majority is enough; and in others, independent leadership is more appreciated than delegating authority. We have a lot to learn as we approach one another. To assume that our method—or even the methods that seem to work with one cultural segment—should be applied to other cultural groupings, within our country or elsewhere on the planet, is a gross misperception.

As we work together on a task, some cultures and some individuals will place a great emphasis on establishing relationships as the basis for a successful outcome. For others, it is natural to simply get to work, allowing the relationships to build as the job unfolds. For either type to expect the other to change is asking a lot. Look around; observe yourself. Find out what you are doing and what others seem to want. Learn to adapt and compromise; put yourself in the other person's shoes.

Because our learning styles are different, so too will be our ways of communicating about issues. Some members of a group might look to logic and library research as their first line of attack, while others will not feel they know a situation until they have visited the people and places under investigation.

Such differences are cause for celebration, because they show just how vast human potential is. Yet obviously they can also create conflict among the sexes and races and cultures—socially, professionally, and intimately. Ultimately, we all belong to the same human race, with the same fears, desires, and needs. Our survival depends on our willingness to understand and be understood.

9.14 Beyond Human Communication

Humankind has long been intrigued with the idea of contacting and communicating with other intelligences. We've devised elaborate systems to probe outer space for signals that might be coming to us and informational plaques to identify our space probes to other intelligences. As for more earthly concerns, many studies have been made and are being made on communication in species other than humans—particularly the higher forms of life such as apes, elephants, dolphins, and whales—in an effort to crack their codes and establish communication with them. Only rudimentary lines of communication have been established to date, and as far as we know, no signals from outer space have been received. However, in trying to solve these theoretical problems we have learned more about our *own* communication processes and thought mechanisms.

There is the distinct possibility that we would have much to learn from extraterrestrial beings, and much to learn from the species that share this planet with us, if we only knew how to communicate with them. In a remarkable series of studies that spanned a decade, John Lilly, M.D., set out to do just that with dolphins. He chose dolphins primarily because the dolphin brain is similar to the human brain in both size and complexity and he felt they would be the logical first choice for trying to establish interspecies communication.

Dolphins communicate almost solely by sonic transmissions. They use sonic and ultrasonic waves to scan their surroundings and to identify objects by shape and distance, and they seem to be able to transmit information to each other. Lilly attempted to analyze and codify their underwater sounds in search of patterns that might indicate language. In another series of experiments, he studied the ability of dolphins to mimic human sounds (dolphins are able to vocalize out of the water). He thought that if dolphins could learn to communicate in the human mode as we were learning to understand their language, there would be a greater possibility for finding common ground.

I once asked Dr. John Lilly what he thought dolphins did with their large forebrains. "Something else," he replied. I asked if there was any way I could get an inkling of what that "something else" was. He said, "Yes: swim with them." I did. It was "something else."

—Roedy Green

After a lapse of several years, Lilly returned to his research, this time using a computer as a language interface. While he was not successful in establishing true interspecies communication, he worked in the full expectation of eventually doing so, to the mutual benefit of humans and dolphins. Lilly's work invites us to speculate on our own modes of communication. We humans receive at least 80 percent of our input *visually;* then, in order to communicate, we must translate our experience into words, which we then generally convey orally. For dolphins, the major input is *aural,* so they need not translate their experiences from one medium to another in order to communicate. Their communication is more efficient and accurate than ours, and less information is lost in the process. If we could communicate as directly as dolphins do, there would be much less misunderstanding and a greater degree of intimacy than we usually experience in our exchanges with each other. Communications would probably resemble those rare moments of contact we share with someone when minds seem to be joined and words are unnecessary.

Superorganisms

Consider now another level of communication, a level where individual units transcend their separateness and join to form a new unit. This new superorganism then functions with a life of its own. Lewis Thomas, in his *Lives of a Cell,* gives the example of ants as a group of individuals combining to create a larger individual. The colony becomes the new organism, taking a shape to which it is automatically restored if it is disturbed, and having long tentacles that reach out to the surrounding area, gathering food and materials to support it. When fish form schools, they are also so closely integrated they function as a great multifish organism. A certain type of slug is created by the union of separate slime mold cells; to complete its life cycle, the slug produces more slime mold cells that form the next generation.

These examples point to uncommon modes of communication and extraordinary levels of intimacy and cooperation. This level of communication is not yet well understood, even though it can be said to apply to everything from the creation of a single cell to the operation of the entire universe. Complex interactions of many separate organisms made up of cells permit you to function as a human being. The town you live in is a collection of human beings; through organization, the town functions as a unit, too. The chain is endless.

9.15 Communication and the Planet

By expanding our concept of communication, we can see how entire superorganisms can result from intimate contact and cooperation. This then provides a basis for considering that perhaps our entire planet is a single organism.

The hypothesis that the planet is a single organism was first suggested by Johannes Kepler hundreds of years ago. It was more recently expounded by James Lovelock in *The Gaia Hypothesis.* (In Greek mythology, Gaia was the earth goddess.) Observing that the planet, Gaia, has systems that can regulate temperature, oxygen concentration, and other variables, he reasoned that the earth is much more than a hunk of rock with different species of plants and animals living on it; it is a whole system made up of many smaller systems, including humankind.

As with any organism, earth's life depends on the integrated functioning of all her components. There are many signs that all is not well, that the planet is ailing. The recent upsurge of volcanic action, earthquakes, and unusual weather patterns may well be messages from Gaia, calling us to pay attention to her needs. If we continue to ignore her communications, there may be even harsher outbursts as Gaia is forced to take more drastic action to regain balance. Our survival may depend upon our listening to her and responding to her needs.

SUGGESTED READING

Alberti, R., and M. Emmons, *Your Perfect Right* (Impact Publishers, 2001).

Avruch, K., and P. Black, *Conflict Resolution* (Praeger, 1998).

Beattie, M., *Codependent No More* (Hazelden, 1996).

Blanton, B., *Radical Honesty* (DPT, 1996).

Bolton, R., *People Skills* (Touchstone, 1989).

Bradshaw, J., *Healing the Shame That Binds You* (Health Communications, 1988).

Campbell, S., *Getting Real* (HJ Kramer, 2001).

Fanning, P., M. McKay, and M. Davis, *Message: The Communication Skills Book* (New Harbinger Publications, 1995).

Fisher, R., et al., *Getting to Yes: Negotiating Agreement Without Giving In* (Penguin, 1991).

Gordon, T., *Parent Effectiveness Training* (Three Rivers Press, 2000).

Hendricks, G., *Conscious Loving: The Journey to Co-Commitment* (Bantam, 1992).

Hendrix, H., *Getting the Love You Want* (Owl, 2001).

James, M., and D. Jongeward, *Born to Win* (Perseus, 1996).

Lovelock, J., *Gaia: A New Look at Life on Earth* (Oxford University Press, 2000).

McKay, M., et al., *Messages: The Communication Skills Book* (New Harbinger Publications, 1995).

Odent, M., *Primal Health: Understanding the Critical Period between Conception and the First Birthday* (Clairview Books, 2002).

Ornish, D., *Love and Survival: The Scientific Basis for the Healing Power of Intimacy* (Perennial, 1998).

Powell, J., *Why Am I Afraid to Tell You Who I Am?* (Thomas More, 1995).

Prather, H., *Notes to Myself* (Bantam, 1983).

Reusch, J., *Therapeutic Communication* (Guilford Press, 1998).

Rogers, C., *On Becoming a Person* (Mariner, 1995).

Rosenberg, M., *Nonviolent Communication* (PuddleDancer Press, 1999).

Seligman, M., *Authentic Happiness* (Free Press, 2002).

Tannen, D., *You Just Don't Understand: Men and Women in Conversation* (Quill, 2001).

Thomas, L., *The Lives of a Cell* (Penguin, 1997).

For an updated listing of resources and active links to the websites mentioned in this chapter, please see www.WellnessWorkbook.com.

NOTES

1. Odent, M., *Primal Health: Understanding the Critical Period between Conception and the First Birthday* (Clairview Books, 2002). See also www.birthworks.org/primalhealth.

2. Hayakawa, S. I., *Through the Communication Barrier* (Harper and Row, 1979), 73.

3. Rogers, C., "Communication: Its Blocking and Its Facilitation," *ETC.* Vol. 9 (Winter 1952), 84.

4. Tannen, D., *You Just Don't Understand: Men and Women in Conversation* (Quill, 2001).

5. This material is well-summarized in "Working on Common Cross-Cultural Communication Challenges," by Marcelle E. DuPraw, National Institute for Dispute Resolution and Marya Axner, consultant in leadership development and diversity awareness. Their overview is posted at www.wwcd.org/action/ampu/crosscult.html#PATTERNS.

CHAPTER 10

Wellness and Sex

Sex is an expression of the vital life force, the élan vital, or, in Eastern philosophy, ki or chi. It is the energy of our aliveness. Sex is also about the preservation of life—a type of communication in which the entire organism attempts to unify itself with another. It depends dynamically upon the input sources that we get from breathing, sensation, and food/fuel for its complete expression, and it is strongly modified by our energy outputs of thoughts, feelings, and messages. Sex may also serve to open us to new levels of meaning in life as well as provide experiences of transcendence.

Where would we be without sex?

—J. Moose

The so-called sexual revolution that began in the 1960s in the United States has certainly had many positive effects on the social climate of the past forty years. It has paved the way for more frank and open discussion of sex and sexual problems, has made it easier to get needed information on sexual matters, and has fostered a somewhat more tolerant attitude toward behaviors and lifestyle choices that in previous times would have been condemned as unhealthy, deviant, or criminal. To get a picture

of how far we've come in our openness about sex, we have only to compare ourselves to the mores advocated in Victorian England. In that cultural environment, words like *leg* or *trousers* spoken publicly in some company would be considered in bad taste, if not downright offensive. The carved legs of pianos were sometimes covered with specially designed cloths, as the bare leg might be sexually suggestive. If a woman was spending the night in a room in which paintings or pictures of men were displayed, these portraits were removed for the sake of modesty.

Clearly, however, the new openness of our times has not solved all our problems. In many cases it has created new ones, for both young and old. Young men and women (some still boys and girls!) are faced with more opportunities and more peer pressure to engage in sex. The widespread availability of sexually explicit material for entertainment, which the Internet, television, and magazines offer, has become a source of concern for parents and a source of difficult personal decisions for lots of us.

Sex still has the aura of being "dirty" or "forbidden" in its presentation today, despite the so-called freedom that we have achieved about sex. Evidently, we still have a lot to learn.

10.1 The Need for Education and Awareness

How would you rate the sex education you received? The role modeling you had for an integrated view of sex? Your level of comfort in speaking about sex? Your degree of self-awareness about your own body?

Young people today enter their adolescence in a world that is plagued with epidemics of sexually transmitted diseases, some of which are literally threatening the survival of certain nations, certain races of people. One in four new infections of HIV in the United States today occurs in people below the age of twenty-two, and HIV infection is increasing more rapidly among this age group than in any other. Kids are experimenting with sex much earlier, and often with multiple partners. By the time they reach age twenty, almost 77 percent of women and 86 percent of men have had sex. Because part of being a teenager is taking risks, many act as if they are invincible—testing limits and questioning authority. The need for preparation for and education about sex and its profound responsibilities is still bypassed by many parents, who assume that their kids "know more than we do" because they are exposed to more. Many are afraid to speak about sex simply and clearly. Sex education is generally left up to school systems. But many schools lack properly educated personnel. Some refuse to mention homosexuality. Others fail to offer specific instruction in the use of condoms. In many schools, these factors add up to making sex education classes a joke for the adolescents in attendance.

Another painful but necessary side of increased openness about sex is that we are hearing about the abuses that used to go undisclosed and undiscussed. We are discovering how common sexual abuse has been and still is! Parents, teachers, priests, psychotherapists, gurus—taking advantage of their power over a child's or a client's life—have misused their positions of authority to gain personal sexual favors. We have learned that others, while not the sexual perpetrators, have been enablers. They stood by or denied the obvious signs that something was amiss. It is no wonder that many today despair at the state of the world, the state of the family, the state of the church. Without consciously facing the truth of *what is,* we will unconsciously repeat it, or encourage its repetition.

Abuses and epidemics aside, a quick glance at the newspaper, an overheard conversation, discussions with friends, perhaps an examination of your own thoughts, will reveal that problems, misconceptions, and fears about sex still abound. Here are a few typical statements:

- *"Before we got married we did it all the time. Now my partner just doesn't seem to have any interest in sex. What's wrong?"*

- *"I must be abnormal. I've never had an orgasm at the same time as my partner."*

- *"If only I _____, then I could please my partner sexually."*

- *"He says he really loves me. So why do I feel like a sex object?"*

The basic problem remains: rather than living sex as a total body-mind experience, we have learned to block off sexual energy or to confine it to our genital organs. It is here that we get "turned on" and here that we hold our guilt, our confusion, our fear. As noted in module 3.14, the needs for caring, and tenderness, and total body involvement are unmet when the focus of sex becomes intercourse alone. The result is disappointment, frustration, and damage to your self-concept.

Despite their education or their best intentions, many still consider sex dirty, part of the "lower" nature, something to be feared, earned, or supplied dutifully; they still consider the body secondary to the mind, a thing you attend to when necessary and keep carefully covered up. Few of us have escaped contamination from the fear, embarrassment, confusion, and anger that surrounded sex in the thoughts and words and behaviors of our parents, teachers, ministers, and friends. The relationship of sex with all of life is hard to discover when it isn't talked about in a balanced, commonsense, and respectful way in school, church, or polite company.

The result of all this confusion is the contamination or blockage of our sexual energy, leading to a range of problems that include the following.

- *Impotence or frigidity*

- *Compulsiveness or sexual addiction*

- *Dysfunctional relationships*

- *Sexual abuse, including rape*

- *Diseases, especially of the reproductive organs*

- *Physical, emotional, and spiritual pain*

Most of us need help—as couples or single people—to accept ourselves as sexual beings, to accept sex as a normal part of life, and to use our sexual expression in ways that enhance life, rather than promote disease, unhappiness, fear, and death.

10.2 Challenge the Myths

As a culture we are preoccupied with sex. Sex sells! Check the latest offerings on the local magazine rack, take a critical look at advertisements, examine the contents of the average TV serial—they all underline the preoccupation with sex. This exaggerated importance assigned to sex has led us in search of the multiple orgasm, the simultaneous orgasm, the twenty-minute orgasm, and the G-spot to prove our potency. It has contributed to the pressures and tensions that many experience in connection with sex. It has led us to develop unrealistic expectations of how great sex is supposed to be, how it will solve all our problems, and how there is one perfect person out there for each of us, a soul mate, waiting to be found. When sex is defined in terms of flawless physical bodies and perfectly compatible relationships, in terms of power and prestige and ecstasy, we are bound to feel inadequate when our own experiences fall short.

In her insightful book, *The New Celibacy*, author Gabrielle Brown asserts, unapologetically:

. . . we've been taught that sex is the road to personal fulfillment. This is one of the most destructive myths about sex. . . . No matter how great an orgasm one has or how great an orgasm one's partner has, sex does not bring fulfillment. And if something more deep and permanent is desired in the expression of love and one does not even experience it, one may feel unfulfilled, even saddened by the sexual act. . . . Many people, believing that sex is the only way to become fulfilled, spend years searching for lasting happiness in sexual encounters. Such is the loneliness of the sexual seeker who continues to search for personal liberation in a series of static encounters. In this fixed pattern of behavior, there is always a feeling of futility, of going nowhere. . . .

10.3 Well-Sex

Having taken this look at some of the challenges and difficult issues involved in sexuality today, let's now consider what the Wellness Energy System has to offer. For those who are sexually troubled, this approach offers some suggestions for dealing with the problems, as well as encouragement for seeking assistance from reputable counselors or therapists. For those who want to enhance the role that sex plays in their lives, this approach supplies some guidelines. In both cases, the key word is *integration*.

Well-sex is the term we've chosen to describe what we think is an integrated approach to sexuality—one that considers the needs of the body, mind, and spirit of yourself and your partner(s). The term *healthy sexuality* or *sexual health* has been used by others for a somewhat similar orientation. Yet, because the word *health* (and, to a lesser extent, *well*) may imply that there is one, natural, good, wholesome sexuality that is medically approved, we urge you to approach all such terms with caution. These designations can be misused to convey disapproval of specific behaviors. Any researchers or authors (including us), as human beings and products of their cultural upbringing and their personal beliefs, are bound to have their own social norms and ideas about sex. These will be reflected in their treatment of the subject, despite their best attempts to remain objective.

Sexual ideas and norms, like health norms, emerge from many sources, including customs, science, medicine, spirituality, and experience. We assume that no single definition of sexual health or wellness will satisfy everyone or represent the diversity of sexual behaviors and attitudes in this culture today, no less in others around the world.

If you want an example of integrated sexuality as we apply the term here, just look at a baby. The infant's body is fully alive; every cell is dancing. If we could capture this energy in motion on film, we would see rivers of energy sparkling all over and swirling all around. The body would appear as a sea of light. The child responds with pleasure to the stroking of its fingers and toes. Here is a clear, unblocked channel. Sexual energy flows throughout every part, head to toe.

Well-sex also depends upon the integrated flow of all the energies discussed in the preceding chapters. For adults, sex is a complex activity involving much more than the genital organs and the physical act of intercourse; it is bound up with feelings and emotions; it involves free use of all the senses; it may be a form of play or recreation. And, importantly, it is influenced by your thinking, as well as by your ability to communicate with yourself and with your partner.

In sexual exchange, we experience the dynamic presence of another human being. At least temporarily we are assuaged of our isolation; we are touched, sometimes held securely; we are excited; we feel energy moving more powerfully; sometimes we feel unified; sometimes we sense that we have transcended our usual limitations and self-definitions. Consequently, we look to sex for affection, or attention, or confirmation of aliveness, and, often, for integration. On one hand, lovemaking in general, and the moments of orgasm in particular, can allow us a temporary respite from the judging, anticipating, and questioning of our rational minds; such moments seem to transport us into another realm. On the other hand, sex can also provide us with a powerful experience of *nowness*—a full-bodied awareness of all that is happening at the moment, rather than any type of departure.

Catherine Chilman, in *Adolescent Sexuality in a Changing American Society*, provides a highly balanced and expansive view of the subject. We think that the components of her definition of sexual health for adolescents, presented below, apply to adults of all ages. We consider them expressions of "well-sex" (although we would substitute *we/our* for *they/their,* add *and others* to *parents,* and include adults).

Adolescent sexual health:

- Involves "increasing ability to communicate honestly and openly with persons of both sexes with whom they have a close relationship."

- Includes "acceptance of their own sexual desires as natural but to be acted upon with limited freedom within the constraints of reality considerations, including their own values and goals and those of 'significant others' in their lives."

- Is characterized by the ability "to form interdependent, rather than dependent or defensively autonomous relationships."

- Develops increasing freedom from "anxieties over their own self-worth and competencies as feminine or masculine persons; they learn to behave and feel in such a way as to experience relatively minor guilt over their own sexuality and that of others."

- Involves growth "towards more egalitarian, less dependent relationships with their parents and a sense of their own gender and sex identity, their own set of values that may be, but are not necessarily, different from those of their parents."

- Involves an understanding "that their sexuality is not a thing apart, but an integral aspect of their total lives . . . thus specific sex behaviors take place within the total context of their life situation and goals."

- Includes, as they mature, the development of rewarding mate relationships and use of either abstention or contraceptive techniques to achieve planned timing and numbers of children . . .

- Does not include the concept that healthy adolescent sexuality involves complete freedom to behave as one wishes so long as contraceptives, including condoms, are used and so long as this behavior is in private with consenting partners, because the "recreational" view of sex "tends to trivialize the depth of the exceptional intimacy and potential involvement of the total self through intercourse."

- Incorporates in the definition "the development of both heterosexually and homosexually oriented adolescents."

10.4 Energy Awareness and Sex

Self-awareness includes physical, mental, and emotional awareness. In the physical domain, awareness is primary in learning to trust and appreciate our body. In sexuality, body trust is something that we grow into by experience. We learn to attend to where, how, when, and with what intensity the energy is moving within us. We listen to the cues the body gives about what it likes and needs to be "turned on" sensually and erotically. We stay present, alert, to ourselves. The primary question becomes, "What is going on in my body now . . . and now . . . and now?"

As a child you easily played with your body; you probably enjoyed the freedom of nakedness and delighted in being held against the bodies of others, stroked, and tickled. There was no shame or fear attached to any of these activities until other people who felt uncomfortable with what you were doing began to give you messages to the contrary. As the sole inhabitant of your body, you knew what felt good to you, and you did it. But at some point you probably gave up on yourself, and began to believe that what was natural and normal for you was not acceptable.

Reclaiming this freedom—the goodness of your body—is the first step in body trust, and the basis for the living of wellness.

To say yes to the body is to say yes to all that moves through you, both pain and pleasure—and sex can be one of the most pleasant experiences you can have. Pleasure can be appreciated as your reward, not for *doing* something, but simply for being alive. The fact that you inhabit a body that is soft, and pliable, and covered with sensitive nerve endings, and requires touch for survival, presents a strong case for allowing yourself to accept pleasure, for celebrating the magnificent creation that your body is.

Self-touch, or self-massage, can be an invaluable aid in learning about the unique sensitivities of your body. Often a concentration on genital involvement leaves vast areas of pleasure and arousal unexplored. Many approaches to sexual therapy include a recommendation that individuals and couples deliberately avoid stimulating the genitals for a period of time in order that the sensations in other body parts can be appreciated.[1] All the fuss and furor, and guilt, and secretiveness about masturbation testify to a fear of the body in general, and of pleasure in particular. For many, the guilt learned in childhood endures. Kids—both boys and girls—generally play with their own genitals because it feels good! Yet, because parents are embarrassed by these behaviors, they often stop the child's touching with slaps, harsh words, and demeaning looks. While our culture encourages pleasure seeking in some domains, and advertises it everywhere, self-initiated pleasure in sex is still considered suspect or somehow inferior. Perhaps it has to do with a work ethic that attaches a price to pleasure, or that presents it as a reward for service. Some of us actually harbor guilt in experiencing joy and other good feelings.[2]

Another side of this self-awareness issue is that many people find that sexual activity in general and physical orgasm and ejaculation in particular, while serving as a type of stress release, can be de-energizing, resulting in an overall energy loss. For this reason, and for many specific purposes, some (actors, musicians, many athletes, and other performers) will refrain from sex before their performance event. Others, like artists and writers, find that temporary sexual abstinence builds energy in such a way that it can be rechanneled into other creative expressions. Celibates in religious community speak of "sublimation" of sexual energy, which means that this powerful life force is not physically expressed but used to expand the heart, turning the person more dynamically toward the very source of love. And, from the East (particularly China and India) we learn about sexual energy management (particularly the conservation of ejaculation) that is claimed to enhance health and longevity.[3]

The idea here is that you learn about *your* energy and become an explorer in the domain of sexual energy and its effects in *your* body.

10.5 Your Mind in Sex

The next step in awareness is to recognize what is going on in your mind. It is commonly noted that the brain is the most potent sexual organ you have, and it can turn you off as easily as it can turn you on. Listen as you "talk" to yourself before, during, and after sex, and you will gain important insights about how your thoughts are creating your reality:

- *Since your thoughts assign meaning to sex, your body will follow suit.*

- *Preoccupations with performance and expectations take you out of the here and now and build tensions.*

- *Your fears can freeze you.*

- *Your guilt and anxiety can stifle your pleasure.*

- *Your judgments can easily lead to dissatisfaction.*

You can use your brain in the service of sex, as you have in other areas of wellness. As you become aware of the "voices" (your own or others) that fill your head, they can serve as cues to come back to the here and now, to focus on the part of the body being touched, to breathe deeply and allow sexual feelings to carry through your whole body, to open all your sensory pathways to increase your pleasure many times over.

For many people, reading erotic literature or watching sexually explicit films can be extremely provocative and helpful in breaking through fear or shame. (For others, these activities may have the opposite effect. Personal preference is always the foremost consideration.) Sexual fantasies, once a taboo subject, now are often recommended for the powerful effects they can have on the body. Allowing yourself to experiment in these areas may be as beneficial as allowing your own touch.

Throughout the process of developing or enhancing awareness in body and mind, remember to appreciate your limits and your degree of comfort, and to be compassionate. Take small, slow steps and celebrate each new awakening.

The scope of this book does not allow more than a brief presentation of possibilities for your consideration. Programs abound that deal specifically with restructuring sexual attitudes, heightening awareness and sensitivity, and coping with sexual blocks or physical problems. If sex is a conflict area for you, you can take the next step by reading some of the resources listed in this chapter, and seeking the support of others in the available programs.[4] Self-responsibility means never staying stuck.

DON'T FORGET TO KEGEL

In the 1940s, Dr. Arnold Kegel, a gynecologist, first introduced a simple exercise (now commonly known as "Kegels") for the P.C. (pubococcygeus) muscles. The exercise was originally used to assist women in regaining bladder control after childbirth.

The P.C. muscles are the support muscle for the genitals in women. Over the years, Kegels have been of great benefit to those with continence difficulties, and as a means, for men, of naturally massaging the prostate gland. For sex, Kegel exercises are invaluable in increasing your awareness of feelings in the genital area, increasing blood flow to the genitals, and thereby helping you to increase your sexual responsiveness. Doing Kegels regularly helps you to gain control over these muscles and thereby helps you gain control over your orgasm.

For a moment, tighten or clench the muscles that you would use to stop the flow of urine when urinating, the same muscle you would use to force out the last drop of urine from your bladder. You are now using the P.C. Each time you tighten and then release that muscle you are doing a Kegel exercise.

Make Kegels a part of your daily routine for health and pleasure. To begin:

1. Tighten and relax the P.C. muscle repeatedly (about ten times in succession), but slowly, holding the tension for three to five seconds each time, then releasing it.

2. Do the above sequence five times a day.

3. Gradually work toward doing the exercises thirty times in succession, holding for three to five seconds each time. Repeat this three times a day.

Depending upon how often you practice, it may take four to six weeks to get your P.C. muscle in good shape.

You don't have to retire to the bedroom or to the gym to do your Kegels. They can be done as you talk on the telephone, listen to a boring lecture, wait in line at the grocery store, or brush your teeth. If you associate doing these exercises with another activity you do daily, you will help yourself to remember them. Some current exercise methods, like Pilates, also encourage Kegel-type awareness and practice. Building strength in the genital area is part of building strength in your body's core. So, don't forget to Kegel daily!

10.6 Awareness of Your Partner

The focus on self-awareness is never meant to undermine awareness of one's partner in sex. Ideally, as we grow in appreciation of our own body's responses and expressions, we become more sensitive to the responses and expressions of our partner. It is not a question of competition for getting needs met, but a recognition that energy flows, and is shared, *between* us, as well as within each of us. The question becomes, How can you capitalize upon the energetic exchange in ways that are enjoyable and satisfying for both your partner and yourself?

How many of us have taken the time to really get to know our partner's body—like which areas are particularly sensitive besides the sexual organs? How many of us can immediately detect a change in our partner's breathing pattern or skin tone indicating a change in the energy flow? How many of us are willing to indefinitely delay our own sexual release or gratification in order to remain focused on our partner's pleasure? Can we stay present to the person we are with rather than putting some fantasy lover in his or her place?

The subjects of timing and degree of desire are big issues in sex for couples. One partner generally wants sex more regularly than the other (high-libido versus low-libido types). One partner requires more time to be turned on. One partner wants more relaxed post-sex time. These are not easy issues to resolve. It is important to recognize that differing desire quotients are normal and natural, because it is easy to think that there is something wrong with the relationship if and when our libido varies from that of our partner. According to Michelle Davis, author of *The Divorce Remedy*, "Unsatisfying sexual relationships are the all-too-frequent causes of alienation, infidelity, and divorce."

Approaching the issue as if "we have a problem" is not the most ideal method. Talking about "what's wrong with our sex life," or nagging that "I want this and you won't give it to me" can create an endless cycle of conversation that goes nowhere, or recrimination that ends in disappointment and separation. Where sex is concerned, acting differently is generally much more effective than problem solving. To speak simply about what can be a somewhat complex issue, the high-desire types can learn to be more sensitive to "courting" or nurturing behaviors, while the low-desire types can learn to "just start" even when they don't initially feel like it. In either case, each partner needs to be willing to act differently without bearing a grudge if the other doesn't change immediately. Patience is always called for, as are respect, kindness, and remembrance of the love that brought the couple together in the first place. When each partner places attention on the awareness and appreciation of the other, it is much more likely that difficulties can be successfully addressed.

10.7 Self-Responsible Sex

Self-responsible sex means accepting that, in most ways, you are the expert about yourself. Just as you may be tempted to give up personal power and deny your own experience in other areas of your life, when it comes to sex it is easy to become confused, if not persuaded, by the opinions of others—your friends, your role models, the media, the poll-takers. On the other hand, part of self-responsibility means recognition of limitations; recognition that we are often blind to our own tendencies and inclinations. It includes taking the initiative in reaching out for help in areas that are problematic and painful. Self-responsibility never means that we deny ourselves support or insight or direct guidance from those we determine are trustworthy.

In observing self-responsibility in sex, you need to examine who and what you are listening to, and question who or what you are believing. Our youth-oriented culture is obsessed with appearances. In so doing, it often dismisses the needs of the elderly and the mentally and physically handicapped, for whom sex is a right or a privilege as much as it is for the young and beautiful. Because the media use sex to sell everything from toothpaste to tractors, they constantly present a distorted view of the subject. Popular magazines inform you of the statistics regarding sexual orientation and frequency of expression; they may lead you to believe that you are abnormal if you fall outside the norm. The fact that, as some of these surveys report, married couples in the United States average X acts of intercourse per month merely indicates that some do it several times a day and others only on their anniversaries. Statistics can be very misleading, even when you approach them with an understanding of how they are gathered.

The research of Kinsey, Masters and Johnson, Hite, and others serves to underline the need to trust your own experience.[5] Their findings demonstrate that individual differences in sexual practice are truly amazing. In fact, there seems to be a wider range of human sexual appetite, capacity, and behavior than of almost any other human trait. Sexual practice often varies as widely as the number of subjects questioned.

Sex is self-responsible when it is informed, consensual, conscientious, and mutually enjoyed. Consensual means that it is freely entered into, not coerced or manipulated; conscientious means that it is not used to prove power, or get favors, or keep the other from leaving. Nonconsensual sex is abuse. It is against the law and against the integrity of the body and mind of the other. Nonconscientious sex often results from childhood associations of sexuality being linked with shame, guilt, pain, or violence.

Finally, sex is self-responsible when the rest of life is self-responsible. What we eat or drink, how we breathe, the exercise we take, the thoughts we program, our sense of spiritual alignment with the source of life—all will affect our ability for and enjoyment of sex. One friend reports that his jogging program did wonders for his sex life. The increased flexibility, improved muscle tone, and controlled use of the breath that come with exercise can certainly enhance sexual vigor. The improved self-concept that exercise encourages is a strong foundation for a healthy sex concept—and vice versa. When people feel good about their sexuality and the expression of it, they are more inclined to want to care for their bodies, and maybe even for their minds and hearts, too.

10.8 Sexual Orientation and Gender Identity

Any claim that leads you to question whether you are "normal" should be held highly suspect and can easily be checked out with a little research or inquiry. Virginia admits that she feels inadequate because she does not have the same desires for sex that her friend Claudia has. What she may not realize is that, in addition to psychological reasons, gender orientation reasons, factors connected with beliefs and ethics, or the nature of her current relationship, there may also be hormonal reasons for her lack of sexual interest. The place to start in such a process is to clearly face the "what is" about our own needs, sensations, feelings, without judging them as bad, wrong, or inadequate.

Virginia is asking the wrong question when she asks "What's wrong with me?" There will never be an answer unless she first addresses the real issue that underlies the question. The real issue is: "Why inadequate? Why guilt for feeling how I feel?"

When I stand up and say that I want to oppose discrimination against people because of their sexual orientation, it is not because I want to seem nice. It is because if I don't, everything I have done in my life will be in vain.

—Anglican Archbishop Desmond Tutu

DEFINITIONS OF SEXUAL ORIENTATION AND GENDER IDENTITY

Sexual Orientation

Sexual orientation refers to one's sexual and romantic attraction. Those whose sexual orientation is to people of the opposite sex are called *heterosexual*; those whose sexual orientation is to people of the same sex are called *homosexual* (or lesbian or gay); and those whose sexual orientation is to people of both sexes are called *bisexual*. The term *sexual preference* is misleading because it implies that this attraction is a choice rather than an intrinsic personal characteristic. Sexual orientation is not necessarily the same as sexual behavior.

Gender Identity

At birth, we are assigned one of two gender identities, usually based on our visible genitals. For many people this gender assignment fits and feels comfortable and they never think about it further. Others do not feel as comfortable with their assigned gender, either because they find the two-gender system too limiting or because they feel more identification with the gender opposite to the one assigned to them at birth. People deal with this discomfort in many ways: sometimes only in personal ways; sometimes in ways visible to others.

Lesbian

A lesbian is a woman whose primary sexual and romantic attractions are to other women. She may have sex with women currently or may have had sex with women in the past. A smaller number of lesbians may never have had sex with another woman for a whole host of reasons (age, societal pressures, lack of opportunity, fear of discrimination), but nonetheless realize that their sexual attraction is mainly to other women. Some lesbians have sex with men and some don't. It is important to note that some women who have sex with other women, sometimes exclusively, may not call themselves lesbians.

Gay

A gay man is a man whose primary sexual and romantic attraction is to other men. He may have sex with men currently or may have had sex with men in the past. A smaller number of gay men may never have had

(continued)

sex with another man for a whole host of reasons (age, societal pressures, lack of opportunity, fear of discrimination), but nonetheless realize that their sexual attraction is mainly to other men. Some gay men have sex with women and some don't. It is important to note that some men who have sex with other men, sometimes exclusively, may not call themselves gay.

Gay is also used as an inclusive term encompassing gay men, lesbians, bisexual people, and sometimes even transgender people. In the last twenty years, this has become less and less common and *gay* is usually used currently to refer only to gay men. The term is still often used in the broader sense in spoken shorthand, as in "The Gay Pride Parade is at the end of June."

Bisexual

Bisexual men and women have sexual and romantic attractions to both men and women. Depending upon the person, his or her attraction may be stronger to women or to men, or they may be approximately equal. A bisexual person may have had sex with people of both sexes, or only of one sex, or he or she may never have had sex at all. It is important to note that some people who have sex with both men and women do not consider themselves bisexual. Bisexuals are also referred to as *bi*.

Heterosexual

A heterosexual man or woman's primary sexual and romantic attraction is to people of the other sex. She or he may or may not have had sex with another person, but still realizes that his or her sexual attraction is mainly to people of the other sex. Some people who consider themselves heterosexual have or have had sexual contact with people of the same sex. Heterosexual people are also referred to as *straight*.

Transgender

People who identify more strongly with the other gender than the one to which they were assigned (for example, women who feel like men, or men who feel like women) are called *transgendered*. Some transgendered people may cross-dress or "do drag" regularly or for fun (and many of these people are comfortable in their assigned gender). Other transgendered people may take hormones of the opposite gender and/or have surgery in order to change their bodies to reflect how they feel inside. These people are also called *transsexual*. Transgendered people may identify as heterosexual, homosexual, or bisexual.

Female-to-male transsexuals are sometimes referred to as *FTMs* or *transsexual men,* and male-to-female transsexuals as *MTFs* or *transsexual women*. Pre-operative (*pre-op*) transsexuals are preparing for sexual reassignment surgery (SRS) and may take hormones. Post-operative (*post-op*) transsexuals have undergone SRS and continue to take hormones, often for the rest of their lives. Some transsexuals (*non-op*) either do not want or cannot afford SRS, though they may still take hormones.

King County (Seattle, Washington) Public Health Department, "Gay, Lesbian, Bisexual, and Transgender Health," www.metrokc.gov/health/glbt/transgender.htm.

10.9 Birth Control

The "informed" part of self-responsible sex includes adequate preparation and protection for disease prevention and birth control. Amazingly, despite education in other domains, many intelligent adults are ill-informed or simply careless about sex. They use no birth control. The responsibility cannot be laid at the feet of either partner—("She's a responsible woman; she must have taken precautions")—but requires the conscientiousness of both or all concerned.[6] The epidemic proportions of venereal disease reflect this same carelessness. With the spread of the AIDS virus, misinformation about how it can be contracted has also spread—along with massive denial about who might have it. Thinking that AIDS is solely confined to the homosexual male population is one of the gravest misunderstandings around. Since 2003, in certain parts of the world the number of women infected with the virus has outnumbered the number of men infected. AIDS affects everyone.

While we may speak frankly about sex in general, there is still an unromantic aura attached to straight talk about preferred methods of birth control, and the health aspects of intercourse. Far from diminishing the excitement of sex, this kind of communication can actually serve to bring the partners closer together, increasing mutual respect and engendering a deeper tenderness.

10.10 Guidelines for Safer Sex

The purpose of "safe sex" guidelines is protection against sexually transmitted diseases (STDs), including HIV/AIDS, herpes, gonorrhea, genital warts, and chlamydia. Except for complete abstinence, no disease-protection method is completely safe as long as any bodily fluids are exchanged. Disease is transmitted through such fluids as saliva, blood, mucus, semen, vaginal fluid, even urine. Basically, the infected fluids have to penetrate the body in some way, and that usually happens through tiny skin wounds or abrasions (not necessarily visible) in the soft tissue (mucous membranes) of the mouth, vagina, tip of the penis, or rectum, or even in mucous membranes of the nose.

The possibility of disease has always been a factor in sex. But, because of changing values and practices—particularly, the number of sex partners engaged with—the likelihood of infection has increased enormously throughout the sexually active population. Many STDs are treated successfully with a variety of pharmaceutical drugs, but with HIV/AIDS the situation becomes much more serious. The introduction of lifesaving drug combinations known as highly active antiretroviral therapy (HAART) in 1997 means that AIDS is no longer an automatic death sentence. The treatments, when administered properly, may cut the death rate by as much as 80 percent. However, in poorer populations, these costly and often complicated treatments are not always accessible, and growing numbers of infected people worldwide are proving resistant to the drugs.

Communication, common sense, and courage are needed for wise sex/well-sex/safe sex—whatever we call it. When alcohol and drug use enter the picture, as is frequently the case in "party" situations when everybody is "feeling good," or in the down times when we are most hurting, depressed, vulnerable, and needing "a friend," our sense of judgment can be impaired and our desire for contact, fun, or affection may override our usual cautions and precautions.

The following guidelines, published by the University of Maryland Medicine Department (2003) for their student population, are fairly standard in their recommendations for safer sex. We offer them here in an effort to increase awareness for adults and younger people as well:

- *If you limit sexual activity to only one partner, who is having sex only with you, you greatly reduce exposure to disease-causing organisms.*

- *Think twice before beginning sexual relations with a new partner. First discuss past partners, history of STDs, and drug use.*

- *Use condoms: a male condom made of latex or polyurethane—not natural materials; a female condom made of polyurethane—particularly if your partner will not use a male condom.*

- *In addition to a condom, always use a spermicide to provide additional protection against sexually transmitted diseases (STDs).*

- *Women should not douche after intercourse— it does not protect against STDs; could spread an infection farther into the reproductive tract; and can wash away spermicidal protection.*

- *Women should have annual Pap tests and pelvic examinations.*

- *Men and women should have periodic tests for STDs.*

- *Be aware of your partner's body—look for signs of a sore, blister, rash, or discharge.*

- *Check your body frequently for signs of a sore, blister, rash, or discharge.*

- *Consider sexual activities other than vaginal, oral, or anal intercourse—techniques that do not involve the exchange of body fluids or contact between mucous membranes, such as those in the vagina, anus, and mouth.*

At the heart of and beyond all safe-sex methods will ever remain self-awareness, conscientiousness, and genuine caring for oneself and others.

10.11 Saying Yes and Saying No

Responsible, consensual sex means allowing yourself permission to say yes to what you want, and no to what you don't.

Yes implies that you have a sense of safety about the encounter; a sense that your needs, wishes, and limits will be respected enough that you can essentially relax and move with the energy that is generated between you and your partner. *Yes* may also mean that you know your own body well enough to be able to kindly or generously guide or help your partner in pleasuring you in a way that works well for you. While it is generally more advantageous to encourage a mood of intimacy rather than turning your sex play into an anatomy lesson, do not assume that the other can read your mind or your body. Placing sole responsibility for your sexual gratification on your partner is one sure way of leaving the encounter dissatisfied. Learning what feels good,

what works for you, may mean practice and experimentation on your own. Self-massage and masturbation skills are being taught by many sex educators and therapists today to help both men and women rediscover their sensuality and unlock pleasure centers throughout the body.

No means allowing yourself to set limits; to say no to any techniques; or to the whole process if you no longer enjoy it or feel good about it. Many times your discomfort is a shared one, and your courage in calling a halt to the proceedings may be a great gift to your partner as well. When people care about each other, they respect each other's limits. Otherwise the encounter can quickly become tense, superficial, or phony. Anger and resentment build when you feel taken advantage of. Intimacy and trust flourish when you accept the other as unique and special. If you find yourself questioning "Will

---

HIV/AIDS PANDEMIC

Of the 42 million adults and children living with HIV/AIDS worldwide, an estimated 30 million, or 70 percent, live in sub-Saharan Africa. In 2003, 58 percent of those infected in the region were women.

The United Nations Security Council has declared that, if unchecked, HIV/AIDS is likely to pose a major threat to economic, social, and political stability as well as human security. It is estimated that there are 15,000 new infections every day, 95 percent in developing countries. An estimated 11.3 percent of infections are occurring in children below fifteen years of age, and 86.6 percent in people in the reproductive age group (fifteen to forty-nine years). Since the beginning of the pandemic, an estimated 21.8 million have died of AIDS, and the disease is now the fourth leading cause of death in the world and the number one cause of mortality in Africa, exceeding the number killed in armed conflict. Over 13.2 million children have been orphaned as a result of AIDS; over 12 million of these are in Africa.

The major mode of transmission is heterosexual transmission (70 percent) and, in some parts of Asia, intravenous drug use. It takes a long time to develop full-blown AIDS; thus many people do not even know they are carrying the virus and so continue to infect their partners.

Sharifah H. Shahabudin, "Gender and HIV/AIDS—The Human Rights and Security Perspectives," UNAIDS and Women Watch, www.un.org/women watch/daw/csw/Shahabudin2001.htm.

this person respect me in the morning?" realize that you are really asking: "Will I be able to accept myself?" Your ability to integrate and to feel OK about your sexual interaction should be your guiding principle.

Many of us learned as children that it was not OK to say no to touch. Remember all those hugs and kisses from aunts, uncles, or grandparents who hugged too tight, or smelled funny, or pinched your cheeks too hard?

In order to learn that they have sovereignty over their bodies, and to learn how to say no when appropriate, children must be allowed to accept and refuse touch, even from relatives. It's hard on a parent if a son or daughter doesn't want to kiss Grandma, but it's more important that children know that we respect their feelings and the fact that they have the right to say no.

Today, sexual abuse is a major problem in North America. It results in demoralization, depression, repression, loss of belief in the ability to protect oneself, and fear of people. The most common age at which sexual abuse begins is three. Heterosexual males commit the vast majority of sexual abuse. Nearly 90 percent of sexual abuse is committed by someone the child knows, not by a stranger.

Many boys grow up thinking that ignoring no—especially from a female—is an expression of their strength and manliness. Many girls and young women were taught to be nice, rather than honest, toward males—which essentially leads them to decide that it's better to be hurt by a male than be perceived of as unfeminine by the male who seeks to take advantage of you.

Many women are reluctant to appear rude because they fear they'll cause someone to be angry. In the context of being approached by a stranger in a public situation, the anger you may cause will rarely be a step toward violence. Indeed, if you are perceived as a rude woman, you are a far less attractive target than a polite woman.

Maintaining sovereignty over our bodies requires that we be wary of anyone, male or female, especially a stranger, who ignores the word no. If we are to maintain the integrity of our body and soul, we need to care less about protocol and politeness, and to practice until we are comfortable saying and doing what needs to be said and done.[7]

Understand that when a man in our culture says no it's usually the end of a discussion, but when a woman says no it's the beginning of a negotiation.

—Gavin de Becker

If young men learn how to hear no, and young women learn that it's all right to explicitly reject, then acts of violence to the integrity and sovereignty of the body will dramatically decline and our sexual wellness will be enhanced.

10.12 Sex as Wholeness

In sexual intercourse we have a brilliant symbol for what we all seek—integration, union, communion. We seek this with others; we also look for it in ourselves.

Whether we are men or women anatomically, each individual is composed of both "male" and "female" energy.[8] Typically, we associate the outgoing, thrusting, rationally involved aspects of our nature with "maleness" (the *yang* in Chinese cosmology) and the inward-looking, nurturing, intuitive elements with "femaleness" (the *yin* force). A whole, balanced person is one who has incorporated the two into one harmonious dance, to whatever degree they naturally exist within us. If there is a definition of healthy sexuality, this is it. The integrated being channels all of life energy.

From this place of wholeness, of personal integrity, one approaches another person out of a desire for *sharing* energy, rather than a need for *taking* what is lacking in oneself. So, if there is any magical formula to be used, or first step to be taken in establishing satisfying relationships with others, it is the realization that you already have within yourself everything that you need for your happiness.

Anita is just such an integrated being. She is a strong and gentle woman. Her power sparkles in her sensitivity. She is happy in living and working alone for weeks, even months at a time. She is happy in living and working with family and friends. She cries as easily as she laughs. She writes poetry with one hand, and a research paper with the other. Her sexuality exudes from every pore and is contagious. She can be celibate for six months of the year without pain. She can make love every night of the week with pleasure. She is a living example of the union of sexuality and wellness.

SHIVA AND SHAKTI

In the essential male-female dichotomy [within the Hindu cosmology], Shiva is pure knowledge, that is, Context. Shakti is content—manifestation, form, and energy. Shiva is unmanifested allness, and Shakti is everything else—everything sensual, alive, moving, created. A weak feminine, therefore, can be related to . . . difficulty acting, doing, or manifesting. Shiva is the strong silent type, not the warrior. Diana, Athena, or Shakti is the warrior. You strengthen the feminine, therefore, by acting. . . . Masculine energy doesn't speak. It *is*. Feminine energy acts: it speaks; it is alive, aggressive, and powerful. Masculine energy just radiates based on wisdom, not based on accomplishment or beauty. The way you strengthen a weak masculine is by resting in pure knowledge—by coming to know, to discover, wisdom. If you are insecure, if you think you don't know anything, the way to strengthen a weak masculine is to find that place in yourself that does know and acknowledge it, embrace it . . . To strengthen the feminine is to use your energy in an optimally productive fashion, not squander it and reinforce the weaknesses. . . . A very practical way to strengthen the feminine through optimal activity is to never leave a project unfinished; another way is through conservation of energy in the use of speech.

Lee Lozowick, *The Alchemy of Love* (Hohm Press, 1996).

10.13 Sex and Love

For too long we have relegated love to a commodity to be earned or won; something that must be held tight. We have guarded it, guessing that there was just so much of it to go around. We have assumed that in loving you, I therefore diminish the quantity of love I have to give others. If any notion needs liberation, this one does.

The great lovers, the great humanitarians of the world, loved and were loved by hundreds of people. They flourished with it. They were all the more energized for it. They tasted the reality that love is the energy of life, the breath of God, the ground of being. They realized that everything they did, every decision they made, either enhanced their capacity to experience love, or diminished it.

The old problem of "charity begins at home" and the idea that "I can't love you until I can love myself" were never considerations for them. They often spent long periods of time, sometimes years, in contemplation. But their looking within brought them in touch with the place where everything was connected. They found no difference between themselves and us. In loving us, they loved themselves. In loving themselves, they loved us.

**Love is not something we find.
Love is something we build.**

—Bhai Sahib

So if love is as natural as breathing, and eating, and working, and playing, it is also as natural as "sexing." If love becomes our "life-support system," then every decision we make, sex included, will be guided by it. We will choose to have sex with one another if it enhances our experience of unification with all that is. We will love each other anyway, whether we have sex or not. We will celebrate the abundance of love that is always available to us if we keep ourselves open channels for the flow of life energy.

10.14 Sacred Sexuality and Tantra

All the theistic traditions teach that the Divine, the Sacred Source, dwells within us, besides being pervasive throughout the universe. Yet, while "God lives in me" may be a basic tenet of faith, it is rarely our moment-to-moment reality. More likely we experience ourselves as separate entities, separate from "God." We place the Divine outside ourselves, and wonder why we feel unintegrated. We are not bad or wrong for doing this; we can't help but perceive ourselves as discrete elements in creation, even though contemporary physics indicates we are all one energy. Without knowing this in our guts, however, we are simply missing a fuller experience of wholeness. Spiritual practice, from all traditions, is about remembering or reexperiencing this wholeness, our lack of separation.

Because everything shares the one energy, everything shares the force of the Divine. Hence, everything is inherently sacred, including the body. Unquestionably, sex can provoke and reinforce this wondrous recognition. Because sex can be simultaneously so physical and even raw, as well as so blissful and heart expanding, it can integrate heaven and earth, body and soul, self and universe. Sexuality has always been inherently sacred, despite what certain institutions have taught or legislated throughout the ages. There have always been groups of practitioners, faith traditions, or wise individuals and teachers who have proclaimed the beauty and truth of the human form; the goodness of human love; the wonder of pleasure; the profound gift of our participation with the Source of Life in the very act of creation. Anyone with the genuine inclination to use the body and lovemaking as an expression of worship, of prayer, of mutual adoration, is already approaching the realm of sacred sexuality. The mysteries of this realm reveal themselves slowly, over time, to those who set their hearts in the right direction.

Sacred sexuality is not about generating better sex, freer sex, more ritualized sex as a way of magnifying our orgasms. Rather, it is meant to fully integrate life and to draw the partners beyond their egos. Through mutual surrender and alignment with the Divine, the partners offer themselves to one another and to God. Their offering is a prayer, an act of universal love, a movement into a more profound communion with the Whole. How does the idea of worshipping your lover strike you? A little strange, perhaps? Yet, this is precisely the meaning of sacred sexuality. The lover or partner is viewed essentially as an embodiment of divine potential, the Beloved itself, or as the cocreator with the Divine in the act of perpetuating life.

When we approach our sexual intimacy as an act of sacred merger, we also heal our sexual wounds. As author Mariana Caplan states so well in her book *To Touch Is to Live:* "Sacred sexuality has the potential to heal the wounds created by false conditioning, body shame, self-denial, and self-hatred, revealing within our bodies the sacred temple where God has always lived, albeit disregarded."

Although it is commonly used today to describe esoteric or sacred sexual practices, the Hindu-Buddhist term *tantra* actually means "continuity." It is about the interconnectedness of all life forms; how, moment to moment, each event unfolds from the next, in much the way that a flower opens. It is an entire way of life, encompassing everything we do, say, think, or intend. In the Buddhist system of graduated levels of spiritual practice, the tantric path is considered a state of high achievement, one that requires the direction and guidance of an experienced teacher, basically because of its difficulties and challenges. Tantra involves the nonrejection of all things. Not the indulgence in everything, but the nonrejection of anything. In other words, it may be easier and less confusing to live with lots of rules about good and bad, and to simply follow them, no matter what. It is more challenging and requires lots more maturity and the ability to maintain balance in one's spiritual practice when one is exposed to things that are easy to indulge in—money, food, alcohol, drugs, sex, power. Yet, each of these things is a vast source of energy. Each of these "substances" may be deeply experienced as sacred, when approached in the right context.

No longer the sole prerogative of the Hindu or Buddhist adept, aspects of tantric sexuality are being taught in workshops and discussed in popular magazines as another exotic panacea for all our sexual woes. While there are definitely advantages to these forms of liberating ourselves from our sexual hang-ups, and while sexual attitude restructuring is invaluable and highly recommended, in most cases it is unfair to call these programs by the name of *tantra*. Sex workshops are to tantra, as playing a tape of Gregorian chant in your car is to adopting a monastic vocation. In casually or exclusively presenting "tantra" or "sacred sexuality" as a primary means of increasing sexual vigor, proponents have adapted the accoutrements of an age-old, sacred lifestyle in ways that may actually undermine the essential meaning of the practice. Consider for a moment that the Dalai Lama is a tantric adept, and those visions of sexual bliss that the word *tantra* conjures up quickly dissolve. Tantra and other genuine practices of sacred sexuality are meant to provide a multifaceted path to self-realization.

10.15 Sex and the Planet

As we look at our world today, we see only too clearly that integrated sexuality is the exception rather than the rule. People who touch their wholeness, who appreciate their own integrity and their union with everything else, do not ravage their own bodies or the body of the earth. Yet this is what we commonly find.

The word *rape* has been justly applied to our dealings with the land. We have stripped our forests and fields, robbed our soil of its fertility through wasteful overuse and poisoning with chemical substances, and erected hard, cold structures anywhere and everywhere at will.

Personal impotency will often show itself in cruel power tactics toward those whom we perceive to be weaker than ourselves. We often seek our own affirmation at the expense of another. In our attempts to experience a sense of our personal power, we have set out to dominate and control nature. Instead of marrying the earth, or establishing an ongoing love relationship with her, we have used her to suit our pleasure, denying her cries for help, disregarding her needs for tenderness and caring.

In war we do the same to a race or nation of people. The enemy becomes an "it"—objectified as evil. Were we to look into their eyes, we could not kill them. So the strategy of war demands that the enemy remain faceless, nameless, different from us. War can't work if we remember that we're all one family, that we breathe the same air, that we share the same energy.

During the 1960s and 1970s we often heard: "Make love, not war." The juxtaposition of these two activities expresses a powerful truth. You won't kill if you really love. To love your enemy is to cease to view them, or "it," as enemy. To love is to desire that others fulfill their highest potential. To love is to leave others free to determine their own lives. It is to revere and celebrate their bodies, their minds, their souls. If we experience the free, unimpeded movement of our sexual energy within, not only shall we not make war without, we shall also not make the ornaments of war, or monuments to our greed, or playgrounds of waste, nor shall we furnish for ourselves apartments in a city of death. Rather, we will kiss the earth, and touch the sky, and clothe our planet in beauty. We will truly love ourselves, and in so doing, revere our primal lover—the earth.

SUGGESTED READING

General

Barbach, L., *For Each Other: Sharing Sexual Intimacy* (Signet, 2001).

Boston Women's Health Book Collective, *Our Bodies, Ourselves for the New Century* (Touchstone Books, 1998).

Brown, G., *The New Celibacy* (McGraw-Hill, 1989).

Chang, J., *The Tao of Love and Sex: The Ancient Chinese Way to Ecstasy* (Viking, 1993).

Deida, D., *Finding God Through Sex* (Plexus, 2002).

Downing, G., *The Massage Book* (Random House, 1998).

Feuerstein, G., *Sacred Sexuality: The Erotic Spirit in the World's Great Religions* (Inner Traditions, 2004).

Fromm, E., *The Art of Loving* (Perennial, 2000).

Hite, S., *The Hite Report: A Nationwide Study of Female Sexuality* (Seven Stories, 2003).

———, *The Hite Report on Male Sexuality* (Ballantine, 1987).

Huxley, A., *Island* (Perennial, 2002).

Inkles, G., *The New Sensual Massage* (Arcata Arts, 1992).

Institute for the Advanced Study of Human Sexuality (IASHS), *SAR Guide for a Better Sex Life* (Multimedia Resource Center, 1525 Franklin St., San Francisco, CA 94109).

Reinisch, J., and R. Beasley, *The Kinsey Institute New Report on Sex: What You Must Know to Be Sexually Literate* (St. Martin's Press, 1991).

Stubbs, K. R., *Erotic Massage* (J. P. Tarcher, 1999).

Zilbergeld, B., *The New Male Sexuality* (Bantam, 1999).

Older People

Gross, Z. H., *Seasons of the Heart: Men and Women Talk About Love, Sex, and Romance After 60* (New World Library, 2000).

Wei, J., and S. Levkoff, *Aging Well: The Complete Guide to Physical and Emotional Health* (John Wiley, 2000).

The Disabled

Sexuality and Information Council of the United States, www.siecus.org/pubs/biblio/bibs 0009.html. This website offers an annotated bibliography of publications relating to sexuality and the disabled.

Sex Education for Parents, Children, and Adolescents

Chilman, C., *Adolescent Sexuality in a Changing American Society: Social and Psychological Perspectives* (University Press of the Pacific, 2001).

DeBecker, G., *Protecting the Gift: Keeping Children and Teenagers Safe (and Parents Sane)* (Dell, 2001).

Haffner, D., and A. Tartaglione, *Beyond the Big Talk: Every Parent's Guide to Raising Sexually Healthy Teens From Middle School to High School and Beyond* (Newmarket, 2002).

Harris, R., *It's So Amazing! A Book About Eggs, Sperm, Birth, Babies, and Families* (Candlewick, 1999).

Richardson, J., and M. Schuster, *Everything You Never Wanted Your Kids to Know About Sex, but Were Afraid They'd Ask: The Secrets to Surviving Your Child's Sexual Development from Birth to the Teens* (Crown, 2003).

Lesbian/Gay Sexuality

Berzon, B., and R. Leighton, *Positively Gay* (Celestial Arts, 2001).

Clark, D., *Loving Someone Gay* (Celestial Arts, 1997).

Newman, F., *The Whole Lesbian Sex Book* (Cleis, 1999).

Silverstein, C., and F. Picano, *The Joy of Gay Sex*, 3rd edition (Harper Resource, 2003).

Spirituality and Sexuality

Feuerstein, G., *Tantra: The Art of Ecstasy* (Shambhala, 1998).

Lozowick, L., *The Alchemy of Love and Sex* (Hohm Press, 1996).

Moore, J., *Sexuality, Spirituality: A Study of Masculine/Feminine Relationships* (Harper-Collins UK, 1991).

Wright, E., and D. Inesse, *God Is Gay: An Evolutionary Spiritual Work* (Tayu, 1982).

For an updated listing of resources and active links to the websites mentioned in this chapter, please see www.WellnessWorkbook.com.

NOTES

1. McCarthy, B., and E. McCarthy, *Sexual Awareness: Couple Sexuality for the Twenty-First Century* (Carroll and Graf, 2002); and Davis, M., *The Sex-Starved Marriage: Boosting Your Marriage Libido: A Couple's Guide* (Simon and Schuster, 2004).

2. Laquerr, T., *Solitary Sex: A History of Masturbation* (Zone, 2003).

3. Friday, N., *My Secret Garden: Women's Sexual Fantasies,* revised edition (Pocket Books, 1998) and *Men in Love* (Dell, 1998).

4. For information on available programs, contact Sexual Attitude Restructuring (SAR), Institute for the Advanced Study of Human Sexuality, 1523 Franklin Street, San Francisco, CA 94109, (415) 928-1133, www.iashs.edu; Masters and Johnson, Relational & Sex Therapy, Sexual Trauma and Compulsivity, 16216 Baxter Rd., Chesterfield, MO 63017, (314) 781-1112; or Albert Ellis Institute, 45 E. 65th St., New York, NY 10021, (800) 323-4758 or (212) 535-0822, www.rebt.org.

5. Hite, S., *The Hite Report: A Nationwide Study of Female Sexuality* (Seven Stories, 2003), and *The Hite Report on Male Sexuality* (Ballantine, 1987); Masters, W., and V. Johnson, *Human Sexuality* (Addison-Wesley, 1997); and Reinisch, J., and R. Beasley, *The Kinsey Institute New Report on Sex: What You Must Know to Be Sexually Literate* (St. Martin's Press, 1991).

6. For information about birth control, contact any local office of Planned Parenthood; call (800) 230-7526 for the office nearest you. Also see www.plannedparenthood.org.

7. For a thorough treatment of this topic, see DeBecker, G., *Protecting the Gift: Keeping Children and Teenagers Safe (and Parents Sane)* (Dell, 2001).

8. Singer, J., *Androgyny: The Opposites Within.* (Nicholas-Hays, 2000), 5.

CHAPTER 11

Wellness and Finding Meaning

The search for meaning is a complex energy output that involves all previous energy forms. It involves these basic questions: Who am I? Why am I here? Where am I going? What do I want? What is real? What is true? Regardless of whether these questions are conscious or unconscious, all life activity, all energy expressions, are colored by them. The ongoing process of addressing these questions encourages a balanced life and provides us with a focal point toward which to direct our energy.

The great and glorious masterpiece of humanity is to know how to live with a purpose.

—Montaigne

Generally, the meanings we assign to our lives flow out of our cultural heritage, together with our relationships with those close to us, the jobs we do, the roles we play, and our religious beliefs. When significant changes take place in our lives—graduation, breakup with a partner, retirement, divorce, the death of a loved one, the last child leaving home—we lose a piece of our identity. When our normal illusions of security are threatened—as in a national emergency, a war, or a natural disaster such as a serious earthquake or flood—we are shaken. We question, "What does it mean?" We may actually feel that we have lost our foundation or our reason for being. Such periods of change are generally times of great stress, anxiety, and unhappiness, even if they are also characterized by acts of heroism and generosity.

A certain amount of worry and fear is built into the process of adjusting to change and working it all out. It is when we become stuck in delaying and evading tactics that problems arise. Some people are thrown into deep depression or beset with feelings of uselessness, emptiness, or boredom. Other people launch themselves on a series of feverish activities, anxiously keeping themselves occupied at all times. Others play Russian roulette, with high-risk behaviors such as overeating, drinking to excess, or taking drugs. And for some, the ultimate solution is suicide.

Finding meaning is probably the most personal and most challenging issue anyone can address, because it requires looking inward and self-searching, which some find a frightening prospect. And this is not something another person can do for you. Because finding meaning is a process, however, there are some helpful guidelines you can follow:

- *Learn to look within and begin to trust what you find there. Listen to your own inner voice, your own wisdom.*

- *Focus on what is instead of living for future breaks or living in the past.*

- *Strive for greater honesty and clarity in your relationships with yourself and with other people; be just who you are, not what you think you are supposed to be.*

- *Make friends with loss, pain, and death, rather than running from them and awarding fear an unwarranted place in steering your life.*

We wish you courage, strength, and joy in your exploration.

WHAT THE FROG TAUGHT US

Today the biology teacher brought a frog, fresh from the neighborhood lake, into the lab. We were going to learn about what makes frogs work—how they digest, eliminate, breathe, reproduce—to discover the essence of "frogginess."

The frightened little thing moved nervously in the teacher's hand, hopped onto the table, gazed wonderingly in all directions, gave an occasional "croak" to the amusement of the class. We were excited. All eyes following the movements, delighted by how closely it resembled the cartoon frogs of our TV experience. We oohed and ahhed and giggled and screamed. Occasionally there was even a moment of reverent silence when one of our crowd, talking quietly, seemed to have established an instant of rapport. The movements of our hands, our bodies, mimicked our tiny subject. We were animated, questioning, intrigued.

But then something changed all that. Under the skillful knife of our instructor, we watched the life force, with the sticky frog-blood, oozing from our victim. The time had come to get down to the real business at hand—to dissect, to label, to describe, to preserve the tiny frog-heart in clear, liquid solutions. We had to watch carefully because tomorrow we would have to do the same. But somehow, we really didn't care. This was not a frog. In pulling back its familiar warty skin it became an objectified mass, a lump of slime. No longer were we amused. This was messy business and the fun had left.

We left the class with a neat list of drawings, a rack full of samples adequately preserved, a full page of notes to be transcribed into our workbooks. But we also carried away a funny taste in our mouths, a tension behind our eyes, and a feeling of sadness that in seeking to understand the parts, we had lost life in the whole.

—Frank Young

What's Important?

By looking at our values today, we catch a glimpse of what is most meaningful to us. Supposing that you needed to escape from where you presently live, and could take along only ten things that you currently have, what would they be?

1. _____
2. _____
3. _____
4. _____
5. _____
6. _____
7. _____
8. _____
9. _____
10. _____

What will be important to you at the moment of your death? What will it take, by way of accomplishment, or attitudes, or possessions, to allow you to die satisfied? Spend a few moments in quiet reflection and then write them down.

_____
_____
_____
_____
_____
_____
_____
_____
_____
_____
_____

II.I **Where Do Meanings Come From, Anyway?**

Meanings are made up in human minds, and perpetuated by common agreement. They vary according to place and time and heritage. Your personal meanings vary with your need, or mood, or what you ate for breakfast. You give meanings to things, just as people in other parts of the world during other periods of history have given meanings to things. Sometimes those meanings are shared. At other times they are vastly different, and disagreement about them causes wars. But in and of themselves, things don't have meaning. Things simply are.

Look at something near you right now—a lamp, a chair, a diamond ring, a scratch on your finger. What does it mean?

For you, the lamp may simply mean something to light your page. For the antique dealer, it may mean a profitable sale. For the child, it may mean something pretty to play with. For your mother, it may mean a recollection of the old homestead where it first stood. Each person will treasure, discard, or ignore the lamp based on the meaning they have assigned it.

The meaning you assign to something can change from one moment to the next. The ring that you wear today and treasure as the sign of external fidelity or friendship may tarnish in the back of your drawer next year. Meanings change because people's lives change.

Since meaning comes from inside of you, finding meaning will be a process of going to the source—*yourself.*

The past
is dead
The future
is imaginary
Happiness
can only be
in the Eternal
Now
Moment

This sunset . . .
This smile . . .
This word you are writing . . .
This pain you are feeling . . .
The question you are asking . . .
This omelet you are cooking . . .

The meaning of life
is the tear of joy
shed at the
sight of
the
well-cooked omelet.

—Jere Pramuk

II.2 The Examined Life

The unexamined life is not worth living.

—Socrates

In our modern, materialistic, media-saturated society, few people take the time to ponder the questions of meaning, yet doing so is crucial to creating a balanced, purposeful, and rewarding life. If such questioning seems important to us, then making it a priority (at least now and again) is a good way to start. For many people, consciously setting aside time for reflective contemplation—a subject we will consider in greater depth in chapter 12—is a must. Journal writing can be an invaluable tool in moving us to greater insight and even clarity. When we attempt to write about something as integral to our lives as "What am I here for?" or "What makes a difference?" we are forced to make our fleeting ideas into something solid, tangible. We take the ruminations and scattered fragments of thoughts and feelings and form them into words that we can look at, read back to ourselves, and ponder.

Talking in depth with a trusted listener, one who encourages us to explore rather than to come up with answers, can be tremendously rewarding. We get to form new questions. If we can hold these questions without judging ourselves as inadequate for not being able to answer them, we increase the breadth and depth of our soul.

Looking at our priorities and values is a much more immediate process. Values and priorities essentially show up in how we live, not in our concepts about how we wish we could live. This is a hard truth to face. If we say that spending quality time with our children is a priority, but we continually put dozens of other tasks ahead of spending time with them, then our priorities are skewed, and our values are questionable. While there are millions of good excuses about why we aren't getting to do the things we say we want to do, excuses don't build satisfying relationships. Acting in line with our values and priorities creates personal integrity and gives meaning to our lives.

Although we may never be completely sure of our purpose on the planet, and may find very few answers to our questions, we must nevertheless be willing to ask such probing questions of ourselves. Then we must be willing to live in the gaps between how we would like our life to be and the reality of how our life presently appears. We have to endure the pain of our misplaced priorities and unlived values before we will make a natural change. We can make being compassionate with ourselves a value and priority throughout the process. Learning to live with our eyes and hearts open in the gaps, filled with uncertainties and questioned priorities, is probably more important than coming up with any definitive answers once and for all—for there may be none. Meaning may be found in the process, not in the result.

The Work is with you and in you in such a way that once you find it in yourself, where it always is, you have it always, wherever you may be, on land or sea.

—Hermes Trismegistus

In contemplating what is truly meaningful to them, many people discover that experiencing and expressing love are central to their fulfillment in life. The challenge is to transform the fear that is so rampant in our culture (often expressed as anger or impatience) into love. This can be a lifelong project that propels meaning and direction into every moment of life. Often, just when we think we may have mastered the lesson, the bar gets moved a notch higher—perhaps to keep us from getting bored?

Your Big Question

Not everyone can relate to the same Big Question or Questions about life purpose. Some people have worded theirs these ways:

What's life all about?

Why am I here?

What am I doing with my life?

Why did God make me?

How can I find happiness?

What about you? How do you express your Big Question or Questions? Spend a moment or two reflecting, and write them down here:

_____

_____

_____

_____

_____

_____

_____

_____

_____

_____

_____

_____

_____

_____

_____

_____

_____

_____

The American public and most of the rest of the world believe that happiness equals pleasure. A life that maximizes the amount of positive feelings and minimizes the amount of negative ones is a happy life.

Happiness Equals Pleasure?

So pervasive is this "hedonic" view of happiness that when I tell audiences that there are two other paths to happy lives—the Good Life and the Meaningful Life—that need not have any positive emotion at all, they are incredulous. "You are redefining happiness arbitrarily," they say.

The hedonic view of happiness convinces us that Goldie Hawn and Debbie Reynolds are the paradigmatic examples of being happy: smiley, ebullient, cheerful, bright-eyed and bushy-tailed.

Two Things Wrong with This Idea

But there are two things radically wrong with this hedonic view. The first is that smiley ebullience is highly heritable and very hard to get more of. This trait is called "positive affectivity" and identical twins are much more likely to share it than are fraternal twins. It is not very changeable, and the best you can hope for from learning skills such as "savoring" and "mindfulness" is to help you live in the upper part of your set range of positive affectivity. The fact that it is normally distributed means that half

the population is not very smiley, cheerful, and ebullient, and not likely to become so—even with carefully reading and diligently doing the exercises in Authentic Happiness.

The second problem with the Hollywood view of happiness, as pervasive as it is, is a very poor intellectual provenance. When Aristotle spoke of the "Eudaimonia"—the Good Life—he was not focused on the positive feelings of pleasure— orgasm, a backrub, and a full stomach. Rather, he was concerned with the "pleasures" of contemplation— which do not reside in orgasmic thrills or sensations of warmth, but in deep absorption and immersion, a state we now call *flow*. And during this state there is neither thought nor feeling. You are simply one with the music.

Three Paths to Happy Lives

So the core thesis in Authentic Happiness is that there are three very different routes to happiness. First, the **Pleasant Life,** consisting in having as many pleasures as possible and having the skills to amplify the pleasures. This is, of course, the only true kind of happiness in the Hollywood view. Second, the **Good Life,** which consists in knowing what your signature strengths are, then recrafting your work, love, friendship, leisure, and parenting to use those strengths to have more flow in life. Third, the **Meaningful Life,** which consists of using your strengths in the service of

something that you believe is larger than you are.

Important New Evidence

Until recently, the idea that there are three routes to happiness, two of which do not involve any felt positive emotion at all, was merely an untested theory. Recent unpublished research shows startling results.

Pleasure doesn't add to satisfaction. One of the studies found that both the Good Life and the Meaningful Life were related to life satisfaction: the more Eudaimonia or the more Meaning, the more life satisfaction. Astonishingly, however, the amount of pleasure in life did not add to life satisfaction.

Eudaimonia predicts satisfaction. The other study found that eudaimonic pursuits were significantly correlated with life satisfaction, whereas hedonic pursuits were not.

Cheerfulness not needed to be happy. The upshot of these two studies, done independently, is that successfully pursuing pleasure does not necessarily lead to life satisfaction, but successfully pursuing the Good Life and the Meaningful Life does lead to higher life satisfaction.

Adapted, with permission, from Martin E. P. Seligman, Ph.D., "Pleasure, Meaning, and Eudaimonia," www.authentichappinesscoaching.com/news/news1.html.

II.3 Listening to Our Inner Voice

The path is the goal.

—Chögyam Trungpa Rinpoche

Today we are bombarded with self-serving and superficial messages from a multitude of often conflicting directions, telling us how to live our lives. Divorced from our own inner voice, our own wisdom, we are easily swayed. We also look to external "authorities"—from teachers to doctors to media advertising to popular songs—to comprehend and assign meaning to our lives.

Some of these authorities have a track record. Great wisdom teachings *have* endured throughout the ages and can be found at the core of most religious and philosophical traditions. Women and men of eminent knowledge and love have spoken about and taught these great truths to their tribes, their followers, their families, for countless generations. Today, we have immediate access to much of this wisdom through books, videotapes, practitioners of all sorts, and groups of all types. Tremendous help and guidance is available to us if and when we seek it. Yet, ultimately, each of us, individually, must face those questions that have formed the basis of philosophy and spirituality throughout the ages.

It is only by looking inward, past and through the multitude of voices that surround us, and growing quiet enough within ourselves, that we can hear, with our heart, what is true for us. Many people today are seeking to connect with their own inner wisdom through meditation, vision quests, retreats. We can also cultivate our ability to listen by simply taking time alone to do something that brings us closer to nature, to our own inner spirit—gardening, walking in the woods, relaxing in the park, or even settling reflectively into a welcoming corner of a coffee shop. As we talk about hearing a voice of wisdom from within, or listening with our heart, it is easy to misinterpret what this experience may be. Actually, many people report that the voice they hear is more of a sense of something. They *feel* "aligned with God," or "in tune with the universe," or "moving in the flow." The words used are sometimes off-putting, but the experience they point to is undeniable for those who have it. If this type of self-exploration is attractive to you, be patient in allowing your wisdom to bubble up, be heard, or express itself in a way that you may not be able to anticipate or describe. Getting quiet may take more time than you might hope or initially have planned. Keep an open heart and mind, experiment, ask for guidance as you feel the need for it. The process of such opening to wisdom *is* an expression of wisdom itself.

At the heart of each of us, whatever our imperfections, there exists a silent pulse of perfect rhythm. A complex of waveforms and resonances, which is absolutely individual and unique, and yet which connects us to everything in the universe.

—George Leonard

II.4 Getting Where You Want to Go

Before you can have any real sense of getting somewhere, you need to know the point from which you're starting, and where you want to go. Goal setting, action, evaluation, and redirection are a set of dynamic tools that can assist you in navigating successfully toward your desired destination. In the absence of these tools, you may well be washed downstream!

Yet many of us resist setting goals and taking the steps that will get us where we want to go. We often take whatever comes along in life with half-hearted resignation, making the "best" of a situation rather than risking the disappointment and frustration we may experience when our hopes and expectations are not met. And then we wonder why a once brightly colored world has become nothing but a blur of grays.

It takes courage to call into question, and to consider changing, some of our most basic behaviors and ways of thinking. Working at the process of goal-setting, therefore, may be uncomfortable. Nonetheless, it is well worth the effort. Even if we don't accomplish all the goals we initially set for ourselves, the very process of formulating goals is energizing and life-affirming. It says to the deeper self, "I'm worth it," and "I can make a difference in the way I live my life."

We recommend a simple exercise that never ceases to surprise us, no matter how many times we do it. To start, you take four blank sheets of paper. On the first you write: "Where/How I Want My Life to Be Five Years from Today." On the next: "Where/How I Want My Life to Be Two Years from Today." On the third: ". . . Six Months from Today." On the fourth: "How I Would Spend the Next Six Months of My Life If I Knew for Sure They Would Be My Last." Give yourself a time limit; say, no more than fifteen minutes to work on each sheet, beginning with the five-year projection, and moving down to the last six months. As you complete each page, cover it, and do the next one without referring to the previous ones. They may connect, or they may be totally different. This exercise is all about generating lots of data that you will later work over in a variety of ways.

To provide this exercise with a wellness perspective, recall now that a life of wholeness is an integration of body, mind, and spirit. Then look back at your lists and note if you have included goals that reflect all of these aspects of being. Perhaps you recorded lots of things about new tasks to be accomplished in a job, or different types of relationships you want to establish, but have written nothing about your state of physical health, your lifestyle habits, or your desires for enhanced emotional well-being. Now is the time to add those. Take two or three minutes to rework each sheet, including these newly remembered aspects. (If you are using a personal wellness journal—see appendix B—record these observations there.)

Read over what you have written and look for things that are repeated or strongly expressed. Note patterns that are emerging. As you write, listen to your internal self-talk that may be undermining the process; saying, for example, "But that can never happen" or "I don't have the money [or courage or time] to do that." Keep moving ahead despite these self-defeating messages.

Put this exercise aside for at least a day, and do it again tomorrow, or next weekend. Compare and contrast the results of the two experiments, and keep asking yourself, "What would I have/do/be if I had no limitations [like time, money, children, etc.]?" So often we use our imagined limitations as defenses against clearly asserting and then setting out after what we really want. The difference between a life of greatness and a life of mediocrity is that the great move ahead with their limitations, while the mediocre stay stuck in them.

The next step is to focus on one or more of your strongest goals, and to draw a road map or timeline with actions or steps that will begin to bring your dream into form. For instance, if you've always wanted to run your own school, you can start today with a trip to the library to find every book available on innovative education. You can make three phone calls and talk to people involved in a similar venture, sign up for an adult education course in administration, and so on. Many people testify to the power of "magnet maps"—colorful collages that depict your dreams as accomplished realities. These maps are placed somewhere they can be seen regularly and serve to keep your vision alive.

Living Will

To My Family, My Physician, My Lawyer, and All Others Whom It May Concern,

Death is as much a reality as birth, growth, maturity, and old age—it is the one certainty of life. If the time comes when I can no longer take part in decisions for my own future, let this statement stand as an expression of my wishes and directions, while I am still of sound mind.

If at such a time the situation should arise in which there is no reasonable expectation of my recovery from extreme physical or mental disability, I direct that I be allowed to die and not be kept alive by medications, artificial means, or "heroic measures." I do, however, ask that medication be mercifully administered to me to alleviate suffering even though this may shorten my remaining life.

This statement is made after careful consideration and is in accordance with my strong convictions and beliefs. I want the wishes and directions here expressed carried out to the extent permitted by law. Insofar as they are not legally enforceable, I hope that those to whom this Will is addressed will regard themselves as morally bound by these provisions.

Signed _____   *Date* _____

Witness _____   *Witness* _____

Copies of this request have been given to _____

_____

_____

II.5 Making Time for Your Dreams

> One can go through contemporary life fudging and evading, indulging and slacking, never really frightened nor passionately stirred, your highest moment a mere sentimental orgasm, and your first real contact with primary and elemental necessities the sweat of your deathbed.
>
> —H. G. Wells

Most of us are so caught up in the busy-ness of life that we put off the things that are most important to us—beginning or completing that project our heart calls us to act on, taking time with friends, children, loved ones. Time stretches out before us and we think that we will do it tomorrow, next week, as soon as things settle down.

The pace of modern life gets faster with each passing year. Unless you take charge and resist the temptation, pressure, or expectation to keep up with it, you will likely never do the thing that you say you most want to do. Getting clear on what your goals are is the first step, but goals are meaningless unless you structure your time so you can pursue them.

Stephen and Ondrea Levine's book *A Year to Live* is an excellent tool to help you accomplish this time structuring, because imagining that this is your last year on the planet brings you to grips with what is most important in your life.

In their work with dying people, the Levines came to a profound appreciation of what death has to teach us. There is nothing like imagining that this is the last time you will see the leaves turn color, the snow fall, or the buds open in springtime, to awaken you to the importance of living each moment fully and keeping your priorities clearly before you.

BEING HERE NOW EXERCISE

At this moment, if you set the alarm to get up at 3:47 tomorrow morning and when the alarm rings and you get up and turn it off and say:

What time is it?

Then say: Now.

Where am I? Here. Then go back to sleep. Get up at 9:00.

Where am I? Here!

Try 4:32 three weeks from next Thursday.

By God,

It is—there's no getting away from it—that's the way it is that's the Eternal Present.

You finally figure out that it's only the clock that's going around. . . .

It's doing its thing but you—
you're sitting
Here,
Right Now,
Always.

—Ram Dass (Richard Alpert),
Be Here Now

11.6 Living in the Now

Looking to the future for happiness or living on past glories is a sure setup for disappointment. Ultimately, we have no assurance of anything beyond this present moment. There really is no future or past—just a continuous progression of "now" moments.

The question then is "What am I to *do* in the 'now' in order to experience meaning?" The secret of happiness, shared by great mystics throughout the ages, is to do just what you are doing, but do it with awareness. Be just who you are, but be it intensely. Look long and lovingly at what is real *right now*.

A classic Zen tale relates the adventure of a monk being chased by a tiger. After running a short distance the man found himself at the edge of a cliff. As the tiger approached, the monk noticed a small tree branch jutting out of the wall of the cliff, just a few feet below him. Managing to catch hold of the branch, he hung there, with the tiger above him, and an abyss below. A mouse began gnawing on the branch. What to do? Just then he observed a tiny strawberry plant within arm's reach. He plucked it, put it in his mouth, and savored it. It was delicious.

Everyone's life has its tigers and its mice and its strawberries. And, while we may not have the attention or the discipline of the monk to stay fully focused in such a difficult, yet wondrous, present, we can begin to notice how often we leave the present moment and begin obsessing about the past or future. Awareness of this tendency is the vital step.

Watching our thoughts (as we discussed in greater depth in chapter 7) and choosing where to place our attention is a skill that we can cultivate.

Some events are easier to stay present to than others. Eating a meal, we can remind ourselves to do nothing else but eat with awareness, enjoying every sensation. Making love, we can remind ourselves to stay present to the body, rather than retreating into fantasy. Taking a walk, we can remind ourselves to look, smell, feel, hear what is around us. We can stop ourselves occasionally throughout the day and simply ask, "Do you know where you are right now, and what you are doing?"

Living in the here and now is a practice, not some concept. It requires our dedicated commitment to learning this practice. Refer back to the chapter on breathing, chapter 2, for many helpful reminders about how to use the breath to keep you present to yourself and your world.

Sometimes, living in the now means that we simply savor what is given. At other times, full awareness of the now means that we take dynamic action. Tenzin Palmo, a Tibetan nun, was snowbound in her hermitage during a great storm that precipitated an avalanche. The situation seemed hopeless. For many hours she sat quietly, practicing meditation and observing her thoughts, her fears. She prepared herself for death. In the midst of her meditation, and with an internal state of great calmness, she heard a voice with a strong demand. "Dig!" it said. She did, and lived.

II.7 Life Is a Mystery

> We stake our lives on our purposeful programs and projects, our serious jobs and endeavors. But doesn't the really important part of our lives unfold "after hours"—singing and dancing, music and painting, prayer and lovemaking, or just fooling around?
>
> —Father William McNamara

Living well and fully experiencing life means squarely facing the question of purpose and meaning. On the other hand, it is important to seek a balance and not get deadly serious about the whole matter, for, as the saying goes, life is a mystery to be lived, not a problem to be solved.

So go ahead and ask the questions, examine motivations, read about the lives of inspiring people, meditate on the ultimate purpose of things, but at the same time live with your questions when you can't come up with any definitive answers. Relax, laugh, and play when things get too serious and you realize that you'll never be finished with learning, changing, and growing.

DIE, DIE, DAYENU

The span of one human life, even if it were eighty or a hundred years, is but the twinkling of an eye in the history of humanity. Everything is transitory. Everything dies. In every moment I am being born and in every moment I am dying. On the inhalation I take in the spirit, on the exhalation I let it go—I expire.

I have no guarantee that there will be any more than there is right now. Nevertheless, I live my life as if I have forever. And in reality I do—but certainly not in this particular manifestation of the physical body, for no one will hold this form forever. All is movement, all is change, all is passing away, all is resurrecting in this moment. To look at death is to look at life. To live with the presence of death is to live with the presence of life. Not in the sense of eat, drink, and be merry, but in the sense of *dayenu*—a Hebrew word meaning "it is enough"; that is, all in this moment is sufficient. If there is no next moment, I leave freely, happily, with deep appreciation for all that has been and is.

—RSR

11.8 Facing Death and Finding Meaning

Paradoxically, for those who seek to understand it, death is a highly creative force and a meaning-filled fact of life. The highest spiritual values of life can originate from the thought and study of death. But before we can use the confrontation with loss, separation, or death as a way of finding meaning, we must repudiate the connection between death and failure. We need to replace death within its rightful context if we are to use it to find meaning in life.

The culture in which we live has emphasized the prolonging of life—often supporting its *quantity* above its quality. A spiritual teacher recently humored his audience by telling them: "Ladies and gentlemen, the point is not who lives the longest."

A cartoon in a major magazine depicted a hospital bed surrounded by monstrous electronic devices attached to a sad-faced patient. One weak arm emerged from under the covers holding a tiny white flag. The nurse, turning to the attending doctor, remarked—"Everything is working, doctor, but Mr. Jones doesn't want to cooperate."

Mr. Jones had had it! He was ready to give up, to surrender rather than to be subject to any more life-supporting technological "miracles." His response causes us to chuckle grimly because we relate to stories of people being kept alive at any cost. And cost it does!

Hospitals are established for the handling of disease and accident and trauma, for remediating conditions and then releasing patients once they can stand on their own. Doctors are committed to keeping us alive—as an inherent value. Consequently, when death occurs it means failure. It's that simple.

But death is not the ultimate enemy, the terminal disease to wage war against, to be eliminated at all costs. Nevertheless, this attitude subtly underlies so many approaches to health and wellbeing. As if by doing the right things—eating the proper foods, taking our exercise programs seriously, keeping infection at bay, improving surgical techniques—death, like the smallpox virus, could be wiped out.

We delude ourselves in believing that medical research will discover a cure for death. It's true that people who watch their diets, exercise, and enjoy satisfying relationships often *do* live longer. Nevertheless, we are all terminal, and death is our natural inheritance.

11.9 Death and Meaning

The poet Khalil Gibran writes of life and death as one; he says that in every moment of life you are dying, and in dying you are preparing the way for new life. You experience living and dying in every instant in small ways. Baby teeth must fall out so that adult teeth may emerge. Skin cells constantly die and are sloughed off so that new cells may take their place. Taking a new job means death to a previous one. Growing in wisdom and truth means death to old patterns of belief.

Always, a dying precedes a rebirth, for life and death are one. As we become increasingly aware of dying and being reborn in every moment, the experience of death that occurs at the culmination of our life becomes just one more familiar transformation to be embraced and accepted. In her many years of work with dying people, Elisabeth Kübler-Ross, M.D., found that almost everyone reaches a stage of resignation and acceptance prior to death. If each death has meant a small transformation, a new life, why should the Big Death be any different?

We may speak easily of the cycle of life, or the food chain, when talking about plants and animals, yet we often retract in horror from the stark reality that we humans are also a part of this cycle. Our bodies will return to the earth to nourish it, to feed our children's children. My thoughts and accomplishments build a foundation that will support the growth of future generations. It is the way of nature. Death is an energy-transforming process; thus, fighting it is a wasteful and irrelevant effort. Relaxing into acceptance of the inevitable eases this natural progression.

The tremendous popularity of such books as *Life after Life,* by Raymond Moody, M.D., indicates a widespread curiosity about what happens after death. It is but one report of a growing body of literature collected from people who have "died" and yet still are alive; people who have gone "beyond and back." These reports have much to say about the lessons brought back from these close encounters with death. And what were the lessons? Simply, that life is given to us in order to learn from *everything.*

In learning, we can grow in love for, and acceptance of, all that exists. We think that learning and loving are the attitudes and behaviors that give meaning to life. These are the things that will endure.

Also there is the fear that there *is* an afterlife, but no one will know where it's being held.

—Woody Allen

11.10 Coming to Terms with Death

Many people claim that they don't fear death. When questioned further, they are quick to add:

- *". . . but I don't like to think of the sorrow it will cause my family or children."*

- *". . . but I'm not ready for it to happen for a long while yet."*

- *". . . but I want to go quickly."*

- *". . . but I don't want to be laid out in a funeral parlor."*

As reasonable as they sound, these statements imply a fear of sorts. Few people express no uneasiness at all about the subject of death.

Looking squarely at any of our fears about death, and being able to talk about them, can supply us with meaningful information about what holds us back from the full experience of life.

If you fear death because you fear the unknown, chances are this is the way you approach life—with fear, avoiding change, minimizing risk, keeping yourself secure in known routines.

To face death consciously, you must face life consciously—embracing your fears, kissing your monsters.

What do *you* fear about death?

- *The unknown that follows*

- *The humiliation of giving up control*

- *The loss of bodily functions*

- *The separation from family and friends*

- *The pain*

- *The sorrow and hardship to family and friends*

- *The surprise, not knowing the time or place*

- *The sense of incompleteness, that you didn't do all you intended to do*

- *The sense of meaninglessness, that you never found out your purpose in being*

- *The unendingness of eternity*

- *The experience of nothingness*

Now look back over the fears of death that you have identified. Ask yourself: How do these fears reflect the ways I live, or fail to live, my life right now? What do fears of death tell me about my real fears of life?

Then have a dialogue with yourself about each fear in turn.

I have been able to function as a catalyst, trying to bring to our awareness that we can only truly live and enjoy and appreciate life if we realize at all times that we are finite. Needless to say I have learned these lessons from my dying patients—who in their suffering and dying realized that we have only NOW— "so have it fully and find what turns you on, because no one can do this for you!"

—Elisabeth Kübler-Ross

II.II **Dying with Dignity and Awareness**

Sooner or later, we all face death. You can take greater responsibility for this experience right now. The largest part of this process entails taking responsibility for your life. There are many facets unique to the death experience that allow you to maintain your personal power and enable to you embrace death with conscious awareness. First of all, face it. This takes courage, but the alternative is being stuck in the fear and withdrawal that drain away the energy needed for living fully.

Secondly, make some choices about it now. Do you currently have a will? (It doesn't matter if you are twenty or eighty; you have no assurance of living beyond this very moment.) How do you prefer to die? Do you wish to be hospitalized in your last days? What alternatives exist for your care outside of a hospital? Do you know about hospice programs for home treatment of the terminally ill? Do you have a living will regarding life-support systems, surgery, pain medication, and the presence of supportive people (see page 273)? Will you donate your eyes or other organs to others? What kind of funeral ceremony do you want? Are you aware of the costs of burial and all that goes with it? What about cremation? Who do you entrust with making choices for you when, or if, you can no longer make them for yourself?

Finally, accept your weaknesses, as well as your strengths, as you confront death. Knowing that death is a transformation, allow your darkness to surface with your light. Give yourself permission to express the emotions that are real for you. Fear, anger, or deep sadness are all a part of who you are as a fully functioning, alive, and aware human being. Flow with and love yourself. Let go. The body, mind, and spirit know when it is time to move on. Trust yourself—trust the process.

HOSPICE

Hospice represents an interdisciplinary, holistic approach to caring for people with a life-threatening illness, either in the patient's home or in a facility. The patient and family together are considered a single unit of care. Hospice combines the skills of physicians, nurses, clergy, psychotherapists, social workers, and volunteers who, together with the family, design and implement the care plan. Care continues for the family after the patient's death.

11.12 **Looking Ahead**

It is essential to your wellness to see your life as an unfolding process rather than a static role merely to be played out. Many people assume that once they have finished school, gotten a job, married, and have children, all they have to look forward to is retirement.

These people age more rapidly and get ill more often. Looking for the lessons offered by every encounter with life keeps your mind active, your heart open, and your spirit alive.

SUGGESTED READING

Andrews, C., *The Circle of Simplicity: Return to the Good Life* (HarperCollins, 1998).

Bach, R., *Illusions* (Dell Publishing Co., 1994).

Covey, S., *The Seven Habits of Highly Effective People* (Simon & Schuster, 1990).

Dass, R., *Be Here Now* (Crown Publishing Co., 1971).

Dominguez, J., and V. Robbin, *Your Money or Your Life: Transforming Your Relationship with Money and Achieving Financial Independence* (Penguin, 1999).

Elgin, D., *Voluntary Simplicity: Toward a Way of Life That Is Outwardly Simple, Inwardly Rich* (Quill, 1993).

Fields, R., et al., *Chop Wood, Carry Water* (J. P. Tarcher, 1984).

Frankl, V., *Man's Search for Meaning* (Washington Square Press, 1997).

Gibran, K., *The Prophet* (Random House, 1923).

Golas, T., *The Lazy Man's Guide to Enlightenment* (Gibbs Smith, Publisher, 2002).

Koch, R., *The 80/20 Principle: The Secret to Success by Achieving More with Less* (Doubleday, 1999).

Krishnamurti, J., *Think on These Things* (Perennial Press, 1989).

Kübler-Ross, E., *On Death and Dying* (Scribner, 1997).

Levey, J., and M. Levey, *Living in Balance: A Dynamic Approach for Creating Harmony and Wholeness in a Chaotic World* (Conari, 1998).

Levine, S., *Who Dies?* (Anchor Books, 1989).

Levine, S., and O. Levine, *A Year to Live: How to Live This Year As If It Were Your Last* (Three Rivers Press, 1998).

Luhrs, J., *The Simple Living Guide: A Sourcebook for Less Stressful, More Joyful Living* (Broadway Books, 1997).

Moody, R., *Life After Life* (Harper San Francisco, 2001).

Pirsig, R., *Zen and the Art of Motorcycle Maintenance: An Inquiry into Values* (Bantam, 1984).

Simon, S., L. Howe, and H. Kischenbaum, *Values Clarification* (Warner Books, 1995).

For an updated listing of resources and active links to the websites mentioned in this chapter, please see www.WellnessWorkbook.com.

CHAPTER 12

Wellness and Transcending

Transcending is the movement in which all energies, once experienced as separate and in individual contexts, are appreciated as one. We come to know that we are one with all that is—and that the "one" that we are is energy. This knowledge inspires both love and self-responsibility, which bring us full circle in the never-ending spiral of wellness.

[We are] that being in whom . . . the universe reflects on and celebrates itself in conscious self-awareness.

—Thomas Berry

At some time or other, each of us has experienced moments of transcendence—often referred to as "peak" (or humorously as "peek") experiences—moments when the body-mind leaps beyond its ordinary limits, moments of supreme joy, of enlightenment, of gazing into the face of the Ultimate. You may simply be looking across the kitchen table at your children and be momentarily overwhelmed with joy. Or you may experience transcendence as the ecstatic high following sex. For a brief time all problems, all worries, disappear. You feel more "together" than you've ever felt before. There are many other examples:

- *Watching the waves at the ocean and losing your sense of time and space; feeling that the ocean is within you, not separate from you*

- *Pushing your body to the limit in dancing or running a race; breaking through the "wall of pain," actually getting a second wind, and then feeling like you could go on forever*

- *The simultaneous breathlessness, excitement, and peace when a realization of unconditional love melts through you, followed by the urgent wish to "be" this love with everyone around you*

- *Total absorption in a piece of music, or blending with the dancers or actors on a stage so that the separate "you" is not your primary fixation*

- *Finding peace even in the face of deep grief, when the larger perspective of the interplay of life and death temporarily replaces a self-centered view*

- *The "Aha!" moment when the solution to a problem you've long wrestled with spontaneously pops into your head*

Then your window is clear, and as you pitch over, getting near horizontal, you catch the first glimpse out the window of the Earth from space. And it's a beautiful sight. . . . And you realize from that perspective that you've changed, that there's something new there, that the relationship is no longer what it was.

—Russell Schweickart, crew of *Apollo 9*, March 1969

Such moments of transcendence leave us changed, generally only for a brief time—since such awareness takes time to soak in and integrate in our being—but occasionally forever. In any case, such moments are usually indelibly etched in our consciousness. They supply us with new energy, joyfulness, and motivation about this business of living. They serve as reference points, opening us to previously untapped possibilities, thus expanding our horizons and creating new options. They often put us in touch with our truest, most peaceful, and most balanced selves. They show us glimpses of the connectedness, the oneness of all things.

The most beautiful experience we can have is the mysterious.

—Albert Einstein

Most of us are quite busy handling daily routines and the immediate problems of life, and many of us are quite comfortable within the confines of the world as we know it. We may not feel an immediate need to reach beyond, to peek through the cracks in the cosmos. Some of us, however, want much more. The aim of this chapter is to pique your curiosity, to help you break through conventional ways of thinking when you are ready for it. This chapter deals with many of the spiritual (or "transpersonal") dimensions of wellbeing.

For some people, spiritual wellness is experienced primarily in participation in an organized religion. For others, *spiritual* is synonymous with the relationship to the natural world, or to the unknown or mysterious, or simply to a reality called "love." The material presented here is for everyone, however. We hope it will stretch your mind and heart, and even inspire you to take a longer and deeper look into yourself and the world (or worlds) in which you live.

Love the world as your own self; then you can truly care for all things.

—Lao Tzu

12.1 Peeking through the Cracks

History is filled with accounts of people who held fast to dreams—even when they contradicted the consensus of society. Often these dreams came in a state of awareness other than the normal waking consciousness. They have occurred in sleep, or in a state induced by trance, or after ingesting drugs, or after running for fifteen miles, or in looking at the earth from the surface of the moon, or in prayer. What the dreamers shared afterward was a new vision of the way things worked, or a new realization of connectedness with all things and everyone.

Mystical revelation and scientific insight from generations of dreamers point to alternate ways of looking at the world. The Hermetic philosophers of Greece and Rome saw thoughts as vibrational levels—energy exchanges that could change the physical universe. Christ challenged the troubled times of his era with a radical message of love, even for one's enemies. The mystics of Judaism followed the Kabbala, a series of teachings said to have been brought to earth by angels. The shamans in widely scattered cultures saw illness as a result of disharmony in the sick person's world. Pythagoras developed a mysticism based on his vision that "all things are numbers." Anaximander described the universe as one large organism supported by the cosmic breath.

If history teaches anything, it teaches that the consensus reality, in almost any age, has been woefully

When Have You Transcended?

Can you recall a moment in your life when this experience of seeing the big picture, or feeling that all was connected and everything was right, happened to you?

_____

_____

What happened?

_____

_____

Were you changed as a result?

_____

_____

How?

_____

_____

inadequate; that those whose minds were open to alternate visions of "the way things are" have been our greatest teachers, our most powerful agents of change. The hard-and-fast view of reality held by contemporaries of Copernicus and Galileo led them to ridicule the dreams these great thinkers revealed.

Perhaps you are ready now to take the next step in furthering your own break with consensus reality. If so, this chapter is built around four theories that depart from traditional thinking:

- *Theory 1: Everything is connected because everything is one.*

- *Theory 2: We shape our own reality.*

- *Theory 3: Everything is in process.*

- *Theory 4: Falling apart is often a prelude to falling together.*

These theories are not really new ideas . . . they have been part and parcel of mystical understanding for ages. What is new is that today they are receiving support from the research of scientists—notably physicists, psychologists, and medical doctors. All are related in some way to the transcendental experience and have implications for wellness.

ALL IS ONE—ALL IS RIGHT

Everything in the universe is connected, somehow. Everything is all right! There is no need to be afraid of anything—even death. I know this surely, so deeply—and it brings utter peacefulness and real understanding.

The moment of awareness—which I only later learned to label a "peak experience"—happened to me in 1968 when I was an Air Force pilot in Vietnam. I was returning to the airfield in my single-person aircraft. It was sunset. On this particular evening, the sun was setting into the horizon directly at the end of the runway. As I lined up to make my final approach, I was momentarily concerned. Flying directly into the sun, it was difficult to see. That was my last conscious thought before "it happened."

Words fail to adequately communicate what next took place. The best I can tell you is that I merged totally with the sun—I was one with the light. There was no longer any sense of "me." There was no separation between Bob and everything that exists. All personal boundaries were completely dissolved.

Nothing mattered. There was no fear. There was no sense of time—no sense of space. All was One and all was Right. My next awareness was that I was on the ground, moving in a perfectly straight path down the runway. "I" had been "gone"—but yet "I" had made a textbook landing. I knew I was completely safe. I had no sense that I had gone crazy. There was simply nothing to fear.

Despite the fact that this happening was totally outside the realm of everything I had ever known, I never doubted it, I never questioned it. I just *knew* it. I walked away feeling that something exciting and powerful had taken place. Yet I felt no compulsion to do anything about it. No sense of "mission" to go out and change myself or anyone else. Nor has there been any need to seek out some way, some means, to bring it about again. It was complete. I was complete. All I know is that I can say with total clarity that I no longer fear death.

_____

From a conversation with Bob Arnold educational/aeronautics consultant, Loveland, Colorado.

12.2 Theory 1: Everything Is Connected Because Everything Is One

> You are not a strand in the web. You are the entire web. You are doing something no mere strand ever does—you are escaping your "strandness," transcending it, and becoming one with the entire display.
>
> —Ken Wilber

In chapter 7, it was observed that we live in a predominantly left brain–oriented culture, one that values the logical, linear, mathematical approach to life, accepting C as the result of adding A and B. Unless the causal connection can be established between things, we all too often dismiss them as coincidental and hence meaningless.

Carl Jung, M.D., the Swiss psychiatrist, popularized the term *synchronicity* to describe the occurrence of two events, in close proximity of time, that have no apparent causal relationship yet appear related. For instance, you are thinking about a friend you haven't seen in ages at the very moment that she calls. Or you are humming a tune to yourself as you turn on the car radio, and are amazed to hear the same tune playing back at you. Or you dial a wrong number, only to discover that the person on the other end is a long-lost acquaintance.

Jung found that such coincidences happen far more often than would be expected by random chance, and increase in frequency for those who are open to them. Regina, who has taught psychology for ten years, notes that many of her students started "seeing" these connections soon after they learned about the concept of synchronicity.

The idea of synchronicity gets strong scientific support from Bell's theorem. Proposed in 1964 and verified in 1972, it was pronounced "the most profound discovery in science" by physicist Henry Stapp in a 1975 federal report. Bell's theorem (anticipated by Einstein in 1935, who was too uncomfortable with it to accept it, causing him to state "God does not play dice with the universe"), proposes that everything in the universe is connected as an indivisible whole. In experiments based on Bell's theorem, it was demonstrated that if paired and identically charged particles "fly apart," and the polarity of one is changed by an experimenter, the other changes instantaneously. They remain mysteriously connected.[1] What this implies is that, as Gary Zukav, author of *The Dancing Wu Lei Masters,* puts it, "There is no such thing as separate parts. All of the parts of the universe are connected in an intimate and immediate way previously claimed only by mystics and other scientifically objectionable people."

> Religion only seems different if you're dealing with a retailer. If you deal with a wholesaler, they all get it from the same distributor.
>
> —Stephen Gaskin

If Bell's theorem is correct—and most experiments do bear it out—it helps to explain many previously questioned psychic occurrences. It doesn't seem logical that a parent would "hear" his or her child crying when the child is 500 miles away; or that I could know what your home looks like when I have never been there or talked to you about it; or that Jim would develop a boil on his knee on the same day that his dad injured his knee on the job;

or that a person who is prayed for, even unknowingly, would heal faster and require less pain medication than one who isn't.

However, if, despite their distance or lack of apparent logical relationship, event A is connected to event B at the subatomic level, is it too difficult to make the leap in saying that ESP, psychokinesis, distant viewing, psychic healing, and "miracles" are merely everyday manifestations of an underlying connectedness? The skeptics among us may dismiss these happenings as mere coincidence. For others, these are meaningful indications that everything *is* somehow related.

A leaf of grass is no less than the journeywork of the stars.

—Walt Whitman

In the 1970s, an English plant physiologist, Rupert Sheldrake, Ph.D., offered a "Hypothesis of Formative Causation" (described in a book by the same name). It proposes that all entities—living organisms as well as inert substances—are each part of a "field" that connects them in some way with every other member of their species or type. He calls these fields *morphogenetic,* which literally means "giving rise to structure or form." Morphogenetic fields do not obey the laws of thermodynamics, and they operate irrespective of distances. Here's how they work: Suppose a mouse in England learns to run a maze. This mouse, in effect, creates a morphogenetic field for the solution of the maze, and therefore sets up a "form or structure" that allows mice all over the world to run the same maze with greater ease. The field becomes stronger with each mouse that completes the maze. This phenomenon and others like it had been observed for years and were the basis of Sheldrake's proposal. This model explains the existence of instincts and habits, which have never been adequately understood, and once again reinforces the appreciation of our connectedness with everything in creation. His hypothesis has withstood many tests, and in time it probably will be considered as important as Darwin's theory of evolution.

OUR FUNDAMENTAL COMMUNITY

So long as we have this worldview in which the earth itself is just stuff, empty material, and the individual is most important, then we're set up to just use it in any way we like. So the idea is to move from thinking of the earth as a storehouse to seeing the earth as our matrix, our fundamental community . . . Darwin shows us that everything is kin. Talk about spiritual insight! Everything is kin at the level of genetic relatedness. Another simple way of saying this is: Let's build a civilization that is based upon the reality of our relationships. If we think of the human as being the top of this huge pyramid, then everything beneath us is of no value, and we can use it however we want. In the past, it wasn't noticed so much because our influence was smaller. But now, we've become a planetary power. And suddenly the defects of that attitude are made present to us through the consequences of our actions. . . . [N]ow, it is the decisions of humans that are going to determine the way this planet functions and looks for hundreds of millions of years in the future.

Brian Swimme, "Comprehensive Compassion," *What Is Enlightenment?* magazine, www.thegreatstory.org/SwimmeWIE.pdf.

12.3 "All Is One" Implications for Healing

If you can accept, or even entertain, the possibility that everything is connected because everything is one, you are immediately presented with alternatives that may significantly affect your life and health. In the early 1970s, neurosurgeon Norman Shealy, M.D., began documenting cases in which psychic healing methods succeeded in both diagnosis and treatment where traditional medical practice had failed. While the terms *psychic healing* or *occult healing*—as Shealy first called it—were objectionable to many then, the activities associated with these methods have become strongly legitimized in the past twenty years. Shealy's work was dynamically augmented in the 1980s and 1990s with the collaboration of Carolyn Myss, a medical intuitive, who began to share her expertise with him—with a 95 percent rate of accuracy. A medical intuitive is a person who "sees" or "knows," by some inner sense, what the psychophysical condition of another is. In the moment of "sensing," the intuitive recognizes that he or she is not separate from the one being examined. The intuitive can then speak from what she sees and feels within herself and can translate that sensing into precise diagnostic terminology that relates to the condition of the other. Together, Shealy and Myss presented their work in the groundbreaking book *The Creation of Health,* which articulated their energy model of health and disease. They found a particular pattern of energy loss associated with every illness they examined, and they described how various stresses led to these diseases. Myss has gone on to publish many other books, including *The Anatomy of Illness,* all of which have been *New York Times* best sellers.

There is no question that there is an unseen world. The problem is, how far is it from midtown and how late is it open?

—Woody Allen

The age-old understanding that all forms of life are different expressions of the same energy is the basis of the whole field of energy "medicine" that distinguishes the work of many alternative practitioners today. In the past thirty years, physicians Brugh Joy, M.D., Richard Moss, M.D., and others, have trained thousands of health professionals to sense body energy fields, and to use a variety of methods (some of which are like a "laying on of hands"), to alter these energy fields, and thus effect healing. Nursing teacher Dolores Krieger, Ph.D., inaugurated a program called Therapeutic Touch, whereby caregivers learn to massage the energy field of the patient, to relieve pain and discomfort as well as the emotional disconnection that causes so much suffering to those who are ill. These and other touch and massage methods have become standard procedure in hospice programs and are currently taught in nursing schools throughout the country.

One of the most remarkable rediscoveries by science in recent years—the power of prayer in healing—is further testimony to the connectedness of all things. For those who believe in and practice prayer, all beings and all circumstances are seen as interrelated. People throughout the world *do* pray for health and healing, and have always done so. Whether from the perspective that God's help is available to those who ask, or from a nontheistic viewpoint that "merit" (a term used by Buddhists) or energy can be shared, vast numbers pray for themselves and for the benefit of others.

The fact that prayer works and can be scientifically verified was brought to massive public attention by Larry Dossey, M.D., in 1993 with the publication of his book *Healing Words.* Because he began his own investigation in the 1980s somewhat skeptically, Dossey was surprised to learn that dozens of highly controlled studies about the efficacy of prayer had already been conducted. Over half of them strongly indicated that prayer was a significant factor in the patient's healing. In one of the most remarkable studies, prayer was tested with heart patients in a modern hospital. The group that were prayed for, even without knowing they were prayed for, recovered more completely and with fewer complications than the "un–prayed for" control group.

The subject of prayer brings us into a vast domain of faith, belief, religion, and spirituality. What we are talking about here, as we consider wellness and transcendence, is the way in which our thoughts—which include our beliefs—connect us within a web of relatedness far greater than our immediate circumstances might indicate. *God* or *Spirit* or the *Universal Energy* are some names we assign to this vast web. In the field of grief counseling, as we mentioned in chapter 11, pioneering researcher Elisabeth Kübler-Ross, M.D., found that people with some religious faith (which essentially translates to some view of reality that transcends their own personal control and management) dealt with their grief work far more successfully than those who had no religion or spirituality in their lives. And more recently, from the International Center for the Integration of Health and Spirituality in Rockville, Maryland, David B. Larson, M.D., unhesitatingly reported, "Statistically, God is good for you."

Reality is what we take to be true. What we take to be true is what we believe. What we believe is based upon our perceptions. What we perceive depends upon what we look for. What we look for depends upon what we think. What we think depends upon what we perceive. What we perceive determines what we believe. What we take to be true is our reality.

—Gary Zukav

A PSALM FOR HELP AND HEALING

Over three thousand years ago, the psalmist King David wrote, or sung: "Out of the depths I have cried unto You O Lord. Lord hear my prayer" (Psalm 130). Using my own words, I continue the prayer:

If you, O Lord, were looking only upon my failings, I wouldn't have the stupidity to call upon You. But I know that is not what You do.

You are a God of merciful forgiveness. And how I need You now, when my own mercy is so thin, my own forgiveness so shallow, my own strength so weak. You are the God of my strength, and I can't seem to muster enough from this poor physical body of mine to endure much beyond this hour. Yet, despite my doubts, my fears, my pain, my fatigue, *I know that Your strength is available to me— through the breath; through remembrance of and gratitude toward You; through the touch or simple healing presence of a friend. Assist me in this time of struggle. Show me what is real, and dispel my illusions. Amen.*

—RSR

12.4 Theory 2: We Shape Our Own Reality

This premise that we do not live in a single, fixed (Newtonian) universe but rather in a domain in which thought (including belief and faith) has power, receives additional support from the most unlikely quarters—the laboratories of the subatomic particle physicists. From them we are finding out that our old concepts of a hard-and-fast, objective reality are simply not true.

According to Einstein's model of the universe, time actually slows down as your speed increases, and light travels in curves! The new physics of quantum mechanics demonstrates that a subatomic particle emitted when an atom is split is not even a "thing"—it is merely a "tendency to exist"; and that it is not possible to *observe* reality without changing it.

Heisenberg has said that the term *happens* is restricted to the observation. What he means by this is that there is *no reality* apart from our observations, evaluations, and judgments about it. A doesn't strike B in a void. It strikes B within the awareness of an observer—otherwise we would not know about it. Furthermore, not only does the observer's skill, computer programming ability, and visual or auditory acuity affect the report—his or her *very presence* has an impact on the process. The observer's energy field is interacting with (and thus changing) the energy field of the whole system. It follows, then, that you are more than a bystander. You have a definite part in structuring your own life, in shaping your own reality.

This view that our energy patterns influence reality and that our thoughts actually shape our bodies has been incorporated into the medical practice and educational approach of many professionals and institutions. The whole field of biofeedback/neurofeedback training, discussed in chapter 7, makes use of mental imagery and verbal suggestion to relieve stress conditions in the body. At the Norman Cousins Center for Psychoneuroimmunology, at UCLA, research is conducted on the effects of psychological and body-mind interventions on immunity and immune-mediated disease, with special emphasis on the role of stress and immunity. Today, cancer treatment programs, both conventional and alternative, almost always include positive self-talk and visualization exercises like those developed in the 1970s by Carl Simonton, M.D., and his associates.[2] While these visualizations may not cure cancer, they have been shown to decrease stress and to help patients cope better (both physically and emotionally) with the side effects of treatment.

Whether in the arena of sports, or in the examples of those who have endured enormous pain and physical deprivation in prisons or concentration camps, we learn that those who succeed most or survive best are those who can manage their minds. Thought and visualization have long been used to maintain a vision of hope, or as a means of transcending current circumstances by remaining focused on some broader reality.

12.5 Beyond Our Limits

Contemporary culture is fascinated with the ability of the human organism to do what seems impossible, as shown by the popularity of Guinness World Records. Every day someone shows us that what we previously thought were our limits are actually only the baselines, offering yet another challenge to be exceeded. In these "X-games," moreover, we find that the mind's role is always paramount. Limited beliefs lead to limited results, and vice versa.

Contemporary spiritual teacher, author, and poet Sri Chinmoy believes in inspiring others to transcend the limitations of the mind and therefore the body. Besides having written over 1,300 books, painted over 135,000 pieces of art, and mastering over 100 musical instruments, he has run 22 marathons and lifted over 7,000 pounds in order to show us that we don't aim high enough. Chinmoy's student Ashrita Furman currently holds the Guinness record for having the most world records—seventy-five. Furman's accomplishments include the fastest somersaulting mile (19 minutes); the most water glasses balanced on the chin (20), and the most consecutive jumps on a pogo stick (131,000). While we may laugh at the examples cited, we would be foolish to dismiss what his activities point to. What they tell us about the power of the body-mind is tremendous. One of the most revealing aspects of Furman's work is that he rarely trained for any of his records. Instead, his preparation would mainly consist of several hours or more in a state of meditation during which he would focus his intention on the task ahead. By the time he was ready to jump, or to somersault, or whatever, he was aligned with an unlimited "higher power" from within himself, and convinced that nothing short of death would allow him to give up.[3]

Michael Murphy, the cofounder of Esalen Institute and a forerunner in the contemporary research and philosophy of human potential, wrote a book in 1991 titled *The Future of the Body*. It draws from ancient and modern records in medical science, sports, the arts, anthropology, psychic research, and comparative religious studies, all pointing to what Murphy terms *metanormal* behaviors and experiences: extraordinary abilities and events brought about through means that generally evade logical analysis, such as the man who can control and actually stop his blood flow even when his skin is deeply punctured.

Murphy had been inspired in his student years at Stanford with the writings of the Indian revolutionary, yogi, and mystic Sri Aurobindo (1872–1950), whose philosophy argued that a new stage was emerging in human evolution; one in which exceptional capacities of body and mind would be observable and even commonplace. And Murphy's ongoing questions have reflected Aurobindo's direction. Are we facing a new evolutionary frontier? he asks. And if so, how then would we live? Murphy's efforts today amount to the creation of programs that challenge and train individuals to bring about greater integration of mind, body, and spirit. He and many others like him are convinced that we can increase the likelihood for breakthroughs in all areas of human life. Such pioneers urge us to change our view of reality and to watch as reality itself changes accordingly.

12.6 Theory 3: Everything Is in Process

As the Greek philosopher Heraclitus said centuries ago, "You can't step twice into the same river." Everything in the universe is in the constant process of changing. All you can do is watch what is happening, and observe what you're left with afterward. Even modern physics is a science of *process*.

Arthur Young, the inventor of the Bell helicopter, presents his own process model in his book *The Reflexive Universe*. He proposes that the universe is not a thing; rather, it is a continual state of evolution from photons of light, through atoms, molecules, minerals, plants, animals ... to conscious beings such as dolphins and humans. These conscious beings are also in process toward more advanced states of development—which brings us back to where we started in chapter 1. Wellness is a never-ending *process* of moving toward the living of your highest potential. It also brings us back to Ilya Prigogene's theory of how dissipative structures change, described in the introduction to this book. Prigogene's theory has much to teach us about wellness.

Dissipative structures are open systems that take in energy from the environment, transform it, and then return (dissipate) energy to the outside world. An important property of dissipative structures is that they are able to resist (dampen) small fluctuations or changes in the energy field around them. For instance, a healthy body (an open system) is able to maintain its equilibrium in the face of minor alterations in diet, exercise, and level of stress.

When these fluctuations or changes reach a certain critical intensity, however, the dissipative structure alters drastically—in some cases completely reordering itself to a higher level of complexity—and a transformation takes place. For instance, the body, when pushed to its limits with strenuous exercise, such as long-distance running, will switch from glucose usage for energy to eating up its own fat reserves. This reordering can mean significant changes in the shape of the physical body.

Solid forms or structures (closed systems, like a rock) can remain relatively stable or unchanged over extended periods of time. Open systems, on the other hand, always possess the ability to change because they constantly channel energy. They are structures in process! Each open system, then, has within it the *potential* for change into a more complex—and often more beautiful and elaborate—structure.

What the caterpillar calls the end of the world, the master calls a butterfly.

—Richard Bach

When transformation occurs it often appears as if things are falling apart. The cocoon that shields the caterpillar looks like a tomb—a dead thing. But within, a magical regeneration is taking place. Far from falling apart, this apparent death signals a falling together— a restructuring, a transformation.

12.7 Theory 4: Falling Apart and Falling Together

Breaking down as a prelude to a higher state of evolution is frequently observed in human beings faced with serious illness and even death. Sickness in the body, disease in the mind, the disintegration of a relationship, can be transforming experiences. At one level they bring us face-to-face with deep questions of personal value, of the meaning of life. They frequently cause a reordering of priorities—a change of job, a dramatic resolution of an alcohol or drug addiction, a lifestyle alteration. On another level, they may unlock doors that have been closed to us for years:

- *Stress reduction techniques that were used to deal with an ulcer become daily practice and result in a changed perception of the world in general.*

- *Massage and deep tissue techniques (e.g., Rolfing, Esalen massage, Swedish massage, neuromuscular massage, polarity therapy, Trager work) and body realignment methods (e.g., Feldenkrais, Somatics, craniosacral therapy, Alexander Technique), which are often undertaken merely as forms of physical therapy, at the same time facilitate the release of long-held emotional trauma stored in the muscles of the body, which leads to profound shifts of consciousness.*

- *Adverse reactions to drug treatment have led people to the investigation of hypnosis for pain control, mental visualization for treatment of cancer, and significant diet changes as an alternative to unsuccessful traditional therapy.*

- *Chronic back pain has led many to the practice of yoga, and yoga has then become a way of life.*

The examples abound. The options increase and so do the possibilities for wellness.

The transcendent view of life as a *process* is the basis for recommendations that we allow the body the freedom to do what it does best. It allows us the healing attitude of compassion as we examine and reassess every aspect of our lives. Realizing that we are in process lets us relax with mistakes, enjoy the paradoxes that life proposes to us every day, and give ourselves permission to be just who and what we are at the moment. And finally, it serves to excite us with the realization that we will never be finished—that there will always be new ways to grow, new doors to open, new cracks to explore in the cosmos.

I *do* think that waking up, enlightenment, can save our world, can save the planet. Because we're doing things that none of us want to see happen. And we're doing it because we're unaware. So if we can wake up and train all of our energies around this, then I have deep confidence that tremendously beautiful, healing things will happen.

—Brian Swimme

12.8 Transpersonal Psychology and Wellness

The realm of the transpersonal is becoming more acceptable today, even in mainstream thinking. Rather than seeing ourselves as merely "a skin-encapsulated ego" as Alan Watts once described us, many are now recognizing the more subtle connections we appear to all have with other life forms. Most people will accept the well-documented phenomenon that pets know things about their owners (such as when they will come home or that they need medical help) in ways that defy all rational scientific conventions. If pets can experience this connection, why can't we? We can! But only if we are willing to question that which has molded our reality to not include the transcendent in our worldview.

A new field of inquiry in psychology has emerged in the last thirty years, called the *fourth force*. (The first was Freudian psychoanalysis; the second, behavioral psychology; the third, humanistic psychology; and now the fourth: transpersonal psychology.) Transpersonal psychology seeks to incorporate the spiritual into the therapeutic process. It grows out of this expanding realization that energy is one; that there are multiple, or alternate, realities that many of us have touched in our transcending experiences; that ancient, religious, and mystical traditions have much to say to the condition of twenty-first-century woman and man; and that a transformation is taking place.

Investigators in this realm are examining areas once scoffed at (and still often exploited by hucksters)—such as mysticism, alchemy, astrology, faith and belief systems, dreams, meditation, prayer, and altered states of consciousness—to see how they relate to body and mind processes. Indeed, the existence of fourth force psychology testifies to a growing need for help in explaining, handling, and using such mystical, transcendent/transformational experiences.

Three of these areas—dream analysis, meditation and intuition—are accessible to all of us, and they will be addressed in modules 12.9, 12.10, and 12.11. They require no elaborate equipment, charts, or intermediaries. You can explore them yourself and reap whatever benefits you can from them.

12.9 Dreams

Dreams are particularly useful tools for developing self-understanding and self-awareness. Because they happen in sleep, in an altered state of consciousness, they often give us the side of the story that is outvoted when the rational, word-oriented brain is in control. Thus, they become a way of looking at a neglected part of ourselves.

There is a universal fascination with the content and meaning of dreams. We know their power because we have all awakened in terror, exhilaration, or sexual excitement as a result of one. Supermarket booklets of dream symbols offer elementary equations (for instance, an ocean means you want to take a trip) that generally leave the seeker dissatisfied. Since dreams are such highly personal experiences, simple explanations will not apply to everybody.

Theories regarding the meaning of dreams range from mechanistic (the mind is categorizing and filing the information of the day) to psychoanalytic (dreams express hidden desires that the conscious mind is afraid to face) to psychic (dreams are modes of spirit travel and ways of

A DREAM JOURNAL

Everybody dreams, every night. We know this because sleep researchers have shown that rapid eye movements (REM) correlate with the state of dreaming. We may not remember our dreams, but since we all experience REM during sleep, we all dream.

You can train yourself to remember your dreams in a number of different ways. The first and most effective is to give yourself the suggestion at night that you will recall your dreams in the morning. Place a pencil and paper (or a tape recorder) beside your bed; this will allow you to note even a few details that may bring back the fuller context the next day. The intention to work with dreams is often all it takes to begin to remember them. Do not become discouraged. For some, this intention and

practice takes several weeks; but in our experience it usually takes no more than a few days. When all else fails, Regina suggests eating an anchovy pizza just before retiring. While it won't make you dream any more, you may wake up repeatedly throughout the night—and remember your dreams better as a result.

Here are some practical suggestions:

- Pick out a special notebook and pen to use for your dream journal.

- Keep the pen and notebook in a clear space, next to your bed. Put it in the same place each night.

- Date the page at the top. Do this at night just before you turn out the light. Let it be a reminder to

yourself: "I am going to remember my dreams."

- Record dreams whenever you awake, during the night or in the morning. Don't wait.

- Write down anything you remember, even one word, or a disconnected fragment, a color, a feeling that the dream generated.

- Write in the first person, in the present tense. For example: "I am in my house and the water is running in the kitchen . . ."

- Describe the dream and the feelings it gave you, but avoid writing your interpretations at this time. That can come later.

- Read up on dreams. See books on dreams in "Suggested Reading" at the end of this chapter.

predicting the future). All of these are probably partially true.

A dream is like a movie, written, directed, and acted out by a whole range of characters in your personal consciousness. The parts you will remember most vividly are the parts that have something to say to you at the moment. You can, therefore, use them to great advantage.

A dream that is not understood is like a letter that is not opened.

—Talmud

Many years ago, Regina was at the point of going back to school to pursue her doctoral studies. She had a dream in which she needed to get to the airport to catch a plane for a very important meeting. These are the details she remembers most clearly: The plane would not take a direct route. To get to her destination, Seattle, she would have to go first from Denver to New Orleans—quite a circuit! The taxi to the airport never arrived, so she had to rely on hitchhiking. As she opened her suitcase, she found it filled with religious objects—rosary beads, prayer books, long black dresses, like the habits she had worn as a nun.

The dream had a powerful impact on her. In writing it down and telling it to her friends, she became aware of how many times she said things like:

- *"I feel pressured."*
- *"I'll be late."*
- *"Why do I have to take such a roundabout route to my destination?"*
- *"I'm not ready."*
- *"I have to get rid of this old junk before I can put in my new stuff."*

The more she dealt with these reactions, the clearer it became to her that these were the same

WORKING WITH A DREAM

Dreams not only provide us with information about ourselves, they can also serve as creative inspiration for poems or stories, paintings or inventions.

Ten Ways to Grow with Dreaming

1. Paint your dream.

2. Write your dream in a three-line poem, capturing its essence.

3. Compose a short story or an essay detailing your dream.

4. Dialogue with your dream characters—one at a time.

5. Dialogue with your dream symbols.

6. Play with the notion that the dream characters and dream symbols are all different parts, different aspects of yourself. Ah, what then?

7. Daydream and finish an unfinished dream in any way you would like it to turn out. Or redream a total dream, changing whatever you want to change.

8. Write down your ideal dream. What would it be about? What elements would it include?

9. Talk your dream out loud. Listen to the words you use, especially the phrases you may repeat. Listen for emotional as well as factual content. Ask yourself: to what situation in your present life do those same phrases and feelings relate?

10. Follow up on the intuitions you tap in dreams. Write a letter to the old friend you dreamed about. Call your mother on the phone when you dream about her. Wear a red shirt on the morning after a red dream. Look for connections all day long.

Happy dreaming.

feelings she had in planning for graduate school. One week after this dream, she withdrew her application for admission—and breathed a sigh of relief.

You can interpret your own dreams. Carl Jung speaks of the "Aha!" experience that accompanies dealing with dream content. "Aha!" means "Yes, that feels good to me," or "That applies to my life now," or "That's just the piece of the puzzle I've been looking for." Although experienced analysts can prove helpful, you are the only one who can generate "Aha!" about your dreams. *So, become your own expert.*

12.10 Coming Home to Ourselves

The stress of living in the twenty-first century on planet Earth requires the programming of safety valves to keep us healthy and happy. From every direction we are bombarded with forces that tend to draw us away from ourselves. The media tell us what we should like and dislike. Pressured jobs preoccupy us and can disturb our necessary sleep. Noises in the environment continually distract us from the task at hand. We can be left feeling like a battered boat on an angry sea—losing touch with what we really want, really believe, and ultimately, with who we *really are.* A daily practice of some spiritual nature, such as meditation, can help you keep your heart and mind open to possibility—even to miracles—and give you support and encouragement when the daily trials of modern life threaten to overwhelm you.

A variety of stress-reduction techniques and meditation forms have become increasingly popular because they work to help us in relaxing, concentrating, and attuning to the deeper, spiritual, creative self.

When we discussed Prigogene's theory earlier, we learned that it is the critical fluctuations that provoke a shift into a higher level of restructuring. Meditation, concentration, and other altered states of consciousness can cause just such critical fluctuations. Normal states of awareness show up on EEG machines as small rapid brain waves. They look something like this:

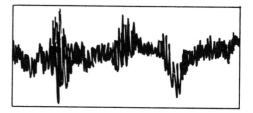

When people meditate, or move inward by other means, their brain waves slow down but also become larger, like this:

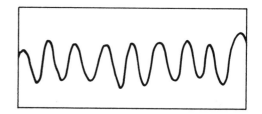

In other words, larger waves mean larger fluctuations affecting the structure. Such states, then, break habitual patterns and, in so doing, open the system to the possibility of a new shift—a leap in consciousness, perhaps. This might take the form of a more gentle approach to life, the ability to flow with contradictions rather than to be overwhelmed by them.

Or it may mean the opening of a new creative potential, since it has been demonstrated that meditation-like techniques enhance personal creativity.

Meditation, from the Sanskrit *medha,* literally means "doing the wisdom." It is a process of locating your center, your temple of inner wisdom, your truest self.

There are many different methods of "doing" meditation, ranging from drumming to chanting to breathing to simply sitting. Should you decide to explore some of them, there are general guidelines that apply to any type of meditation practice. They are presented here to help you on your way.

- *Be clear about what you want from a meditation practice. If you are using meditation as a means to relax and center yourself—essentially, as stress reduction—any one of a number of approaches will do. You can learn from books, from tapes, from friends, or from formal classes. If you want to practice meditation as a spiritual or religious discipline, it may be invaluable to have a teacher or a tradition with which to associate yourself. Meditation can take you deeply into yourself, and often you will appreciate the guidance of one who has walked this path before you.*

- *Make this your express intention. Set aside the time (perhaps ten or twenty minutes each morning and each evening) and prepare a quiet, private place for yourself. Although quiet or solitude isn't a prerequisite—you will eventually learn to meditate no matter what circumstances you are in—it does help in the initial stages to eliminate most of your usual distractions.*

- *Eliminate side trips. Meditation is an exercise of the right brain, the intuitive, spiritual, spontaneous side of you. As you meditate, the logical*

left brain will be busy trying to distract you. ("Remember to call Harry tonight." "This is a waste of time." "I wonder what the kids are doing now.") You will need to learn to set these distractions aside.*

- *Select a centering device. Most forms of meditation practice make use of some centering device to keep you on course. The most common is the focus on the breath. It can be a sound that is repeated, a word or song, or an object, like a candle or picture. It can be a repeated bodily movement. Once you choose a centering device to use, stick with it. Constantly dropping one approach to experiment with another form confuses the body-mind, so it never has a chance to learn to "rest" deeply.*

- *Ask for help. In many cities and on campuses around the country there are groups and organizations devoted to the teaching of meditation techniques. While it is not essential, joining such a group can be very helpful. Moreover, there is an intensified energy that develops when people meditate together.*

The more faithfully you listen to the voice within you, the better you will hear what is sounding outside.

—Dag Hammerskjold

Finding a center, a home, a place of balance, makes anything possible. The universe, from this perspective, is viewed as friendly, and our place in it is experienced as blessed. Life energy emanates from the center, and all that shares this energy is found there as well. Being there means being in harmony with ourselves, with our brothers and sisters, with our environment, our planet, our universe.

APPROACHES TO MEDITATION

A Candle Meditation

Light a candle in a semidarkened room. Place it about eighteen inches from you at eye level. Look at it. Become absorbed with it. As thoughts arise, bring your attention back to the awareness of the candle and flame. Try not to verbally analyze or describe what is taking place. Simply be with it.

Close your eyes and find the image imprinted on your eyelids. Stay with it. As it fades, open your eyes again and see the candle again. Do this for fifteen or twenty minutes.

Breath Awareness Meditation

Assume an upright posture, with a straight—but not rigid—spine. As you inhale, become aware of how breath enters, and aware of what (if anything) "moves" in the body as the breath progresses. Notice at what point the inhalation is completed. Gently keep your attention poised as inhalation becomes exhalation. Now watch as exhalation happens, noting what moves. Breathe normally without trying to change anything. The point is to simply be aware. Each time your mind wanders to another subject, simply bring it back softly to awareness of the breath. Do this for fifteen or twenty minutes.

Walking Meditation

You can do this at any time—either spontaneously as you walk to work, or formally in your room or garden—either barefoot or with shoes on.

Simply concentrate as fully as possible on the sensation of walking. Feel your heel contact the ground. Then attend to the ball of your foot and your toes as they come into play. Realize the motion involved in lifting your foot and preparing it for the next step.

You may wish to add the use of a word, or phrase, or affirmation so that you walk in step with an established inner rhythm.

Chants

Using your voice to repeat a song or chant is a doubly effective way to center yourself. Even greater is the effect when several people together chant the same sounds. Almost every religious tradition makes use of chants or hymns as a means of orienting the human with the realm of the Infinite. If you don't know any chants, hymns, or sacred songs, try making up your own refrains for these:

Peace, peace, peace, peace,
May peace fill up my heart.

All is One, All is One
All is One, All is One.

Truth and beauty are now
living in the temple of my soul.

See Appendix A for some beautiful recordings of chants and music for meditation.

12.11 Intuition and Wellness

> The intellect has little to do on the road to discovery. There comes a leap in consciousness, call it intuition or what you will, and the solution comes to you, and you don't know why or how.
>
> —Albert Einstein

Merriam-Webster's dictionary defines *intuition* as "quick and ready insight"; and "the power or faculty of attaining direct knowledge or cognition without evident rational thought and inference." It is derived from the Latin *intueri,* "to see within." It is a way of knowing, of sensing the truth without explanations.

Think of how many times in the last few months you've "known" or "sensed" something, but because you dismissed it and/or didn't act on it you lost out on some beneficial or helpful consequence. Or because you *did* act on it, something good came of it. The incidents can be minor or major. Maybe you were in the midst of an excessively busy day, but something told you to call a friend or colleague . . . for no good reason. Maybe you disregarded the inner "call" and learned later that your friend could have used some help at precisely that moment. On the positive side, while you may rarely enter contests or raffles, one day you do because you just *know* that you are going to win . . . and that is precisely what happens! Small examples, but many of us find them occurring regularly.

This chapter, and in fact this whole book, affirms that we humans know a lot more, and are capable of being a lot more than we generally imagine. Just as medical intuitive Carolyn Myss can sense when something is off in a person's system even before tests can verify it, most of us know when things aren't right with our health. We simply may not acknowledge to ourselves (or to anyone else) that we *do* know. We're afraid, perhaps. We may know when certain foods are not working for our overall health and strength, but we may not want to admit that truth because it might mean a major dietary change. We know when something is missing or something is not right in the emotional, intellectual, and spiritual domains as well. We also generally have an intuition about what that something is connected to, even if we are afraid to speak such a truth to ourselves because we are afraid of the implications. Where physical health is concerned, because our doctors or caregivers rarely ask us what *we* think is going on, we aren't challenged to listen deeply within to offer some of the valuable clues that could be a part of our healing process.

One of the advantages of our age is that we are seeing many old dualities dissolving—like the duality of communism versus capitalism; of science versus art; of spirituality versus psychology. Yet, other dichotomies—like the hard-and-fast duality of "healer/patient"—still hold us prisoner unless we take a stand to the contrary. Certainly, many fine doctors and healers *do* have more experience and training than their patients typically have, and their expertise should be respected. Yet, we know that the best healers among us will call upon the patient's own self-knowledge to accomplish a transformation; body, mind, emotions, and spirit all aligned and working together to the benefit of the whole.

Those who have a broad view of human possibilities will all affirm the same thing: intuition (called by many different names) can be nurtured and developed. We can learn to see more, to feel more, to sense more, to know things about ourselves and the world we live in—things that would benefit us all.

What we now overlook or dismiss as irrelevant or unimportant often holds precious clues to self-knowledge that are there for the taking, if we know where and how to look. In developing intuition we develop self-knowledge and self-appreciation, and self-appreciation allows us to develop self-trust. And genuine self-trust (not inflated egoism) creates a greater sense of awe at the mystery of this life in which we are all engaged.

When the scientist listens, the artist imagines, the mathematician calculates, or the poet waits for the muse to guide fancy into word pictures, each is praying for divine guidance. And each receives as much guidance as he or she is capable of perceiving.

—Ernest Holmes

How do we develop intuition? Well, we begin by acknowledging that such a thing exists. Openness to it is the first step. If we find that we are telling ourselves a story of "this can't happen for me," or "I'll never get this," we might watch that tendency for negative thinking, and simply divert it before it becomes entrenched in us.

Second, we watch for the arising of "intuitive knowings." We pay attention to what happens in our own mind or body when various situations, especially decisions, are presented to us. Instead of immediately trying to think out the solution to something, we can attune our other senses to get promptings or clues about which direction to move in.

Third, we allow ourselves time to wait; time to let this new knowledge emerge, according to its own schedule. Artists call this "waiting upon the muse."

Fourth, we might pray for guidance and help in "knowing." Many people find that a morning period of meditation is a time in which to rededicate themselves to serving God, or the Good, or Divine Spirit, or simply the relief of the sufferings of others. Once their overall orientation is set for the day, they then proceed to ask for their "work orders"—for example, "What needs my attention today in order to further the overall good?" In a period of silent attention, they allow whatever is being asked to rise to the surface of consciousness.

Where health and wellbeing are concerned, we hope that you will use everything you know to further your wellbeing. Take the risk of telling your caregiver what you sense is going on. Remember that radical honesty with yourself is one of the most challenging tasks you can set for yourself. It is so easy to fool ourselves, to postpone facing something we know but won't admit. Be gentle with yourself in the process. Use one or more of the modalities suggested throughout this book—dream work, journal writing, prayer, meditation, visualization—to help you to access what you already know. If you don't speak your intuitions to somebody or act on them, at first, why not try just writing them down when they occur? When you begin to see how often they prove to be true, you may be more inspired to start trusting them.

Intuition is not a startling gift that is the province of a few psychics. It is less about divining the future than it is about entering more authentically into the present. Intuition is always operative, so common that it often evades conscious recognition.

—Joan Borysenko

TRANSCENDENCE AND THE QUEST FOR ENLIGHTENMENT

The subject of wellness is integrally connected to the subject of "waking up" or "enlightenment," as it is called in many spiritual traditions. In fact, throughout this chapter we have hinted at a type of consciousness that is universal, cosmic perhaps, and one that is certainly not limited by the notion that we are, have ever been, or could ever be *separate entities,* or that we could manage our lives alone, apart from everything else that exists.

While many people think of this quest for enlightenment as being largely a self-obsessed "navel gazing" endeavor, the fact is that mystics and sages throughout time have pointed to the necessity of microcosmic understanding (or self-knowledge) as a prelude to understanding the macrocosm. They point out that the two merely mirror and reflect one another—a view that contemporary science would affirm.

Attempting to change the world "for the better" when our own minds are plagued with confusion and uncertainty can definitely feel like a futile gesture. At the same time, however, we must recognize that enlightenment may not really be equivalent to some state of perfection—some magical place of total balance and harmony. Rather, to be "awake," as many of the greatest teachers and sages have always indicated, is to be fluid and receptive to *all* that life has to offer—including the states of confusion and uncertainty that dominate our consciousness for periods of time.

Our goal then, in wellness as well as in the quest for enlightenment, should probably not be about achieving some static state of nonreactivity. Rather, wellness will be about learning to ride the waves, and gaining ever-greater clarity about what is optimally called for moment to moment.

Here's what Buddhist teacher and writer Pema Chödrön has to say about this:

There's a common misunderstanding among all the human beings who have ever been born on the earth that the best way to live is to try to avoid pain and just try to get comfortable. You can see this even in insects and animals and birds. All of us are the same. A much more interesting, kind, adventurous, and joyful approach to life is to begin to develop our curiosity, not caring whether the object of our inquisitiveness is bitter or sweet.

Pema Chödrön, *The Wisdom of No Escape and the Path of Loving-Kindness* (Shambhala, 1991).

12.12 Transcending . . . Slowly

If the road to enlightenment were not littered with land mines and other obstacles, it probably would have become a superhighway by now. The gradual (or even sudden) awakening into the more spiritual dimensions is not an easy process, as the busy-ness of modern life makes it very easy to avoid exploring the deeper layers of the Iceberg Model.

Many other factors have cut us off from our most intuitive roots, from our connection to the Spirit. We have never established as firm a bond with our mothers and fathers as have most tribal peoples. We have suffered the normative abuse of children by modern child-rearing practices: high-tech births, cribs, circumcision, artificial baby milk, being isolated in strollers rather than being carried in arms or a sling, and being left to cry alone in a separate room. No wonder we often feel alienated, with no place in our hearts to call home. Few of us even know what we are missing unless we have studied the behavior of people who *are* deeply connected, and there are fewer and fewer of them to study as the seductive glitter of Westernization spreads like a cancer around the globe.

Awakening to God is often conceived of as a victory because of the illusion that there is something to attain, that there is a battle to be won. Actually, enlightenment is a defeat because all one does is become ordinary.

—Lee Lozowick

Given the difficulty of this path of spiritual exploration, confusion and paradox can be anticipated at every turn. We must learn how to strive for ideals yet not be too hard on ourselves when we fall into the gap that lies between them and our present reality. Learning to function while in this gap is perhaps the most important skill we can learn, along with how to give generous amounts of love to others and ourselves.

We advocate the approach summed up in the statement that "simple is best." If the ideas in this chapter have seemed remote to you, please don't feel left out. Our orientation betrays years of spiritual searching, for better or worse. Transcending need not be cosmic or spiritual at all. In fact, ageless wisdom supports that we are truly in harmony only when we are experiencing the simple and ordinary of life *as* the simple and ordinary of life.

Transcending is about moving from complexity to greater and greater simplicity. Therefore, each time you make even a tiny step in eliminating excess baggage from your environment, from your diet, or from your mind, you are moving toward greater wellness. Each time you pose a new question, open a new door, willingly challenge any limit you have placed upon yourself, you are, in a sense, transcending.

SUGGESTED READING

Benson, R., *The Relaxation Response* (Avon, 2000).

Brennan, B., *Light Emerging* (Bantam, 1993).

Chödrön, P., *The Wisdom of No Escape, and the Path of Loving-Kindness* (Shambhala, 1991).

Dossey, L., *Healing Words* (Harper Mass Market, 1997).

——, *Prayer Is Good Medicine* (HarperCollins, 1997).

Foundation for Inner Peace, *A Course in Miracles* (1975).

Jung, C., *Man and His Symbols* (Laure Leaf, 1997).

Leonard, G., *Mastery: The Keys to Success and Long-Term Fulfillment* (Plume, 1992).

LeShan, L., *How to Meditate* (HarperCollins, 1995).

Levine, S., *A Year to Live: How to Live This Year As If It Were Your Last* (Three Rivers Press, 1998).

Mitchell, S., *Tao Te Ching: A New English Version* (HarperPerennial, 1992).

Moore, T., *Original Self* (HarperCollins, 2000).

Murphy, M., *The Future of the Body* (J. P. Tarcher, 1993).

Myss, C., and C. N. Shealy, *The Creation of Health: The Emotional, Psychological, and Spiritual Responses That Promote Health and Healing* (Three Rivers Press, 1998).

O'Reilly, M. R., *Radical Presence: Teaching as Contemplative Practice* (Heinemann, 1998).

Ram Dass, *Still Here: Embracing Aging, Changing, and Dying* (Riverhead, 2000).

——, *Be Here Now* (Crown, 1971).

Schulz, M., and C. Northrup, *Awakening Intuition: Using Your Mind-Body Network for Insight and Healing* (Three Rivers Press, 1999).

Sheldrake, R., *A New Science of Life: The Hypothesis of Formative Causation* (Inner Traditions, 1995).

Wilber, K., *A Brief History of Everything* (Shambhala Publications, 2001).

Wilson, R. A., *The Cosmic Trigger* (New Falcon Publications, 1993).

Zukav, G., *The Dancing Wu Li Masters* (Bantam Books, 1994).

For an updated listing of resources and active links to the websites mentioned in this chapter, please see www.WellnessWorkbook.com.

NOTES

1. Ferguson, M., *The Aquarian Conspiracy* (J. P. Tarcher, 1980), 171.

2. Simonton, C., S. Matthews-Simonton, and J. Creighton, *Getting Well Again* (J. P. Tarcher, 1978). Contact the Simonton Cancer Center, P.O. Box 890, Pacific Palisades, CA 90272, (800) 459-3424, (310) 457-3811, www.simontoncenter.com.

3. "'I am not the body; I am the soul'—Breaking Limits with Sri Chinmoy: An interview with Ashrita Furman by Elizabeth Debold." *What Is Enlightenment?* magazine (Fall–Winter 2002), 65–77.

Selected Music for Wellbeing

People have long used music for many purposes, including relaxation, healing rituals, and spiritual inspiration. Music reduces stress and stimulates creativity. Because it can provoke all the emotions, it can assist us in grieving, or provoke ecstasy and dance.

In recent years, music has reemerged as a healing modality; it is now being used and recommended in treatment centers for cancer and other life-threatening illnesses, in hospices and related "transition" programs, and even in conventional hospitals. Music therapy has taken its place beside art and dance therapy.

A wide range of music, recordings of environmental sounds, and chants from a variety of religious traditions are now easy to acquire. Whatever your need or condition, you can find music that will assist you in your healing, your practice, or simply your overall wellbeing.

Whether you are looking for music to accompany your yoga exercises, to enhance your immune system, or to uplift your spirits, the choices are enormous. This listing highlights a few of the many excellent music resources and musical selections available. Consider it a jumping-off point for further investigation. Links for many of these resources (and updates as well) can be accessed directly at www.WellnessWorkbook.com.

Websites

For education about music and healing:

> www.healingmuses.org

> www.healersway.com

For purchasing music and other music resources:

> www.fourgates.com/music.asp

> www.backroadsmusic.com

> www.healingproducts.com

> www.nature-music-therapy.com

> www.amazon.com

Educational Resources

Music as Medicine: The Art and Science of Healing with Sound by Kay Gardner. Using twenty-three years of experience in the field, this educational series explores the unseen relationship between brainwaves and music; music therapy techniques; the law of octaves; the nine healing elements of music; simple exercises for finding your own tone; and much more. Gardner teaches the major elements and techniques within the science of sound healing, and explains how they are used to "entrain" (synchronize) the body to harmonize with the hidden vibrations of the universe. She unravels mysteries of music's therapeutic role through the ages, and shares new research into how sound vibrations affect the chakras and auric fields that many believe surround us. The result is this twelve-session curriculum—complete with exercises—on every phase of Gardner's pioneering system for creating melodies, rhythms, and harmonies with the power to heal. Six audiocassettes.

Healing with Great Music: How the World's Great Music Can Inspire Your Heart and Your Health by Don Campbell. Ancient Greek philosophers believed that the human soul could be perfected through sublimely composed music. This astonishing concept is actually being mirrored by research that points to the links between sound and a balanced, energetic life. Explore these findings and the phenomenal effects of sound on the human body-mind with Don Campbell, author of *The Mozart Effect* and the founder of the Institute for Music, Health, and Education. Learn how music can help orchestrate improved health by its effects on awareness states, movement, the imagination, language development, and even specific functions of the body. Two audiocassettes.

Body-Mind Healing Music

Sound Body/Sound Mind by Andrew Weil, M.D., and others. A multifaceted sonic tool for health, relaxation, and wellbeing. Dr. Weil and brainwave expert Anna Wise have designed a sound/brainwave frequency schematic. Soothing music from Mozart, Mahler, Bach, and Brahms has been rearranged to complement the frequency score. Performed by Arcangelos, this recording facilitates deep, self-directed healing through pulse-entraining rhythms, timbres, and melodies combined with clinically tested sound-wave technology. *Sound Body* opens with a brief meditation by Dr. Weil before a sixty-minute sonic journey in which your brain is coaxed into subconscious brainwave states conducive to self-directed healing. *Sound Mind,* the companion album, explores sound healing. Dr. Weil speaks on music and sound in health. Anna Wise explains frequencies, and Joshua Leeds elaborates on psycho-acoustics. Double CD and sixty-four-page booklet.

The Magic of Healing Music by Deepak Chopra, M.D. Music, through its vibratory impulses on the human heart, can be a subtle yet powerful healing force, restoring balance to the mind and body. These melodies and rhythms are designed to create harmony between the environment and the body, mind, and spirit. *The Magic of Healing Music* provides nourishing, harmonizing sounds to help balance the basic forces of nature that govern our lives. Double CD.

Cho Ku Rei by Weave. This music, designed for Reiki healing, is equally effective for bodywork, meditation, simple relaxation, or nighttime listening. Warm melodies, plenty of space between the musical passages, and an overall sense of wellbeing fill this recording. Single CD.

Healing Journey by Emmett Miller, M.D. Many people find this beautiful recording perfect for any illness or imbalance—physical, mental, or emotional. It features the music of Raphael, a symphony composed specifically to enhance Dr. Miller's imagery and performed by world-renowned artists. Guided by Dr. Miller's voice, you can relax deeply in a safe place, contact and gently awaken your inner healer, and guide the healing energy to the part of you that thirsts for it. Side two, *Breathing Music,* presents the same musical tapestry without words, to nurture and support your inner journey. Single audiocassette. Other selections from Dr. Miller can be found at www.drmiller.com.

Treasures of the Heart: Keepsakes of the Harp by various harp musicians. The harp is one of the most characteristic instruments of a timeless healing tradition. In ancient times, harpists used three properties, or strains, in their music, each property having a different effect. The "sleep strain" lulled people to sleep, the "sorrow strain" caused people to weep, and the "joy strain" encouraged people to laugh. These three harp strains are still properties of harp music today—music that can lull us into a restful state, bring tears to our eyes from its beauty, or enliven us and set the foot tapping. Playing the harp confers a special privilege upon all harpists— the ability to unlock the doors of the soul. Nineteen accomplished therapeutic harp practitioners use their healing art to take you on a journey of peace and restoration. These tunes will fill you with images of lively places, contemplative sanctuaries, and pastures of melancholy. Single CD.

Chants and Healing Mantras

Christian

Women in Chant: Chants by Women in Praise of the Divine by the Benedictine nuns of Regina Laudis. The nuns of the Regina Laudis Abbey invite you to enter their sacred cloister and into the divine mystery embodied within the spiritual cycles of a woman's life—the virgin, the bride, the spouse, and the mother. Recorded for the first time is a complete repertoire of prayer in song to the Four Virgin Martyrs and Our Lady of Sorrows—a celebration devoted solely to the praise of womanhood and the Divine. For the women of Regina Laudis, this is much more than a musical performance: it is the highest form of prayer, a deep and abiding contemplative practice "with the power to communicate to listeners the life of God as no other music does." Twenty-four hymns, antiphons, and other works in the original Latin. Single CD with accompanying booklet.

Vox de Nube: A "Voice from the Cloud" by Ní Riain. Nóirín Ní Riain and the monks of Glenstal Abbey continue a thousand-year-old tradition: giving voice to mystical hymns of praise, inviting us to link heaven and earth. For its rare examples of Western liturgical chant, this recording is certainly important. As vocal music, it thrums with mystical vitality. Nóirín's singing is startling in its clarity, blissful, and evocative of profound spiritual grace. Single CD.

Buddhist

Drops of Emptiness: Songs, Chants, and Poems by Thich Nhat Hanh, Sister Chan Khong, and the Monks and Nuns of Plum Village. In the Vietnamese Zen tradition, mindfully chosen music and words can serve as "soothing droplets" to cool the heart. Recorded on location at Plum Village in France. These deeply felt works include poetry of legendary Zen Master Thich Nhat Hanh and the Vietnamese folk songs and Buddhist hymns of Sister Chan Khong. One review wrote, "Sister Chan Khong . . . sings poems and prayers with the power of the angels. . . ." Single audiocassette or CD.

Sacred Mantras for Peace and Happiness by the Monks of the Tolu Tharling Monastery: Music for Reflection and Relaxation from the Far East. Some of the most loved and sought-after mantras from India and Tibet; some of the proceeds go to support the monastery. From the liner notes: "Music and religion have always been two of humanity's great refuges from the travails of reality and, at best, towards a higher consciousness. Appreciation of the two in combination should not be the sole preserve of the enlightened." Double CD.

Chants to Awaken the Buddhist Heart by Lama Surya Das and Steven Halpern. A mixture of ancient Buddhist mantras with Western styles, this musical selection is a historical collaboration between chant master Lama Surya Das and composer Steven Halpern. Innovative musical arrangements encompass traditional and Sanskrit chants, while rich instrumentals show flavors of hip-hop, Indian raga, and a dash of Jimi Hendrix–style rock. Single CD.

Jewish

Sacred Chants of the Contemporary Synagogue. This live recording features New York mezzo-soprano Cantor Rebecca Garfein in a 1997 Berlin Jewish Cultural Festival concert, documenting the first female cantor to sing in Germany as a soloist. Breaking a new barrier for women with this concert, Cantor Garfein is accompanied by New York organist Arnold Ostlund Jr. and Berlin's nine-voice Pestalozzistrasse Synagogue Choir. Cantor Garfein is the musical leader of the Riverdale Temple in Riverdale, New York. The cantorial music featured on the CD is operatic in character, featuring some of the most popular prayers sung in modern synagogues in the United States. Highlighted on the CD are Ravel's memorial *Kaddisch* and Kurt Weill's *Sabbath Kiddush*. Also featured is Max Janowski's *Avinu Malkeynu*, a well-known prayer sung as part of the High Holy Day liturgy. Single CD.

Indian/Hindu

Magical Healing Mantras by Namasté. Twenty-five musicians, united from around the world, use their voices, guitars, flutes, sitars, tablas, and a tarang to create this memorable East-West musical fusion that is both exotic and familiar. The healing and transformational powers of these seven Sanskrit mantras are available to all who listen. This recording features the Gayatri Mantra, and will calm the mind with tones meant to bring peace and healing to the listener. Single CD.

Door of Faith by Krishna Das. Original songs, invocations, and Sanskrit prayers, recorded with violin, cello, organ, trumpet, piano, and guitar, merge into a semiclassical fusion of Sanskrit and Hindi verses with Indian music. This recording allows listeners into their own world, whether practicing yoga, meditating, or decompressing from the stress of the workaday world. Single CD.

Healing Mantras: Sacred Chants from India by Shri Anandi Ma and Dileepji Pathak. The yogic healing arts of India—a tradition that dates back at least 5,000 years—postulate that all illness is the result of a disturbance in the *prana,* or human energy field. On this CD, Shri Anandi Ma, respected master of the Kundalini Maha Yoga lineage, chants three mantras specifically to reestablish balance on the level of the prana. These chants can impart a powerful healing impulse to the entire human system—body, mind, and spirit. Accompanied by Shri Dileepji Pathak on tamboura, flute, and violin. Single CD and fourteen-page booklet.

Sufic/Islamic

Sufi Chants from Cairo by La Confrerie Chadhiliyya. Sufism began as early as the eighth century. Works like this serve to help the practitioner gain direct experiential contact with God, using techniques that heighten concentration and spiritual awareness. Sufis who practice rituals such as *sama'* or *dhikr,* or who participate in the whirling dances made famous by Turkish dervishes, will especially appreciate these recordings. Others will appreciate the expressive Arabic poetry and Koranic detail that is offered. Poetic and rhythmic, making use of Asma'u l-Lahi l'husna (the beautiful names of God) in various modes, this recording demonstrates techniques that inspire many and are works of linguistic beauty for all. Single CD.

Meditation/Relaxation

Music for Zen Meditation: Shakuhachi Flute Compositions by Riley Lee. Riley Lee creates a quiet pathway to an inner peace with soothing solos and duets. Tracks such as "Sea Breezes," "Under the Stars," "Divine Ecstasy," "Whispers of Eternity," and "Soaring with the Eagles" are a few of the twenty-two selections. Don't let the title limit your imagination. Yoga practitioners, meditation students, massage therapists, healers, and people who love beautiful, gentle, uplifting, and soothing sounds all have responded well to this title. Double CD.

Timeless Motion and *Fragrances of a Dream* by Daniel Kobialka. *Timeless Motion* contains a unique rendition of Pachelbel's Canon in D, a soothing classic, plus two original compositions, *Timeless Motion* and *Lullaby*. *Fragrances of a Dream* features compositions by Erik Satie, plus a distinctive rendition of Bach's Air on a G String (as popularized by Procol Harum in *A Whiter Shade of Pale*). Bernie Siegel, M.D., says, "I found years ago that music creates a healing; I find Kobialka's to be the best available." One CD each.

The Silent Path by Robert Haig Coxon. One of the first and most enduring titles recommended to massage practitioners from coast to coast, this combinination of gentle keyboards, Tibetan gongs, and orchestral instruments such as oboe and flute makes for deeply moving, peaceful music. Coxon adds a few Pachelbel-like touches along the way. This title can be played for years without losing any of its appeal. Single CD.

Classical, European

Classical music, particularly pre-twentieth century, may express struggle and conflict, but the outcome is always redemptive rather than hopeless. Instead of causing you to separate or disassociate from your body, these musical compositions encourage an alignment within you, helping you to harmonize yourself with the natural healing rhythm of your own body and the healing energies of the earth.

The pre-Baroque and Baroque periods offer much music that is soothing, full, rich, and harmonious. There are many recorded collections of this music that offer favorites like Pachelbel's Canon in D and compositions by Vivaldi, Scarlatti, Handel, Monteverdi, and Palestrina. Almost anything by J. S. Bach is wonderful. Start with any of the *Brandenburg Concertos;* these contain a tremendous variety of moods and feelings, from joy and serenity to deep sorrow. And, if you have about four hours of listening time, experience the *Saint Matthew Passion.*

Listening to music that expresses pure sorrow can be transforming of one's own sorrow. Beethoven, in particular, transformed his grief and sorrow into works of great beauty and redemption. For a mood of happiness and contentment, listen to his Sixth Symphony; for pure joy, his Ninth Symphony ends with the famous "Ode to Joy."

The music of Wolfgang Amadeus Mozart generally inspires a sense of magic, joy, and delight and offers much to choose from: symphonies (start with the *Jupiter* Symphony), violin concerti, piano concerti, operas, sonatas for almost every instrument, and more. If you weren't fortunate enough to have seen *Amadeus* in a 70-mm movie theater, rent it from your video store.

Many excellent recordings of Chopin's music are available, particularly his nocturnes for piano, which are dreamy, contemplative, and restful.

Mahler's symphonies are great. For delightful, life-giving sounds listen to his Fourth Symphony.

Almost anything written for violin is usually heart-filling. There are violin concertos by Bach, Mozart, Beethoven, Mendelssohn, Bruch, Tchaikovsky, and many other composers. The cello, too, seems to resonate deep within the body. Choose from among many wonderful compositions written for the cello. String quartets, especially those of Beethoven, can also be uplifting.

The Mozart Effect

Music for the Mozart Effect #1: Strengthen the Mind. For intelligence and learning: It is designed to "charge the brain"—to achieve the kind of effect documented in the innovative research done in the early 1990s by Frances H. Rauscher, Ph.D., at the University of California at Irvine, which found measurable IQ increases after listening to certain Mozart pieces. Use it before and while studying and reading. Single CD.

Music for the Mozart Effect #2: Heal the Body. Designed to soothe and relax your body, and reduce mental and emotional stress, this recording is great for unwinding at the end of a busy day and will help you achieve a state of calm and tranquility in the face of the pressures of life. It is also good for quiet times or relaxed, romantic dinners, or for gently floating toward sleep at day's end. Includes selections from the String Quartet no. 16, Piano Concerti no. 20 in D Minor and no. 21 in C Major, Concerto for Flute and Harp, Sonata no. 1 for Organ and Orchestra, and the "Posthorn" Serenade no. 9. Single CD.

Music for the Mozart Effect #3: Unlock Creative Spirit. Designed to help you access your creative voice. Personal expression, be it in the form of journaling, drawing, painting, or simply letting the imagination run free, is an important part of mental and spiritual health. Mozart can provide a pathway to your personal creativity, unlocking waves of images and impressions and amplifying the expressive inner voices. Includes selections from Twelve German Dances, String Quartet in D Major, Symphony no. 4 in D Major, Piano Concerto no. 1 in D Major, and the Piano Variations on "Ah, Vous dirai-je, Maman." Single CD.

Nature's Creatures and Sounds

Dolphin Song by Bjorn Melander. Dolphin songs joined together in harmony with the relaxing, peaceful tones of the harp and flute. Experience a connection with these great mammals' consciousness and you will be filled with their joy and playfulness. Single CD.

Whale Song by Bjorn Melander. *Whale Song* harmonizes the beautifully gentle sounds of the flute and keyboard with recordings of songs from wild orcas (killer whales). This recording will take you on a journey to experience the wisdom and grandeur of the whales. Single CD.

Individual environmental sounds. Environmental sounds, such as the sounds of ocean waves, the rainforest, thunderstorm, and bird song, are excellent for relaxation and for encouraging sleep. Find many choices at www.nature-music-therapy.com.

Music for Dying and Other Transitions

Graceful Passages: A Companion for Living and Dying. A two-CD set with a fifty-six-page gift book, featuring an introduction by Ira Byock, M.D., and foreword by Sam Keen. The project consists of music with timeless messages and prayers for those facing life-threatening illness, preparing for dying, or meeting other transitions. The spoken-word portions are by Elisabeth Kübler-Ross, Ram Dass, Thich Nhat Hanh, Rabbi Zalman Schachter-Shalomi, Arun and Sunanda Gandhi, and other mentors and guides. The stirring and heartfelt music is by Emmy award–winning composer Gary Malkin. Many other artists contribute to the music tracks, which underscore the narrative and spoken-word portions, and appear as a collection of instrumental-only selections on the second disc. This inspired blending of words and music opens hearts and serves as "soundtracks to your soul"; it is a powerful tool for the grieving as well as a mirror for the aching heart. Double CD and book.

Before Their Time (vols. I and II) by various artists. A collection of songs and music written in memory of people who died young. Featuring original performances by the singer-songwriters and composers, this benefit album was produced by the father of a young man who took his own life. A music resource for people mourning the death of someone close, the music on *Before Their Time* brings comfort, healing, and hope, wrapped in a wide variety of musical styles, ranging from classics by internationally known artists to a début song and performance. *Before Their Time* was produced with grants and donations from foundations and individuals, and all sales of the album benefit suicide prevention and hospice organizations. Extensive liner notes include song lyrics and notes on each selection—many by the artists themselves—plus essays about surviving suicide, music's powerful role in the healing process, SOS (Survivors of Suicide), and hospice bereavement support groups. Includes a listing of Web links to related sites. Each volume is a single CD.

APPENDIX B

A Personal Wellness Journal

What Is It?

A Personal Wellness Journal is a notebook, diary, scrapbook, or computer file. It is *personal* because it is private and confidential. It is a wellness journal because it is used, either in conjunction with the *Wellness Workbook,* or separately, as a means of enhancing your health and overall wellbeing. It is a *journal* because it is a dated, written record.

What Should the Journal Be Used For?

Use your journal for anything and everything you wish, and especially for responding to the exercises suggested and the questions raised in this *Workbook.* For instance, we and our friends, students, and associates have used the journal:

- *To keep notes from wellness-related lectures or workshops*

- *To summarize wellness-related books or articles*

- *To record memorable quotes*

- *To list the questions that arise about health and wellbeing*

- *As a scrapbook in which to store special articles, cartoons, and pictures that pertain to wellness*

- *For poetry writing*

- *As a dream diary*

- *To chart an exercise schedule (as suggested in chapter 5)*

- *To track how various food, meals, times of eating, and quantities affect overall energy and mental clarity (as suggested in chapter 4)*

- *To record goals, inspirations, and prayers*

What Should I Use for My Journal?

Use a form that feels comfortable for you. Some may prefer to keep their journal on their computer, but if you like the idea of a book, choose one that suits your taste and personality. Hardbound or softbound is up to you. If you travel a lot, a hardbound journal is essential, as softcovers tend to fall apart more easily. Regina suggests using a book whose pages can't easily be removed. It helps to keep the sloppy work and the perfect work together in one place, to give a whole picture of yourself. The page size should be large enough to allow for an occasional sketch, or a complete letter (Regina recommends a book that is at least eight inches square). A tiny book might discourage you from expressing yourself fully.

Is There a Standard Way to Keep a Journal?

There are some guidelines for keeping a Personal Wellness Journal, but there is no one right way—there is only *your* way.

- *Be honest with yourself. Dare to admit to your journal what you might be afraid to admit to someone else. Converse with yourself as if you were a most trusted friend. Address yourself by name, if you care to: "Yes, Nathan, things are tough right now . . ."*

- *Avoid self-editing and self-criticism. You will do yourself a big favor if you write quickly and avoid reading over your entry until you think it is complete. Since so much of our unhappiness is often the result of feeling inadequate, many people have the tendency to stop themselves from producing something out of fear that it will be unacceptable. However, you may be amazed at how easily and prolifically you can express yourself when you put the critic to rest for a while. Just do it!*

- *Don't be limited by writing or speaking logically in only full sentences, or even in words. You may really enjoy challenging yourself with different modes of expression. If you usually write only narrative, try poetry for a change or draw with crayons for a few days. Try making an audio recording in which you talk or sing to yourself, or just make sounds that feel good or express your feelings.*

- *Date all your work. This is a valuable way of charting your progress.*

- -

SUGGESTED READING

Adams, K., *Journal to the Self: Twenty-Two Paths to Personal Growth* (Warner, 1990).

Cameron, J., *The Artist's Way: A Spiritual Path to Higher Creativity* (J. P. Tarcher, 1994).

Rainer, T., *The New Diary: How to Use a Journal for Self-Guidance and Expanded Creativity* (J. P. Tarcher, 1979).

Capacchione, L., *The Creative Journal: The Art of Finding Yourself* (New Page, 2001).

Sark, *Sark's Journal and Play!Book: A Place to Dream While Awake* (Celestial Arts, 1993) or any of her other titles.

For an updated listing of resources please see www.WellnessWorkbook.com.

Index

Beyond This Book

This book is about personal growth. It is also about changing our existing attitudes and behaviors. Many of our cultural norms subtly reinforce feelings of powerlessness, alienation, or isolation, and often reward illness and nonresponsibility. Although you may be excited by many of the ideas and feelings you experience reading the book and taking the Wellness Index, they will likely have little lasting influence as long as you live your life in an environment where there is little support for these values.

In making life changes, a supportive network of like-minded people is of tremendous value. One highly effective way you can use this workbook is by meeting regularly with a group of friends to share and discuss the ideas and exercises in the book.

Safe spaces allow people to experience an atmosphere of openness, trust, and honesty. Such spaces can be created wherever there is a group of caring and committed people. It may manifest as a support group that meets regularly at someone's home or at a community space or church. It could be a group of like-minded people at your place of work, or it could be a whole community working together to understand and respect each other's commonalities and differences.

Supportive environments are so rare that most people don't even notice when they don't have any. Those people have either never experienced a supportive environment or dismissed the rare experience as an oddity and never considered it as a possible norm for their life.

We are convinced that people grow and evolve more readily with regular access to a supportive environment. If you have one, rejoice and let us know about it. If you don't have a support group, we urge you to find or create one.

Other resources that can help with lasting lifestyle improvements are wellness coaching and the Wellness Inventory Online. For current information and ideas for support, visit www.Wellness Workbook.com.

About the Authors

John W. Travis, M.D., M.P.H., completed his medical degree at Tufts University and his preventive medicine residency at Johns Hopkins University. He began his career in wellness in the 1970s while serving with the U.S. Public Health Service's Division of Health Services Research, where he developed one of the first computerized health risk appraisals.

In 1975, he gave up the practice of sick-care to open the world's first wellness center, the Wellness Resource Center, in Mill Valley, California. This work attracted international attention culminating in an appearance on *60 Minutes* with Dan Rather in 1979. When the Center was transformed into a nonprofit educational consulting group, Wellness Associates (see the opposite page), John began to present programs around the world for helping professionals interested in the Center's approach—a paradigm of egalitarian partnership focused on enhancing wellness—rather than the authoritarian medical model of fixing "problems."

Out of this work he discovered that authoritarian cultures remain in power through their self-perpetuating, non-nurturing treatment of pregnancy and childhood. Realizing that infant wellness is the precursor to adult wellness, he cofounded the Alliance for Transforming the Lives of Children in 1999 (www.aTLC.org) together with his wife, Meryn Callander, and eleven other professionals. By addressing the critical role of the early years of life in optimizing human development, aTLC takes John's initial wellness work to the foundations of wellbeing.

Besides the *Wellness Workbook,* his publications include the "Wellness Inventory" (1975, 1981, 1988, 2002); *Simply Well: Choices for a Healthier Life* (1990, 2000), coauthored with Regina; *Wellness for Helping Professionals: Creating Compassionate Cultures* (1990); and *A Change of Heart: The Global Wellness Inventory* (1993), coauthored with Meryn Callander.

Together with HealthWorld Online, he has produced the Wellness Inventory Online (see www.WellnessWorkbook.com). This is available for individual use as well as for licensing by hospitals, health spas, and corporations that care about their employee's state of wellness.

In 2000, John, Meryn, and their daughter Juniper moved to E. Gippsland, Victoria, Australia (Meryn's homeland). John spends several months each summer traveling in the United States to facilitate the aTLC network.

Regina Sara Ryan is a wellness consultant and managing editor for a small publishing company. She also serves as a graduate advisor in the fields of religious studies and human development at Prescott College, in Prescott, Arizona. Regina is the coauthor of *Simply Well* (with John) and the author of numerous books, including *After Surgery, Illness, or Trauma: 10 Practical Steps to Renewed Energy and Health; The Woman Awake: Feminine Wisdom for Spiritual Life;* and *Praying Dangerously*. She lives with her husband, Jere Pramuk, and a small community of friends in Paulden, Arizona.

Wellness Associates

Wellness Associates is a nonprofit educational organization dedicated to enhancing personal and planetary wellbeing. It is the successor to the Wellness Resource Center founded by John in 1975. Our commitment is to support people in developing and sustaining the awareness and skills needed to create new cultures—cultures wherein norms supporting personal integrity, authenticity, and partnership replace the existing cultural norms of domination, submission, and competition. A major focus is on fostering a shift from the current culture's emphasis on authoritarianism and domination to one of partnership and cooperation.

More recently, John and his wife, Meryn Callander, created the Wellspring Online, a part of Wellness Associates that focuses on infant wellness and the prevention of many conditions that lead people to seek wellness programs as adults. The Wellspring Online features extensive synopses of books about optimal human development and wellness of children along with reviews of nonviolent children's books.

John is now offering public presentations around the world on the subject of "Why Men Leave," based on his own experience of being poorly attached as a child and the subsequent dissolution of his first marriage.

As part of his work with aTLC (see John's biography) and from the perspective of our gifts arising from our wounds, John both illustrates how the aTLC *Blueprint of Principles and Actions* fosters the optimal development of children by more fully meeting their early nurturing needs, and details how wellness rather than violence, addiction, and depression can be passed to future generations.

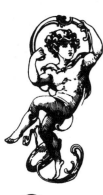
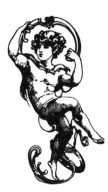

GRAND CERTIFICATE

This GRAND CERTIFICATE hereby certifies, thoroughly and completely, beyond any shadow of a doubt, that _____, in the Month of _____, in the Year 20___, in the Town of _____, in the State (or Province) of _____, in the Country of _____, in the Best of All Possible Worlds, thoroughly and completely, beyond any conceivable shadow of a doubt, and beyond any inconceivable shadow of a doubt, with all the Angels and Spirits of the Cosmos attending and watching over benevolently, and with the Higher Intentions of the Universe in harmonious musical and occipital accord with the movements of the planets and all persons pursuant and participant to the above-named and heretofore specified person, beyond any imaginable shadow of a doubt, and beyond any unimaginable shadow of a doubt, blah, blah, in which all inhabitants and participants in the County of yadda-yadda to which a testimony of conclusions and the reasons stated and explicit as well as, yet by no means limited to harmonious physical and psychic yuk-yuk and therefore to the rights, ranks, privileges, insignias, and yawn, burp, to which and to wit, and that we, the undersigned do recognize you,

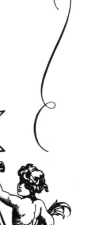

to be a
WONDERBARUS PERSONUS
and hereby entitled to the degree of WONDERFUL PERSON (W.P.),
in all manner, shape, form, and transportation.

_____ W.P.   _____ W.P.

_____ W.P.   _____ W.P.

_____ W.P.   _____ W.P.

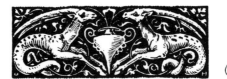

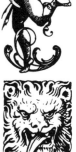